Journal of The American Academy of Psychotherapists

VOICES

THE ART AND SCIENCE OF PSYCHOTHERAPY

The psychedelic experience is a doorway to a higher state of consciousness.

—Alan Watts

Journal of the American Academy of Psychotherapists

VOICES

THE ART AND SCIENCE OF PSYCHOTHERAPY

Psychedelics and Psychotherapy VOICES 2024: Volume 60, Nos. 1-3

Book Reviews

Cover Design: Mary de Wit
Cover Image: *Inner Life of Your Shadow by agsandrew,* iStock
Design and Production by
Mary de Wit | in2Wit®, llc

Published three times per year.

AAP Web Site: www.aapweb.com

Poetry

Images

Calls for Papers

Voices

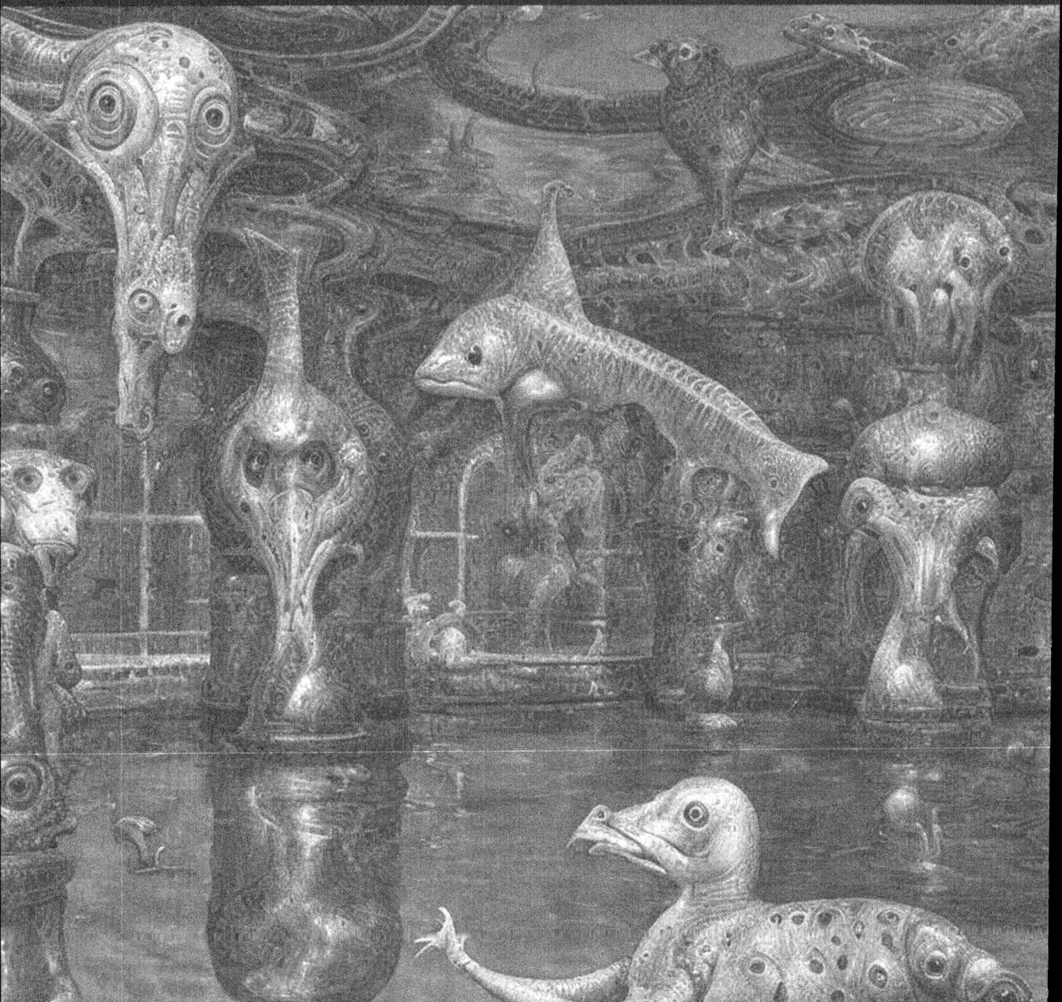

Carla Bauer

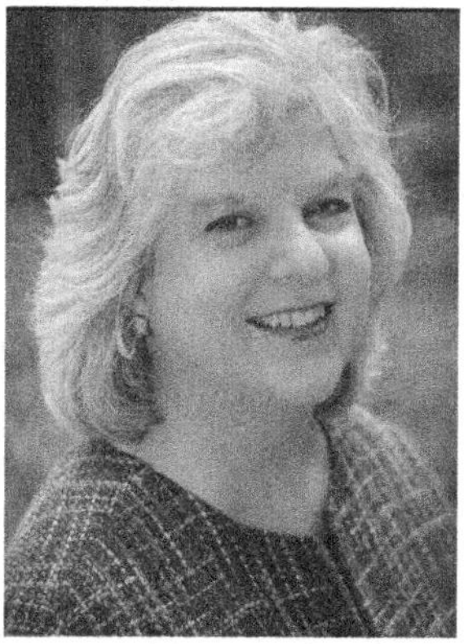

Carla R. Bauer, LCSW, is in private practice in Atlanta, Georgia. A second career therapist, she brings over 25 years of corporate experience, as well as an earlier journey in theological studies, to her understanding of people and their struggles. Psychoanalytically trained and drawn to attachment-based and relational orientations, she seeks to help clients free current dynamics from the grip of early life wounds. When she can't be on the beach, the colors of the beach are on her! As editor of *Voices* from 2019-2024, Carla has offered her voice to the American Academy of Psychotherapists. She looks forward to seeing what is next for her voice.
crbauer01@bellsouth.net

Editorial 1

And What a Trip It's Been!

Our theme, *Psychedelics and Psychotherapy: Healing and Transformation,* takes us on a journey into the mysteries of psychedelic-assisted psychotherapy. Long viewed as unconventional, even forced underground as in large part illegal, this field is enjoying a strong resurgence in popularity, often referred to as the third psychedelic renaissance. Testimonies abound of healings of long-term traumas, treatment-resistant depressions, substance addictions, and existential angst that remained elusive after conventional therapies but emerged profoundly out of psychedelic experiences. Observing this trend, it was clear that we needed to do an issue on this cutting-edge topic. Even so, I hesitated, recognizing that I lacked any knowledge on the subject from which to source or evaluate submissions—I could assess whether well written but would I know whether what was written held merit? When guest editors Steve Eichel and John Rhead agreed to bring their experience with psychedelics to an issue, I knew the time was right. They would know where to source material from credible voices—though never did I imagine that they would bring in over 50 submissions or that one issue would become a triple! I know a lot more about psychedelic-assisted therapy now, after the many re-readings over the course of editing this issue. (This 9-month issue gives all new meaning to the midwifery/birthing sense of bringing each issue into the world!) Hopefully readers will likewise come away from this issue feeling enlightened.

For this issue, authors were asked to consider how psychedelics have impacted them and their views of self, life, and psychotherapy, as well as how psychedelics have impacted their clients, whether used recreationally or within a therapeutic clinical context. Authors were asked to contemplate the therapeutic benefits as well as potential dangers associated with psychedelic-assisted therapy and to consider multicultural and multi-ethnic aspects of psychedelic experience, research, and treatment.

Authors emerged from diverse cultures, most from beyond the Academy and new to *Voices*, and submissions spanned from personal accounts of psychedelic journeys to professional practice with psychedelic-assisted therapy to spiritual and existential dimensions of the psychedelic experience to macro societal issues related to psychedelics. Receiving such a wealth of material, we decided to run a double issue—which when viewing an aggregated layout we recognized as actually a triple. Wow! Given the growing curiosity about this field, we decided to include a wider mix of voices, including some more traditionally academic pieces in addition to the experiential voice that is the hallmark of *Voices*. Understanding the scope and impact of psychedelic-assisted therapy is perhaps best derived from the blend of subjective, often poignant, accounts of personal experience and more objective information.

Our guest editors start us off: Steve Eichel writes of how both his own and a client's impactful journeys with psychedelics primed his interest in a *Voices* issue on the theme; John Rhead speaks of his early career involvement in the psychedelic research of the 1970s and of his lifelong interest in the spiritual dimensions of the psychedelic journey. Pioneer researchers James Fadiman and Bill Richards then share the personal experiences that launched their respective careers in psychedelic research, with Fadiman also introducing his current work on microdosing and Richards offering some best practices for effective therapeutic use of psychedelic substances.

Several authors share personal healing journeys with psychedelics. Rebecca Neisler narrates her personal odyssey from adolescent experimentation with LSD to later transformational healing of childhood trauma through ayahuasca. Vanessa Nguyen recounts how a plant medicine journey brought healing to deep-seated grief and intergenerational trauma. Cathy Roberts traces her interest in mind expansion from childhood imagination to her recent journey with ayahuasca. Brandon Sklar shares how psychedelics opened access to dissociated memories from childhood and thus to his deeper feelings, allowing him to work therapeutically with his inner child. Marilise Blignaut offers two pieces portraying her personal healing journey through first unguided recreational micro- and macro-dosing of psilocybin, then guided ketamine- and MDMA-assisted psychotherapies, emphasizing that as powerful as they are, psychedelics are not a quick-fix; the key to lasting change is in the therapeutic work of integrating the experience. Brodin Anderson recounts how a panic attack while conducting a therapy session led to recognition of his own complex PTSD and to transformational psychedelic treatment for long-buried pain. Lauren Parente describes how ketamine-assisted therapy broke through her treatment-resistant depression, uncovered a buried sexual orientation, and unleashed new creativity. Lisa Noeth shares how she found healing through ayahuasca for her negative body image and the intergenerational trauma from growing up first-generation Filipino American; she advocates for policy changes supporting the integration of psychedelic therapy as a viable alternative treatment for mental health issues and addiction. Michael Conti tells how his journey with MDMA healed the shame associated with his split-off sexuality, bringing self-acceptance, increased emotional regulation, and freedom from sexual compulsivity.

Several authors wrote of the professional impacts of their personal experiences with psychedelics. Denise Rue narrates her healing journey with psilocybin and its transformational impact on her work as a therapist. Rachael O'Donnell tells of her journey from recreational use of psychedelics to personal and professional transformation through ketamine-assisted psychotherapy. Mary Gresham recounts her journey into the field of psychedelic-assisted therapy in addressing the existential anxieties of aging and life transitions. Elizabeth Hoke describes the role of psychedelics in addiction recovery, sharing both her personal journey and her subsequently refocused practice in ketamine-assisted psychotherapy. Valeria McCarroll relates how her experience with psychedelics left her with reverence for the soul midwifery role of the psychedelic guide and the somatic embodiment of this soul journey. Nina Izel expresses how the spiritual, intergenerational, and relational dimensions of healing through ayahuasca changed both her personal life and the focus of her practice. Shannon Gendron shares the vivid ayahuasca journey that led to reconnections with her body, Self, and Unitive Consciousness, freeing her to openly live her pansexuality, from which she built a practice serving the queer community.

Other authors focused on their professional practices in psychedelic-assisted psychotherapy. Laura Hutchins describes her professional transition from addictions specialist to ketamine-assisted therapist, exploring some of the values, challenges, and best practices in this work. Physician Adekemi Oguntala explores the role of shame born of relational wounding underlying many medical and psychological conditions in teens and the power of psychedelics combined with internal family systems (IFS) therapy in healing shame and relational trauma.

Some authors presented case studies illustrating their clients' healings through psychedelic-assisted therapy. Heidi Dalzell relates her own story of healing childhood and present-day grief through a psychedelic journey as well as clinical vignettes of two clients who similarly found healing for childhood trauma and eating disorders through ketamine-assisted psychotherapy. Tali Silver offers a rich psychoanalytic analysis of a case in psilocybin-assisted therapy. Pierre Bouchard and Alyssa Gursky present a clinical case study demonstrating the intersection of psycholytic and somatic therapies with polyvagal theory in healing developmental trauma through ketamine-assisted psychotherapy.

Psychedelics have been widely used in addressing existential issues such as professional burnout, potentially terminal illness, and fear of death. Oncologist Jason Konner recounts how a journey with ayahuasca brought transformative restoration to severe physician burnout. Physician Rob Cole describes his personal journey with melanoma and how psychedelics and cannabis supported his walk with the fear of death. "Anonymous" recounts her facilitation of an underground MDMA treatment with a client facing a stage 4 melanoma diagnosis, work she hoped would come out of the legal shadows soon for broader accessibility. This piece is particularly poignant on the heels of the FDA's recent decline of the anticipated approval of MDMA treatment. Deborah Servetnick writes of the life-transforming role psilocybin and LSD played in her healing from both stage 3 cancer and the brutal side effects of chemotherapy.

Several authors explored spiritual aspects of the psychedelic experience. Steve Eichel interviewed dreams and hypnosis specialist Deirdre Barrett, who shares her early experiences with psychedelics and some thoughts on the parallels between these different types of altered states of consciousness. Ewa Tracz presents ethnographic interviews from her academic work in Poland exploring the spiritual dimensions of psychedelics. David Doane offers an expanded view of psychedelic experience that includes both substance-assisted and non-substance experiences of altered states of consciousness that have the power to shake us to the core. Mackenzie Amara gives a rich Jungian perspective on how psychedelics contribute insight into the human condition and the change process of therapy. Psychedelics researcher Leor Roseman created an imaginary interview with 20th century theologian Martin Buber, using excerpts from Buber's *I and Thou* to explore the spiritual and relational dimensions of psychedelic work. Marilyn Clark writes about the power of music to enhance the psychedelic journey as well as to open up non-ordinary states of consciousness independent of substances.

Addressing some of the macro issues around psychedelic-assisted psychotherapy, Sian Seligman draws from her experience as an Asian American to explore the benefits of psychedelics in treatment of race-based trauma, stressing the importance of including BIPOC populations in the research and development of culturally-sensitive treatment protocols. Shaina Fawn explores the history of cultural appropriation of Indigenous psychedelic rituals and advocates for decolonial practices that include all voices in the current psychedelic renaissance in the United States.

In a timely feature as we approach the anniversary of the tragic events of October 7, 2023, in Israel, with attacks particularly targeting psytrance music festivalgoers, Adriana Kertzer, Pinni Baumol, Madison Margolin, and Hadas Alterman document the wide-spread multi-faceted mobilization of therapeutic interventions by the Israeli psychedelics community in response to the trauma of those attacks.

Original poetry by Brodin Anderson, Marcela Bonancio, Allison Hammond, and Danielle Sukenik and original art by Deirdre Barrett, Marilyn Clark, and Lisa Noeth give further expression to the psychedelic experience. Compelling book reviews by Stephanie Ezust and Mary Gresham round out our issue.

Thank you to our guest editors for bringing in such a bounty. And thank you to all who responded to their call for sharing your voices and enlightening us.

Turning the Page

After 6 years, this issue concludes my term as editor—and what a trip it has been indeed! I had no idea what to expect as I stepped into the role, never having done anything like it before, but I knew it would stretch and grow me. And it delivered. Steering *Voices* through the upheavals of the pandemic and the concurrent waning of authorship within the Academy certainly held its challenges. But notwithstanding those, serving as editor has been such a rich experience! In its own way, a self-altering journey. It brought the discovery of skills I didn't know I had and the development of different parts of myself and new ways of expressing my voice, as well as the pleasure of nurturing so many other voices into publication, from both within and beyond the Academy. I have been reflecting on some of what *Voices* has meant to me over the years—as a reader, a writer, and as editor: intentionality toward personal and professional growth (developing our "person of the therapist"), critical reflection on our clinical work, community connection, and extending the Academy's voice into the broader psychotherapy community. It has been an honor to serve these endeavors.

It is with very mixed feelings that I put down the editorial pen, as it were. It feels rather like leaving behind a part of myself, and I can't fully imagine no longer being in this role. But it is time to channel my energies back into my clinical practice and other endeavors. Time to write a new chapter in my life. Even as I know I will miss much about editing *Voices*, I look forward to seeing what emerges when there is space.

Time, too, for a new *Voices* chapter, one perhaps better led by someone with different skills and interests, bringing new ideas for reaching broader readership and author participation in a changing world. With a new editor yet to be identified and new directions to be determined, *Voices* sits at a crossroads. It is difficult to pass the baton with no one on the receiving end—an incomplete pass—but a team of our former and associate editors are working together to produce a 2025 issue while the editorial board continues to explore future directions: Thank you, Molly Donovan, Jonathan Farber, Hallie Lovett, Penelope Norton, and Barry Wepman for providing a bridge.

One other known change: our amazing layout artist, graphic designer Mary de Wit, is retiring with this issue, after supporting *Voices* since 2003. Though she is somewhat hidden behind the scenes, it is Mary's artistic touch that gives *Voices* its visibility—in layout styling, original composition of many image pages, and creation of our stunning covers. She has also been an invaluable second set of eyes to catch what mine missed and incredibly dedicated to delivering on our deadlines. I could not have asked for a better partner in this venture and cannot imagine doing it without her. From myself and on behalf of the *Voices* team and the Academy, our heartfelt gratitude and best wishes to you, Mary!

My gratitude, too, to the editorial review board—members continuing and those stepping down after many years of dedicated service—and to all who have written during my term, some writing as a personal favor to me. I could not have done this without the support of all of you.

Voices had to say another, very sad, goodbye this year with the untimely passing of Editor Emeritus Tom Burns. Tom's voice was quiet but often profound. It is much missed. Words are inadequate to express the deep hole he leaves in the editorial team and in the Academy at large—and beyond.

One regret I hold is for authors who put their voices out here in vulnerability without feedback. If you read something in *Voices* that speaks to you, let the authors know. Keep voices connecting! ▼

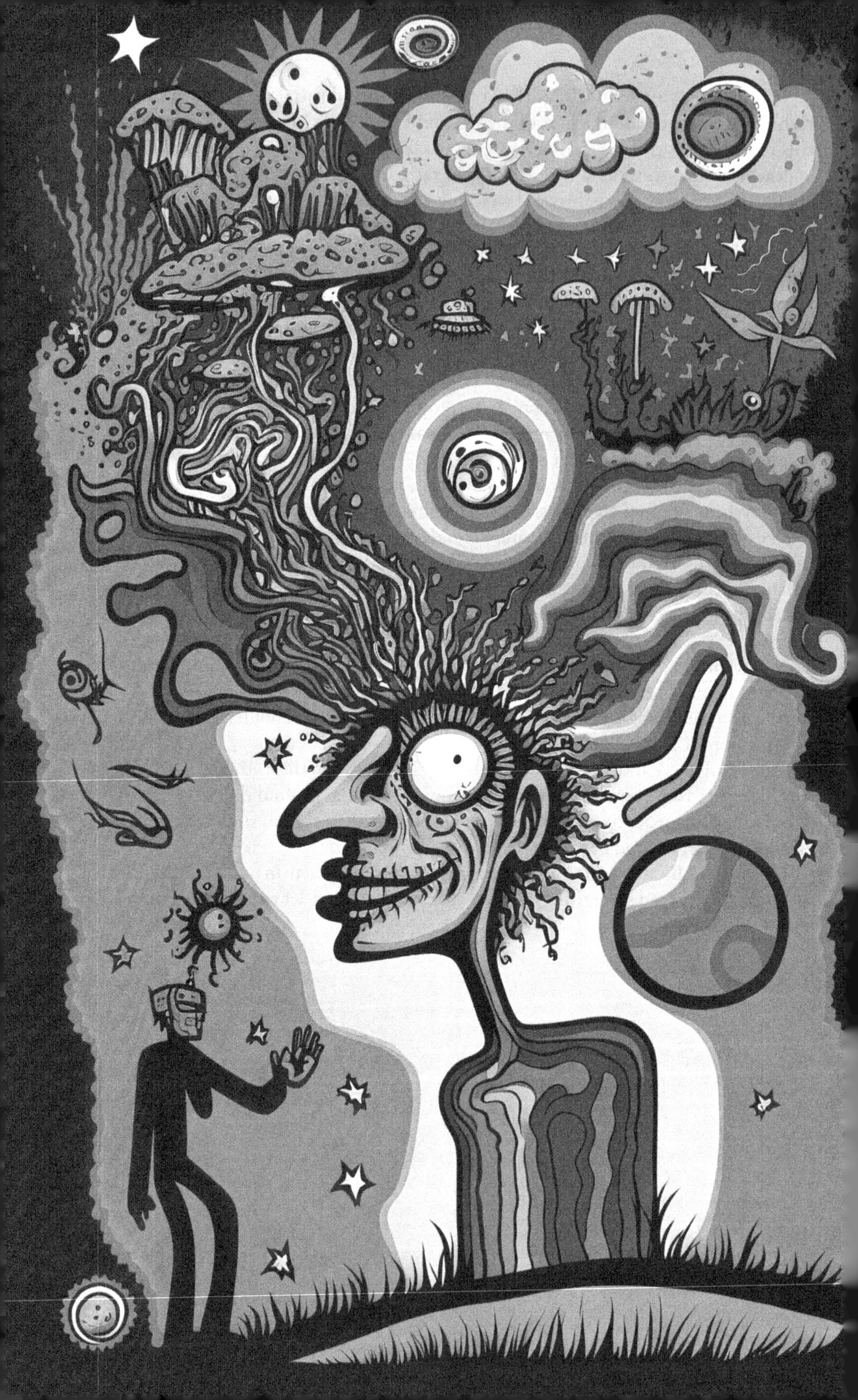

Steve Eichel

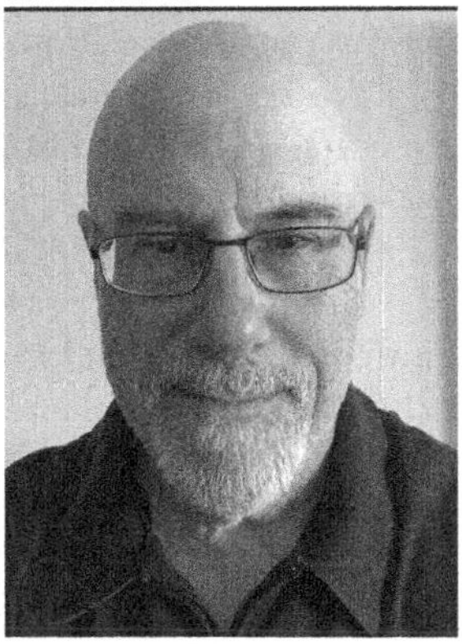

Steve K. D. Eichel, PhD, ABPP, CST is a licensed and board-certified counseling psychologist with a part-time independent practice. His subspecialties include clinical hypnosis (he is a former president of the Greater Philadelphia Society of Clinical Hypnosis), EMDR, and sex therapy. He lives in Newark, Delaware, with his wife Terri, stepson Tristan, five cats, and a mellotron.
steve@dreichel.com

Editorial 2

I Asked: "How Did I Get Here?"

...and I still haven't found what I'm looking for...
—Bono/U2

I didn't know what I was looking for.

I began taking LSD in the fall of 1972 when I was a freshman at Columbia University. I had had one previous psychedelic experience; on the day before Halloween in 1971, I took what I was told was mescaline. What I took was a capsule that consisted of a greenish crystalline powder that, whatever it was, launched me into a vibrating, swirling world of colors and motion. Retreating to my basement, I put on an album by the rock group The Move and began having visions that I later discovered were quite well-described by Aldous Huxley (1954) in his autobiographic, psychedelic masterpiece, *The Doors of Perception*: Magnificent and intricate, glowing geometric shapes of every color, hue, and shape floated in the air around me, moving in time to the music.[1] The geometric patterns very closely resembled those often depicted in Aztec and Mayan drawings. It was delightfully dreamlike; I was ecstatic. Later, I sat in our living room with my mother, watching *The Man from U.N.C.L.E.* I remember talking with her excitedly about how intricate a worldwide law enforcement organization must be...U.N.C.L.E. had to make a complex and wonderful pattern. That evening, I went to a Halloween party in Branchburg, NJ. I still felt the glow from earlier that day; everyone was magical. I eventually left that party for a much smaller gathering at a friend's house nearby; it was

1 Huxley had taken mescaline, which I took as evidence that my drug was indeed mescaline.

at that gathering that I got close to the young gal who would eventually become my first serious romantic relationship.

I did not experience anything close to a craving for psychedelics. Psychedelics and even marijuana were just not that popular in my small town at that time, despite what was going on in most urban areas. Then came college. In New York City. That's when things got weird.

I no longer recall the first time I took LSD. I remember it came in a barrel-like pill (unlike the blotter and windowpane forms of LSD), and the first several trips I took that fall were recreational and usually tied to concerts and other musical venues. I tripped solidly for the March 23, 1973, Pink Floyd concert at Radio City Music Hall. I have almost no memory of that show. Or the Mahavishnu Orchestra's performance at Madison Square Garden's Felt Forum that same spring.

Then I got serious. I began taking bigger doses. I changed suppliers; I was now taking LSD made by the son of a Nobel-prize winning chemist who taught at Columbia. It was pure (the barrel pills contained amphetamine) and reliable. Because the pills and the supplier were from Berkeley, California, these pills were known as "Berkeley double-domes." Each pill reputedly contained the standard LSD dose of 300-350 micrograms. [2] They were powerful. The second to the last time I took acid, I had an out-of-body experience.

It was not enough.

At the time I could not know, let alone explain, what I was looking for. I only knew I was coming close to it when I tripped, but the brass ring always seemed just out of my grasp. I'd hallucinated plenty, including going up on the roof of Carmen Hall (my old dorm) at night, where the stars and other lights were transformed into flying, diamond-encrusted dragons and other monstrous beings. (They frightened me, and I quickly left the rooftop for the relative safety of my room.)

On a weekend night in late April, I took two Berkeley double-domes: 600-700 micrograms. And smoked hashish to launch the trip a little more quickly.

By around 4:00 a.m., I was in the ER of St. Luke's Hospital with my dorm floor's R.A. (Columbia called them "counselors") having what felt like a psychotic break.

It seemed like I had to wait hours before being seen, and I tried hard to avoid looking at all the bleeding people (they looked like they had knife wounds) who were also in the ER. It wasn't until 3 years later that I learned none of what I experienced in the ER was real. I had been seen almost immediately, and there were no other people in the ER that night. What was real, despite claims to the contrary, was that I was rapid-tranqued, probably with Valium or possibly an antipsychotic. Within an hour I was almost completely down from my trip. I was released around 8:00 a.m.

Of course, what I had (intermittently) experienced was complete ego dissolution. Time ceased to exist; every split second seemed to exist forever, independent of the next moment. I was completely unprepared for the experiences so perfectly described by Timothy Leary, Ralph Metzner, and Richard Alpert/Ram Dass (1964) and Aldous Huxley (1954) before them. When I took a survey of religion class at Barnard (taught by the brilliant and famous scholar of Gnosticism, Elaine Pagels) in my senior year, I was finally exposed to excerpts from *The Tibetan Book of the Dead*. That was the first time

2 300 micrograms was the recommended dose for a full-blown acid trip.

I realized what I had experienced: a profound spiritual experience. Still, at the time, if you asked me how I felt about my last acid trip, I would have told you it was one of the worst experiences of my life.

The events following my brief hospitalization were a whirlwind. My university was notified by St. Luke's, and I was put on academic probation for a year contingent on (1) getting therapy over the summer, and (2) no further incidents. I remained almost completely drug-free my sophomore year (I did smoke weed when my friend Brian and I hitchhiked to Florida over Spring break).

Therapy that summer was a revelation. I'd never been listened to like that before. The psychologist I saw pinpointed my issues at that time, which included guilt about a relationship I knew I had to end, my difficulties with independence and adjusting to college, the usual family crap, etc. I do not recall ever discussing my actual psychedelic experiences. When I returned to college that fall, I was sober and happy to not be involved in a relationship. I focused on my studies, especially now that I was able to begin taking classes in my major, political science.[3] But the questions raised by my LSD experiences never really left. In my sophomore year I took my first psychology class; by the second semester of the following year, I had changed my major to psychology. In 1976, I began graduate training in counseling psychology; in early 1977, I spontaneously recovered a traumatic memory that had unconsciously impacted on my last exquisitely intense relationship. That spring I began a long-term therapy with a psychiatrist recommended by one of my professors: Meyer Rohtbart.

I had an opportunity to take LSD again in the early 1980s. I declined; my 1973 experience left me with a combination of respect and fear for the powerful drug.

In March, 2020, I began working with Brian, a new patient who reported a significant psychological breakthrough using ayahuasca (dimethyltryptamine, aka "DMT"). Brian (age 32) suffered from multiple addictions and compulsions. He met the criteria for alcohol dependence and reported he was spending a daily average of 7 hours watching online pornography. He was engaging sex workers and exposing himself in public while driving; the last time he exposed himself the woman took a picture of his license plate, and he was arrested. As a result of these behaviors, he lost his job and his wife and was facing criminal charge as a sex offender. He tried ayahuasca out of desperation, prior to engaging in therapy. The drug made him connect emotionally with the ongoing sexual abuse (by his father and his uncle) he had experienced as a child. He confronted his mother for the first time (father and uncle were deceased), as well as his drug-addicted sister, who he learned had also been molested. Brian tripped two more times, each time becoming more emotionally engaged with his history of trauma. By the time he came to see me, he was completely sober from all his compulsive/addictive behaviors. By the time we terminated therapy in late 2022, he had almost 3 years of complete sobriety. He was working and went through an amicable divorce. He was not in a steady relationship but was content to date casually (he was successfully negotiating ethical nonmonogamy). He had stopped using ayahuasca, but was present for his sister's first two trips, in the hope it would have the same impact on her self-destructive behavior. It did not.

I did not take another psychedelic until just prior to the pandemic. A part-time musician I knew gave me some "magic mushrooms" (psylocibin). The first time I tried

3 Columbia's required core curriculum pretty much filled all the typical freshman's course schedule.

"shrooms," the experience was marred by violent vomiting, even though I'd made a tea out of them as instructed. The second time I did not vomit, however I was very unpleasantly nauseous for several hours. The same friend then gave me psylocibin-infused chocolate. Although I was still nauseous initially, for about an hour, I eventually tripped and had a very emotionally intense and productive experience. An extremely painful family-related issue seemed to have finally been processed to the point where the associated memories no longer cause me deep anguish.

My patient's experiences, along with my own, are what prompted me to approach the *Voices* editorial team about the prospect of an issue focused on psychedelics in psychotherapy. Editor Carla Bauer suggested I invite "psychonaut" (Blom, 2009) John Rhead to be my co-guest-editor. And one *Voices* issue soon became a triple issue!

References

Blom, J. D. (2009). *A dictionary of hallucinations.* New York: Springer.

Huxley, A. (1954). *The doors of perception.* New York: Harper Perennial.

Leary, T., Metzner, R., & Alpert, R. (1964). *The psychedelic experience: A manual based on The Tibetan Book of the Dead.* New York: Kensington.

> Psychedelics are illegal not because a loving government is concerned that you may jump out of a third-story window. Psychedelics are illegal because they dissolve opinion structures and culturally laid down models of behavior and information processing. They open you up to the possibility that everything you know is wrong.
>
> —Terence McKenna

John Rhead

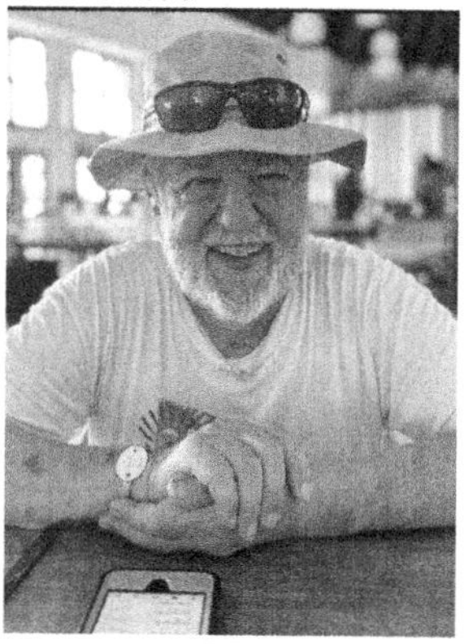

John Rhead finished his PhD in 1971 and immediately began his first job as a psychologist—doing research with LSD. About 1975, he entered therapy with a therapist who always had a copy of a very odd journal, *Voices*, in the waiting room. One thing led to another, and a few years later John joined the American Academy of Psychotherapists. A few years after that he joined the editorial board of that odd journal. The rest is history.
jrheadphd@gmail.com

Editorial 3

A Young Cowboy's Journey on the Psychedelic Bronco

I was born in 1945, in Utah, and grew up in Colorado, the middle of three children. My father was a not-very-devout Mormon and my mother was a wide-ranging spiritual seeker who believed deeply in the power of prayer. I was (and am) a geeky scientist who likes to tinker with things and who was (and is) also very interested in the human psyche and the mystical world. I went off to Dartmouth uncertain about whether to major in psychology or math, and after taking one course in each chose psychology. When I began to read about the burgeoning research (mid '60s) with LSD, I decided to try it. As far as I know I was the first to do this at Dartmouth, and I was very lucky in terms of how well it went, given my totally inadequate preparation and setting. To say the least, my interest was sparked.

By the time I graduated in 1967, federal restrictions were closing off most psychedelic research, but I was fortunate enough to get accepted into psychology graduate school at Stanford. There was a still-surviving psychedelic research group near the campus where I planned to do my doctoral research. However, just as I arrived at Stanford, they were closed down. I considered cancelling my graduate school plans until Jim Fadiman gave me the following advice: "Go ahead and get your PhD from Stanford without ever even whispering the word 'psychedelic' until the ink is dry on you diploma and see what opportunities there may then be to get involved with psychedelic research." I took his advice, and 4 years later was driving across the country in my '51 Chevy (with my ink-dry diploma and towing my motorcycle behind me) to start work at the Maryland Psychiatric Research Center (MPRC, the only remaining psychedelic research facility in the country) with Stan Grof, Bill Richards, and others. Early in that road trip I suddenly had an ecstatic experience in which I shouted out in elation (alone in my car, thank goodness), "I did it!!! I got a f---king PhD from f---king Stanford, and I am going to go get paid by the state of Maryland to do psychedelic research!!!" This manic outburst lasted a few moments and then resolved into a sweet peacefulness at the idea that I had not actually done these seemingly impossible things, but that I had merely surrendered to my calling, which took care of the details and had me on the road to the MPRC and work with psychedelics.

I worked at the MPRC from 1971 until the psychedelic research was ended in 1977. It was clear that all the members of the research team were there more or less with the same sense of purpose and enthusiasm that I had. During the day, Monday through Friday, we did everything but wear white lab coats as we conducted our scientific research. Evenings and weekends were more informal, as we explored different techniques and medicines to alter/expand human consciousness. Learning to facilitate psychedelic journeys of course required that all of us have our own psychedelic experiences as part of our training. I was amazed and delighted to be paid by the state of Maryland in general for being part of this amazing team (I would have gladly paid for the privilege) and particularly tickled when I realized many years later that I was actually on the clock while taking LSD myself.

Since leaving the MPRC in 1977, I have been on the faculty of the University of Maryland School of Medicine, directed a program at a private psychiatric hospital, been a mental health team leader at a special school for emotionally disturbed youth, consulted at a prison, and built my private practice. When I gave up everything but the private practice about 30 years ago, I declared myself retired. I was doing what I love and find meaningful and getting paid at the same time—sort of like my 1971 experience in my car. My private practice focusses largely on the kinds of existential and spiritual issues addressed by psychedelic experiences. I tend to agree with Roland Griffiths, one of the world's foremost psychedelic researchers, when he said at the huge Psychedelic Science conference in Denver in June 2023, "My vision for the future is that we come out with a coherent set of ethical understandings, worldwide, and across cultures that we can agree on—that thereby the human species flourishes and doesn't extinguish itself" (Moscow, 2023).

I think I have had some ideas for a long time, perhaps planted there when I was very young by my mother, that are consistent with Roland's vision. There is some way in which individual humans can come in contact with a profound mystical truth or vision about the meaning of their lives and the meaning of life in general. Such contact with the mystical realm can guide individual lives and can, perhaps by something like contagion, guide our entire species in a better direction. I believe that psychedelics, used well, are one way to facilitate this process.

Reading the articles that have been submitted has reinforced this belief. It also has brought to my attention how amazingly congruent most of these articles are with the fundamental principles of the American Academy of Psychotherapists (AAP)—that psychotherapy is largely about a relationship between therapist and client, and that the most important part of a therapist's training and lifetime continuing education is their ever-deepening exploration of their own inner world. The author of one of the articles, who had no familiarity with AAP, mentioned how important Carl Rogers had been in

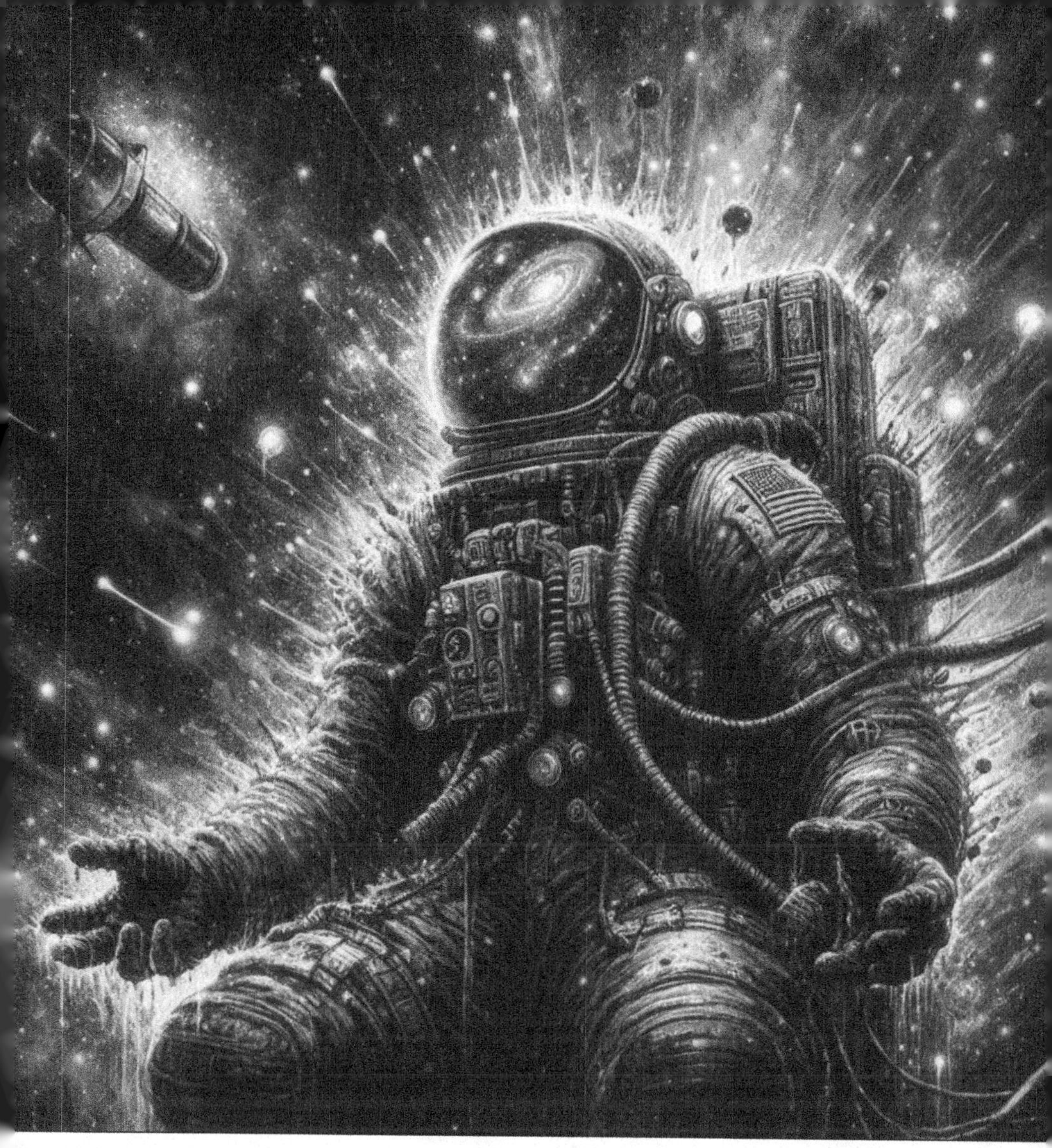

his own evolution. He seemed quite delighted to learn that Rogers was a founder, and first president, of AAP.

It has been an honor to contribute to this issue of *Voices* and an inspiration to see what has been birthed here.

References

Moscow, J. (2023). Psychedelics and spirituality: Exploring the intersection at Psychedelic Science 2023. *Lion's Roar*. https://www.lionsroar.com/psychedelic-science-2023/

▼

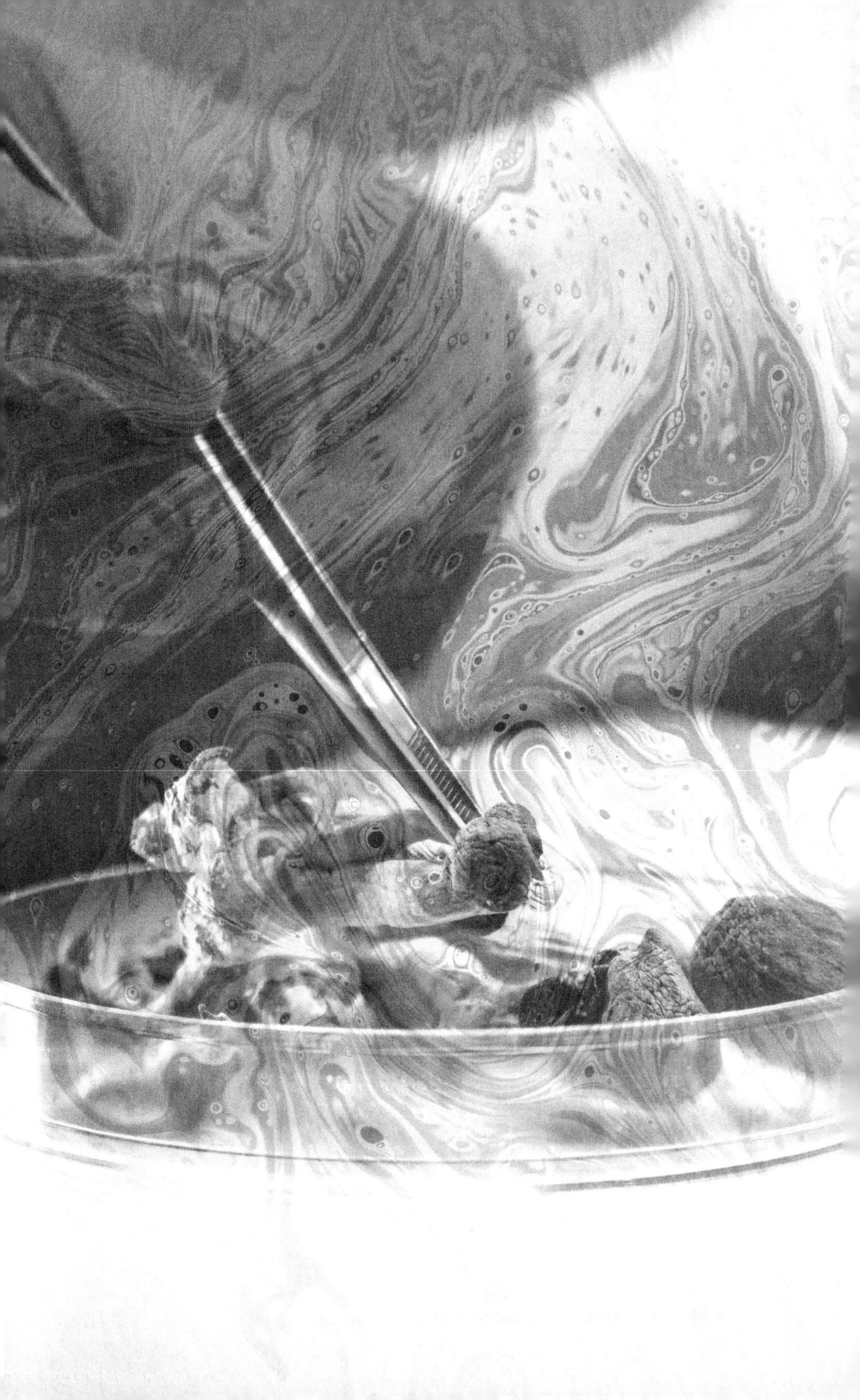

James Fadiman

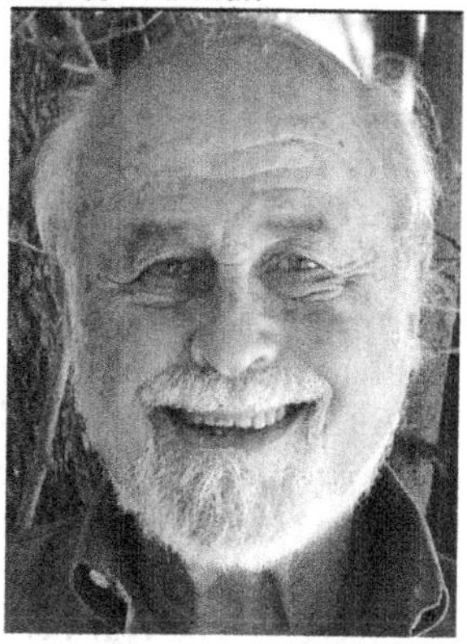

James Fadiman, PhD, has been involved with psychedelics for over 60 years. He developed modern microdosing, including the use of protocols, specific dose ranges, and time off. He is the author of *The Psychedelic Explorer's Guide* and (with Jordan Gruber) *Microdosing for Health, Healing, and Enhanced Performance.* He has taught at three universities, ran his own management consulting firm, co-founded the Institute of Transpersonal Psychology, and served as the director of the Institute of Noetic Sciences.
jfadiman@gmail.com

Articles

Why I Am Not a Psychotherapist: Psychedelics and Other Reasons

I WAS LIVING IN PARIS IN 1961, AFTER GRADUATION FROM COLLEGE, WHEN MY FRIEND AND FORMER PROFESSOR, RICHARD ALPERT, (LATER KNOWN AS RAM DASS) spent an evening with me on his way to Copenhagen to present (with Tim Leary and Aldous Huxley) the first public presentation of their psychedelic work at a psychological convention.

As we sat in a sidewalk café, he said, "The greatest thing in the world has happened to me, and I want to share it with you." I sat back, expecting a story. Instead, he shook a pill from a small bottle and placed it in my hand. Without any idea of what it was, I took it. After a while, the street lights became brighter, colors more intense, and as I listened to the snatches of conversations between people passing behind us I suddenly realized that, although I'd lived in Paris for close to a year, my French had never been good enough to understand such conversations. More than a little shaken, I confessed that everything was too much. He said it was too much for him, too. I said, "But you didn't take anything. "I've never been in Paris before," he answered.

We withdrew to my 4th floor walkup, and over the next few hours a number of understandings I had about who I was and what was important in the world melted away. No visions, no hallucinations, no therapeutic epiphanies, but whatever I'd taken reorganized my worldview. I had been given a moderate dose of Sandoz psilocybin, (equivalent to 1 gram of a cubensis mushroom), what he had been taking and giving to others for most of the prior year.

Several months later, having taken psilocybin once more with Richard, I was better to be around, unafraid of closeness, and open to a level of bonding that I had never felt before. I'd become an inadvertent member of a secret society that knew that a great deal of what concerned people was illusory.

Prior to those occasions, I had experienced the world through the lens of intellect. Now, I had begun to experience the world and especially other people energetically. My beliefs about spirituality, little more than vague atheism, still remained untouched. My interest in psychology, if anything, had diminished. I had been shaken awake, but had not had what I would later understand to be "a psychedelic experience."

A letter from my draft board abruptly ended my leisured period of discovery. It told me to get ready to be inducted, maybe to go to Vietnam. There were few alternative choices: take up residence in Canada, become an instantaneous conscientious objector, or enroll in graduate school. I enrolled.

Accepted the year before by Stanford, I reinstated my acceptance, packed, shipped my belongings, and flew to San Francisco—ill-prepared, disinterested in school, and missing my Paris world but grateful that I would not be crawling through mud cradling my M1 carbine.

Astonished, just 6 weeks into my graduate career, I met Willis Harman, was introduced to an off campus psychedelic clinic, and was invited to have a session with them. Instead of sharing doses of psilocybin, eyes open, conversing and bonding as I expected, I was given 400 micrograms of LSD (a lot). As people's voices reverberated, the outside light became painfully bright and I was unable to speak. I was grateful to lie down, put on eyeshades and headphones, and hear, watch, and taste music.

Whatever feelings "Jim Fadiman" had about the onrush of inner experience were pushed aside by the music, and the flood of changing visions surpassed his capacity to process, appreciate, or understand them. The filters necessary to maintain a separate identity became at first transparent, then vanished. The actuality of being part of an infinitely connected greater reality, eternally in motion, not limited by time or space, became self-evident. No sense of surprise, just recognition. Over the next few years, I discovered that my realization had been described not only by seers, visionaries, and mystics across civilizations and religions but also by physicists, biologists, and poets. Jim Fadiman was a subset of my fuller identity. While he had no capacity to retain what that meant, he remembered that it was so. It was as if one's little finger awakened to an understanding, not only that it was part of a larger body but equally aware of the millions of cells within it coming into being, dying, and being replaced and full awareness of the complexity of the entire circulatory system and the constant dance between the finger's activity and cascades of energy coursing through parts of the brain. Too much to retain, only the memory of having known it.

Yet, whatever I'd experienced and however I held it, by late afternoon I moved in and out of being a draft-dodging first-year graduate student in psychology, saturated with knowledge I couldn't share with anyone who'd not had this experience. I was still at the mercy of my professors, who would see my revelations as psychopathology and would either hospitalize me or let me be shipped off to Vietnam.

I looked to my guides. Relief: They knew what I knew. They would help me. And they did.

I still remain fascinated by how it was possible that a few millionths of a gram of anything could open so many doors so quickly.

Fortunately, I came to recognize that each part of the larger unity had its own function and that it was not dishonest of me to continue to act as if I were interested in psychology. I continued to be quiet, polite, and apparently a diligent student, taking notes, writing papers, and sharing almost nothing with my peers.

Reflecting on that now, except for my roommates, also first-year psychology students, I made no friends during my graduate student years that I've kept in touch with, partly because I had no interest in the psychology but also because I kept my larger identity to myself.

While a psychology student by day, most evenings, I tried to make sense of what was the central defining experience of my life. I read the *I Ching, The Tibetan Book of The Dead,* the *Gita, The Life of Milarepa, The Perennial Philosophy* (a compilation by Aldous Huxley), *The Teachings of the Desert Fathers, The Kabbalah,* collections of western mysticism, and the works of St. Francis, St. Teressa, and more.

I sat in on dozens and dozens of individual sessions, as lives transomed in a single day. I did 60 3- to 4-hour interviews of people 6 months after their sessions, for an intended dissertation. Jack Hilgard, a past president of the American Psychological Association, cautioned me, "If you do your dissertation about psychedelic therapy, you will never have an academic career." He meant it as a warning, I took it as a relief. He was terribly right. Stanford remained disinterested, while all over the bay area and the country, millions of people took LSD themselves and created a counterculture.

Attempts to Become a Psychotherapist

A year or so after I graduated, I interviewed for a position at the San Francisco State University Counseling Center—specifically because of my psychedelic experience. However, when the administration realized that hiring me would force them to admit that psychedelics were already a problem, they told the center to withdraw the offer. A few years later, I accepted a position to be the first counselor for students at the still highly experimental new campus of the University of California in Santa Cruz. The intension was to gradually replace the informal counseling being offered by faculty wives. When the heads of each college recognized that students' issues would be protected by confidentiality and no longer shared freely with administrators, the offer was withdrawn.

Given that I knew that I was connected to everything, and everything was connected to everything, I might have noticed that as my attempts to be a psychotherapist were taken away from me even before I started, maybe I was not to be a psychotherapist.

A few years later, when I was offered a similar position at the Stanford counseling center, specializing with students with troubling psychedelic experiences, or altered states in general, I took it. I loved working with students with drug experience focused issues, and they appreciated being understood and sometimes even helped. But there were not enough to fill my hours, so I also carried a normal caseload of undergraduates becoming independent of their parents, sex-obsessed students, and graduate students coming to the realization that they had become hyper-specialists, but they didn't like the field they were in and saw no way out.

I began to recognize that I could hardly bring myself to pay attention to my conventional clients. Listening to them, after those years of supporting accelerated life changes boosted by psychedelics, spoiled me for the pace and depth of conventional counseling. Worse yet, the days I spent at the counseling center used up my capacity to be present. On those evenings, I had nothing left to share or to appreciate with my wife and children. I lacked the patience, the focus, and the stamina for the satisfaction of one-on-one talk therapy. When I finally realized that I needed to quit, my wife's only comment was "I've known that for months."

Finally released from the illusion that I was cut out to be a psychotherapist, I shared my realizations by helping to establish the Transpersonal Association and the *Journal of Transpersonal Psychology*. Later, with Robert Frager, we established a Graduate School of Transpersonal Psychology. Our graduates have done well, but transpersonal psychology is still rebuffed by conventional psychology, still seeking acceptance by the traditional sciences.

For self-understanding, reflections upon one's childhood and discovering the origins of personal issues, psychotherapy is remarkable. But integrating the depth and intensity of that initial psychedelic experience and some later ones have been better served by working within older and more sophisticated systems of consciousness.

Microdoses

In 2010, Robert Forte told me about microdoses. He had learned about them from Albert Hofmann, who said they were wonderful for thinking while walking in the woods. He also said that had Sandoz listened to him about the effects, there would never have been a market for Ritalin. I shared the low dose possibilities with some local psychedelic-wise friends who immediately tried 10 micrograms. They all reported excellent feelings and intended to do more. The research side of me could not resist.

A microdose is a sub-threshold dose of a classic psychedelic (LSD or psilocybin). Microdosing is taking a small amount (5-12 micrograms of LSD or 0.05-0.4 grams of psilocybin -containing mushrooms) on an intermittent schedule (1 or 2 days between doses) for 4 to 6 weeks, then taking 2 to 4 weeks off before using again, if needed. Sub-threshold means that there are no characteristic psychedelic effects at those doses, and people maintain their normal work and social habits. Brain imaging studies show the same patterns as high dose effects but with far less amplitude. Research studies show that, in general, people have improved moods and improved cognitive capacities, with few if any negative side-effects. Therapists report that clients who are microdosing make better progress than prior to microdosing. Animal studies show reduced inflammation, increased neuroplasticity, and improved social behaviors.

Results from 81 countries (individual reports, surveys, and peer-reviewed research) report a high safety profile and improvements in normal functioning of physical and intellectual skills as well as improvements in physical and mental conditions (Fadiman & Gruber, 2025). Some early research that questioned if there was any effect except expectation and placebo still comes up in some media coverage. For details or questions on specific conditions, a good resource is the subreddit community "microdosing," with 240,000 members.

I have microdosed intermittently over the past decade, sometimes for fatigue but more often to improve focus or flow, especially when writing first drafts of professional articles or books. The manuscript for a book on microdosing to be published in 2025 includes first person reports of improved functioning in healthy individuals and improvement in a wide range of health conditions including chronic pain, ADHD, recurring migraines, and treatment-resistant depression.

In what seems to me an example of divine sense of humor or irony, after being fixated and attached to the upper reaches of psychedelic experience for decades, having no interest in recreational use, and almost none in psychotherapeutic intervention, only focused on the transcendental experience of awakening, I've spent the last 15 years working with microdoses of psychedelics. Microdoses are defined as having no classic psychedelic effects: no visual distortions, no visionary experiences, no awareness of past lives, and no being eaten by giant anacondas. In short, microdoses evoke none of the amazing physical or sensory changes that are at the center of the psychedelic renaissance.

In terms of psychotherapeutic efficacy, however, if one's goal is not to discover one's divinity or immortality, etc., but to be freed of the suffering of depression, anxiety, physical pain, and mental confusion, microdosing is apparently not only as effective as high doses but as effective as psychotherapy and psychopharmacology as well (Fadiman & Gruber, 2025).

If microdoses have only 1/4 of the effectiveness that we've seen in the first 50,000 cases, they may relieve a wide range of conditions currently not well treated by Western medicine.

While I have benefited personally from working with a psychotherapist for some months, being a therapist for hospitalized veterans, and a practicing psychotherapist at a university counselling center, my focus now is researching whether easier, less costly, and swifter methods are viable alternatives.

References

Fadiman, J. & Gruber, J. (2025). *Microdosing: For health, healing, and enhanced performance* [In press]. New York: St. Martin's Essentials.

Psychedelics are catalysts for a deeper understanding of the mind and consciousness.

—Stanislav Grof

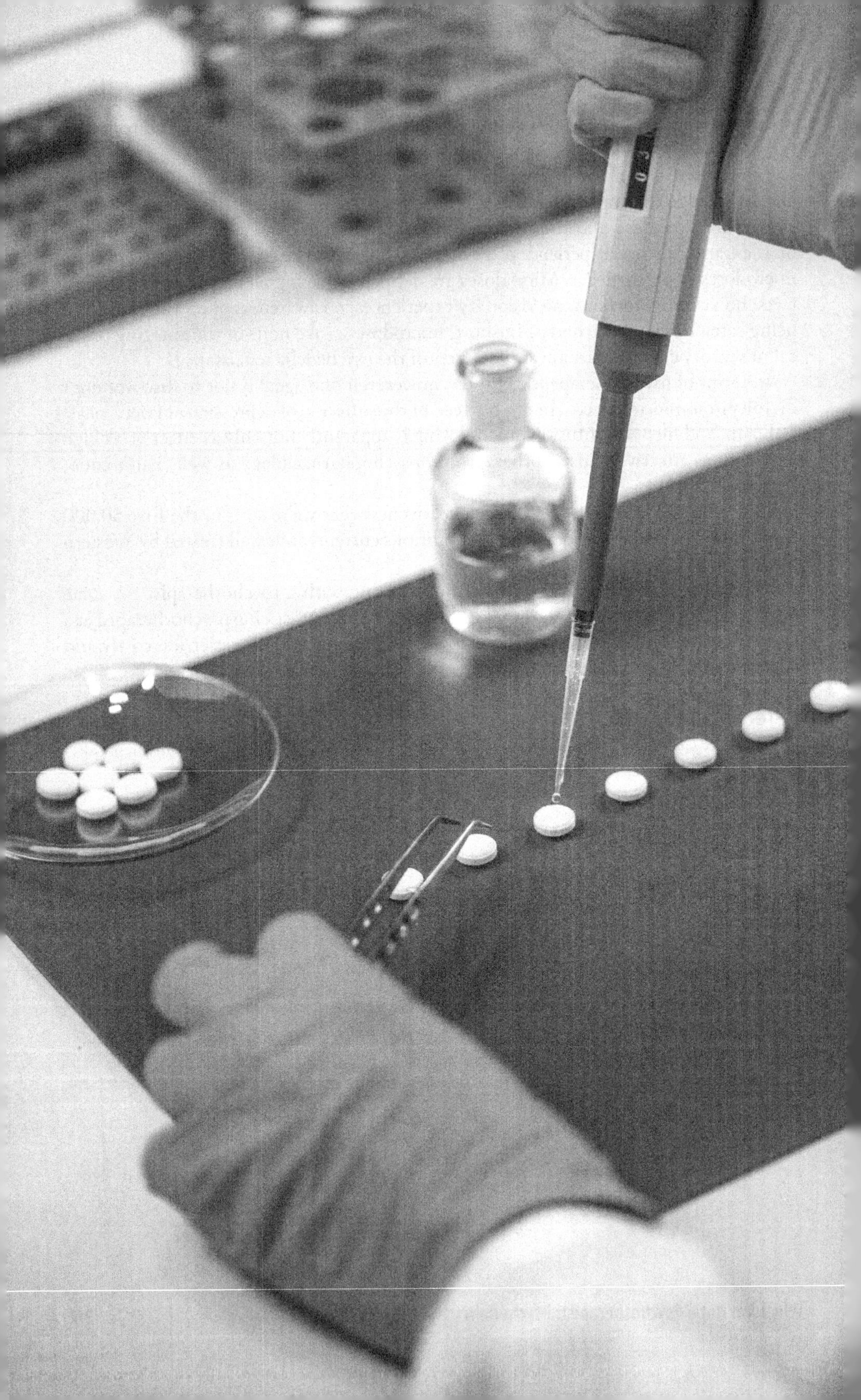

William A. (Bill) Richards

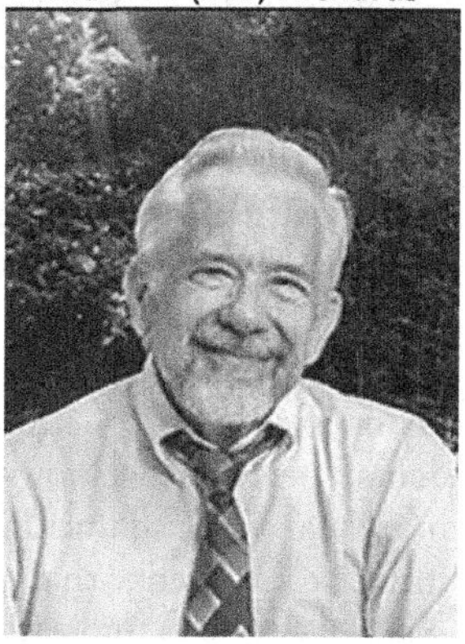

WILLIAM A. (BILL) RICHARDS, STM, PHD, author of *Sacred Knowledge* and a psychologist in the Johns Hopkins Center for Psychedelic and Consciousness Research, has contributed to psychedelic research since 1963. From 1967 to 1977, he implemented projects at the Maryland Psychiatric Research Center; in 1999, he and Roland Griffiths initiated the rebirth of research at Hopkins. At Sunstone Therapies, he currently focuses on integrating psychedelic therapy into palliative care.
richards3@earthlink.net

Fundamental Factors in Safe and Effective Psychedelic Therapy

ONCE UPON A TIME, I WAS A 23-YEAR-OLD GRADUATE STUDENT who had left the Yale Divinity School for a year of study in Germany at the University of Göttingen. Not only were psychedelics legal and uncontroversial at that time, I had yet to hear the word *psychedelic* and had no idea what *psilocybin* might be. I was, however, committed to the development of my own psychological and spiritual life, even to the extent of going without breakfast on some days to record my dreams from the night before.

Two of my new friends told me about an interesting research project going on in the *Nervenklinik* (mental hospital) around the corner from my dormitory. It entailed receiving some new drug that was purported to give access to memories from early childhood. One friend reported a vivid memory of sitting on his father's lap, which was profoundly meaningful as his father had been killed in World War II. The other claimed to have seen a hallucination of SS men marching in the streets. I had never seen a real hallucination, so this sounded intriguing. Curious about my early childhood psychodynamics, notably my oedipal complex, I hiked over to the clinic and inquired whether I also could participate in the research project.

I was given a cursory medical interview to establish that I was in decent mental and physical health and didn't get drunk too often, declared acceptable, and then led to a small basement room, dim and drab, with a cot, an end-table and a narrow window overlooking the hospital garbage cans. There a friendly medical intern about my age, wearing a spiffy white coat and stethoscope, gave me an injection of a short-acting derivative of psilocybin

(13 mg. of CZ-74), and, though looking in on me periodically, basically left me alone for the next 4 hours.

Drawing on the piety of my Methodist childhood, I affirmed trust that God would be with me if any potentially traumatic memories awakened. I then became aware of very beautiful neon-like geometrical designs in my visual field, multi-dimensional, unfolding, and inviting my participation in and through energetic forces that flowed through them.

They reminded me of Islamic architecture and Arabic script. Gradually, yet suddenly, my usual state of consciousness in the everyday world merged into the vivid transcendental awareness we now call *mystical consciousness*—an eternal state of being that felt more real (or fundamental) than my usual awareness, filled with beauty, joy, love, and intuitive knowledge that seemed independent of time and space. Awestruck, I (my usual sense of ego/self) underwent what we call psychological death and rebirth.

In the midst of this unexpected epiphany, as workmen emptied the metal garbage cans outside of the window, I registered tinkling temple bells. When the intern entered, asking me to sit up on the edge of the cot so he could test my knee reflexes, I complied with thoughts of compassion for the infancy of science. Now, 60 years later, I realize that in many ways my subsequent personal and professional life has been footnotes to this unexpected awakening. It led to study of the psychology of religion, comparative religions, music, and clinical psychology. I found myself pursuing research with psychedelics in Göttingen in 1964, in Boston in 1966 (Pahnke & Richards, 1966), and then at the Spring Grove Hospital Center (which morphed into the Maryland Psychiatric Research Center) from 1967-1977 (Richards et al., 1972; Richards et al., 1977; Rhead et al., 1977; Richards & Rhead, 1977). Psychedelic research in the United States then became dormant until dimethyltryptamine (DMT) studies began in the early 1990s (Strassman, 2001). In 1999, Roland Griffiths and I were able to initiate its rebirth with psilocybin at the Johns Hopkins School of Medicine (Griffiths, et al., 2006, 2008, 2011, & 2017; Johnson, et al., 2008; Garcia-Romeu & Richards, 2018), where it continues to this day. I now also contribute to psychedelic research at Sunstone Therapies in Rockville Maryland (Agrawal et al., 2023). Throughout these decades of career research, I have often reflected upon that first psychedelic experience.

During this journey, I have had the opportunity to participate in the implementation of studies using LSD, DPT, MDA, MDMA and psilocybin, both with well-functioning mental health and religious professionals and with persons suffering from addictions to alcohol or narcotics, depression, anxiety, and other forms of psychological distress, notably cancer patients coming to terms with the lives they have lived and the approach of death. During approximately 38 years of research activity, my colleagues and I have experienced the privilege of working in significant depth with a rich variety of persons: adult men and women aged between early 20s and mid-80s from different educational, occupational, and racial/cultural backgrounds. Most were encountered in the context of individual psychotherapy, though some participated in ayahuasca groups in South America or, recently, group interventions with cancer patients. From this vantage point, I offer the following perspectives and recommendations.

The Critical Importance of Interpersonal Grounding

There is no question that safe and effective psychotherapy with psychedelic substances almost always requires more than simply receiving a drug or piece of blotter paper, drinking a tea, or chewing on some plant material. The psychedelic molecule may indeed provide an opportunity, giving access to a vast array of alternative forms of human consciousness, but how one responds to that opportunity depends not only on the molecular structure, dosage, and purity of substance but also on the recipient's ability to choose to relinquish the usual controls of the ego and to enter into the experiences choreographed by his/her own mind regardless of their nature and content. In research settings, for decades, this attitude has been encouraged with the mantram, "Trust, let go, and be open" (TLO). This decisive, courageous attitude for most persons seems to be most easily expressed in the context of a human relationship where a significant degree of unconditional acceptance and support has been established. This is especially critical in sessions with moderate or high dosage when the recipient may feel as though he/she is dying or going crazy as transitions in consciousness are occurring. If one seeks to escape from the emerging experiential content or to somehow censor or control it, the "nightmare sequence" usually occurs, typified by fear, panic, confusion, and sometimes paranoia. Such bad trips are extremely rare when an effective therapeutic alliance has been established in advance.

There appears to be a profound principle being expressed in the therapeutic alliance, often acknowledged in concepts such as the bejeweled net of Indra in Hinduism or the brotherhood of man or family of humanity in Western religious thought. Viewed as more fundamental than the usual everyday awareness of most of us, this sense of belonging or inter-connectedness within the mind, though often forgotten, remains a common discovery when mystical forms of consciousness are becoming manifested. In the framework of transpersonal psychology, one might note that in Latin *trans* means both above/beyond and between/across. When a person thinks, "I can do this on my own and don't really need anybody," some psychedelic sessions may prove to be safe and perhaps life-enhancing, but eventually it appears probable that very challenging content will eventually emerge and be difficult to explore in constructive ways without interpersonal grounding. In my own experience, my introduction to psychedelic experiences described above was indeed positive and occurred without an established therapeutic alliance. I would note that my mental state at the time was one of openness, that I chose to trust/entrust, and that the dosage happened to be relatively low Yet, in a subsequent experience under similar conditions I experienced acute psychological distress which, though intellectually instructive as an experiential seminar in psychosis and paranoia, did not prove to be facilitative of personal development.

Preparatory Psychoeducation

Just as if one were to go skiing or scuba-diving for the first time, it is wise and sometimes imperative to receive some basic instruction on how to navigate within alternative states of consciousness before embarking on a psychedelic-assisted journey. Such instruction is easily provided; it frames the *psychological set* that maximizes the positive, healing potential of psychedelic-assisted excursions into the mind. It also enhances the therapeutic bond. The essence of such preparatory instruction is expressed in the following six principles or guidelines:

1) *Being present, accepting, and exploring the content that emerges, irrespective of its nature.* During the period of psychedelic-assisted access to mental processes, many different experiences may occur. Some may be beautiful and inspiring; others may entail suffering, perhaps involving the confrontation and reliving of trauma, or intense encounters with guilt, shame, fear, anger, or unresolved grief. My impression is that each human mind is endowed with a certain wisdom that knows how to best choreograph the emergence and resolution of conflicts and healing processes. The task of the therapist is to be a facilitator, akin to a midwife who supports the person as emergence occurs, not to be a mechanic intent on fixing or repairing with various interventions. Thus the person who receives the psychedelic is supported in exploring and valuing whatever may emerge rather than judging whether it is good or bad, interesting or boring, transcendental or mundane, etc. The motivation for using a psychedelic to potentially accelerate and deepen the therapeutic process is expressed in a willingness to move into and through any suffering that may be encountered as an intrinsic part of an acknowledged desire for personal and perhaps spiritual development. From this perspective the dark night of the soul, as expressed by St. John of the Cross in the 16th century, is not a symptom of failure or a distraction but rather an intrinsic part of the spiritual journey.

2) *Readiness to rapidly confront* any manifestations within the field of awareness that appear potentially frightening is of fundamental importance. If a monster/dragon/bogeyman appears, one is prepared to meet it, perhaps acknowledging initial fear but then asserting curiosity and a desire for understanding: "Are you ever scary! But, why are you here? Where did you come from? What are you made of? What might I learn from you?" One is prepared to dive into the pupil of the eye if the threatening image has eyes, akin to diving into a swimming pool. The assumption is that it is your very own monster and that it appears in order to teach you something intrinsic to the healing process. In the religions that employ *ayahuasca* (South American psychoactive brew) there is the tradition of confronting the great anaconda serpent if it should appear. If one tries to flee and escape from it, panic and paranoia will reliably occur. Rather, one dives into its mouth and looks out through its eyes. In becoming the anaconda, perhaps one owns his/her own *shakti* (cosmic energy or life force: kundalini, elan vital, chi, etc.) and affirms/accepts the strength, empowerment, and creativity that the symbolic image may manifest.

   Another metaphor for teaching this attitude that has been employed in many psychedelic research sites is the invitation to imagine going into the basement of one's life. One boldly announces, "I'm coming down," and descends with one firm step after the other, carrying a bright search-lamp, and perhaps affirming trust in the company of the therapist. One searches out the darkest corners one can find and brightly illumines them, essentially affirming, "If there's anything down here that's contributing to my anxiety or depression, I want to know what it is." This proactive, courageous intention typically leads through abreaction but eventually culminates in an awareness that there is nothing to fear.

3) *Turning off the intellect* can be especially challenging for well-educated persons who tend to rely on the defense mechanism of intellectualization. A common response to the opportunities afforded by the action of a psychedelic substance is essentially to say to oneself, "Stop! What's going on here? Let me find some concepts, words, or labels to console myself before venturing any more deeply into my mind." This is the point at which some persons, if wearing an eyeshade, may lift its edges to reorient themselves in the room.

An established way to prepare for this defensive tendency is to essentially bribe the intellect in advance, perhaps on the day prior to the psychedelic-assisted session. Essentially one says, "You're a wonderful intellect, so bright and clever. You guided me through graduate school and into my profession and have such a rich vocabulary. However, during the action of the psychedelic, you go out and play. I promise that, when you come back in at the end of the day, there will be many new experiences to reflect upon. At that time, you can draw on your knowledge of depth psychology, comparative religions, philosophy, and even quantum physics and choose the words that you find most helpful as you articulate and begin to integrate your experiences."

As classically expressed by the psychologist of religion, Rudolf Otto (1917), our mental processes may be viewed in three categories: the rational, the irrational and the non-rational. It is this third category, often called intuition, that best reflects the most profound insights that occur in some psychedelic sessions. It is expressed well in a verse from the Taoist scriptures, the *Tao Te Ching:* "Those who know do not speak; those who speak do not know."

4) *Accepting and exploring somatic sensations* may not only decrease potential physical discomfort, but may facilitate the encounter with and resolution of important psychological content. As has become increasingly recognized by therapists who specialize in the resolution of trauma, memories, and concomitant emotions often appear to be stored within or correlated with muscular tensions. If one focuses upon a particular sensation that seems to be demanding attention, often a memory will awaken, and a sequence of potential resolution will occur. As well expressed by Bessel van der Kolk (2014), "The body keeps the score." Thus a sensation that seems to command attention may be much more than an undesirable side-effect of a psychedelic substance; it may be an invitation to insight and healing.

   Practically, this orientation is often helpful when dealing with nausea, perhaps the most common psychosomatic symptom that may occur during a session. One is instructed in advance that, should nausea occur, one should immediately "dive into her/his stomach"; when the sensation is accepted, it often immediately vanishes. Should the sensation be persistent and one reports a need to spit something out, experienced therapists will invite the person who has ingested the psychedelic to briefly sit up and vomit/spit into an emesis basin, held at the person's mouth, typically without even removing the eyeshade or headphones if they are already in place. It is no big deal and there's no need to interrupt the session to attend to the transient symptom.

   Sometimes, as is recognized in communities that employ ayahuasca or peyote, the purgation is experienced as cleansing or purification, even to the extent of *La Purga* (vomiting and diarrhea together). When one lies back down, the inner journey continues to open up, and the somatic distress is left behind. It is noteworthy that with well-prepared persons nausea often doesn't occur at all. When it appears it often may be understood as a symptom of anxiety and an attempt of the everyday self (ego) to resist or control emerging content.

5) *Normalizing physical contact,* which may be sought for reassurance, connection, or occasionally for safety, is an important part of preparation for a psychedelic-assisted session. Demonstrated, discussed, and rehearsed, usually on the day prior to the session, it may provide potent interpersonal grounding especially during unexpectedly rapid transitions in consciousness or the emergence of challenging psychological content. It may supplement the steady, reassuring voice of the therapist. Usually limited to reaching out for the hand of the therapist or accepting a touch on the shoulder or arm, such connection for many persons can provide the nonverbal support required to channel anxiety constructively and encounter psychological con-

tent that otherwise might remain inaccessible. This good touch can sometimes be of critical importance; although the body on the couch may look the same throughout the day, the content being experienced may range from that of a pre-verbal infant through many stages of development, even to the unitive consciousness of a spiritual master. Such human warmth and spontaneity can be communicated sensitively and effectively. The person who has received the psychedelic can reach out at any time and the therapist can initiate supportive touch when his/her intuition prompts such behavior. Touch is never sexual; sessions may be video-recorded in settings where legal back-up or supervision is desired.

6) *Entering into music* that has been thoughtfully selected to provide nonverbal support, especially during the initial ascent and the most intense portions of a medium or high-dose session, may well significantly enhance the safety and efficacy of a psychedelic experience. Generally, the use of a well-designed playlist that has been found effective with diverse people is wise as it frees up the therapist from playing disc jockey and enables the therapist to be more fully present with the psychedelic voyager. The usual musical preferences of either therapist or voyager may not be important during the intense phases of a session, especially when the sound is experienced as a vehicle of transport and support and when consciousness has expanded beyond the usual limits of everyday awareness. Critique of music may be a common defense, especially when potentially stressful content is emerging during a session. When one is encouraged to "hate it with passion," resolution of conflicts tends to occur, and the very same music may be experienced as beautiful (Richards, 2022).

Concluding Comments

Although the use of psychedelics by humans may be traced to 1500 BC, if not to the dawn of civilization, and (like mushrooms) has appeared and vanished in many societies over time, they are now on the verge of integration into Western cultures in medical, educational, and religious contexts (Richards, 2016). The hope I share with many is that this integration will proceed in fundamentally safe and responsible ways. Different people may well require different degrees of preparation, session guidance, and integrative support. Some with severe conditions of poor mental health may require extensive relationship-building and guidance in order to potentially experience the effects of psychedelics in beneficial ways and may be well advised to focus on milder meditative, psychotherapeutic, or psychopharmacological approaches of personal or spiritual development. Continuing research will help establish if, when, and how psychedelics may prove helpful to persons with significant psychotic tendencies or histories. However, we already have substantial data that are supportive of their beneficial use with a variety of mental health conditions. Further, they may well become recognized as powerful educational tools as we continue to explore the nature and mysteries of human consciousness. Their potential role in what we call religion or spirituality is being increasingly recognized. As Abraham Maslow (1966) stressed during the birth of humanistic and transpersonal psychology, true science is on the frontiers of knowledge, stretching to attempt to incorporate new concepts and language, which is where we find ourselves in psychedelic research.

References

Agrawal, M., Richards, W., Beaussant, Y., Shnayder, S., Ameli, R., Roddy, K., Stevens, N., Richards, B., Schor, N., Honstein, H., Jenkins, B., Bates, M., & Thambi, P. (2023). Psilocybin-assisted group therapy with cancer diagnosed with a major depressive disorder. *Cancer, 130* (7), 1137-1146.

Garcia-Romeu, A., & Richards, W. (2018). Current perspectives on psychedelic therapy: Use of serotonergic hallucinogens in clinical interventions. *International Review of Psychiatry 30*(4), 291-316.

Griffiths, R., Richards, W., McCann, U., & Jesse, R. (2006). Psilocybin can occasion mystical-type experiences having substantial and sustained personal meaning and spiritual significance. *Psychopharmacology, 187*(3), 268-283.

Griffiths, R., Richards, W., Johnson, M., McCann, U., & Jesse, R. (2008). Mystical-type experiences occasioned by psilocybin mediate the attribution of personal meaning and spiritual significance 14 months later. *Journal of Psychopharmacology, 22,* 621-632.

Griffiths, R., Johnson, M., Richards, W., Richards B., McCann, U., & Jesse R. (2011). Psilocybin occasioned mystical-type experiences: Immediate and persisting dose-related effects. *Psychopharmacology, 218,* 649-665.

Griffiths, R., Johnson, M., Richards, W., Richards, B., Jesse, R., MacLean K., Barrett, F., Cosimano, M., & Klinedinst, M. (2017). Psilocybin-occasioned mystical-type experiences in combination with meditation and other spiritual practices produces enduring positive changes in psychological functioning and trait measures of prosocial attitudes and behavior, *Journal of Psychopharmacology, 32*(1), 49-69.

Johnson, M., Richards, W., & Griffiths, R. (2008). Human hallucinogen research: Guidelines for safety. *Journal of Psychopharmacology, 22,* 603-619.

Maslow, A. (1966). *The psychology of science: A reconnaissance.* NY: Harper & Row.

Otto, R. (1917/1932). *The idea of the holy.* NY: Galaxy.

Rhead, J., Soskin, R., Turek, I., Richards, W., Yensen, R., Kurland, A., & Ota, K. (1977). Psychedelic drug (DPT)-assisted psychotherapy with alcoholics: A controlled study. *Journal of Psychedelic Drugs, 9,* 287-300.

Pahnke, W., & Richards, W. (1966). Implications of LSD and experimental mysticism. *Journal of Religion and Health, 5,* 175-208.

Richards, W., Grof, S., Goodman, L., & Kurland, A. (1972). LSD-assisted psycho-therapy and the Human Encounter with Death. *Journal of Transpersonal Psychology, 4,* 121-150.

Richards, W., Rhead, J., DiLeo, F., Yensen, R., & Kurland, A. (1977). The peak experience variable in DPT-assisted psychotherapy with cancer patients. *Journal of Psychedelic Drugs, 9,* 1-10.

Richards, W., & Rhead, J. (1977). Psychedelic drug-assisted psychotherapy: Present perspectives, promises and problems. *Journal of Altered States of Consciousness, 3,* 97-98.

Richards W. (2016). *Sacred knowledge: Psychedelics and religious experiences.* NY: Columbia University Press.

Richards, W. (2022). Music in psychedelic research: The continuing legacy of Helen Bonny. *Journal of the Association for Music and Imagery, 18,* 83-93.

Strassman, R. (2001). *The spirit molecule.* Rochester: Park Street Press.

Van der Kolk, B. (2014). *The body keeps the score.* NY: Penguin Books.

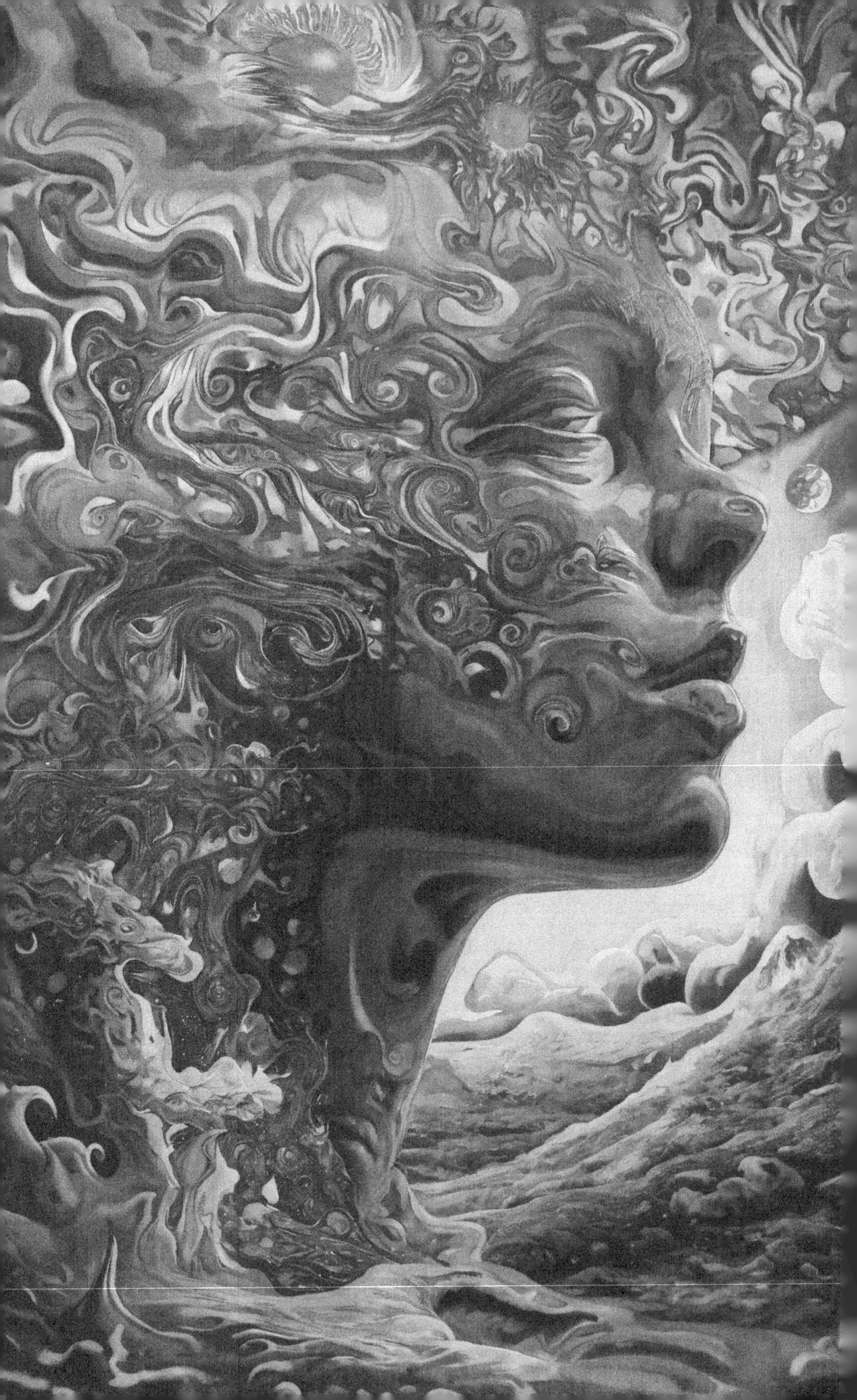

Rebecca J. Neisler

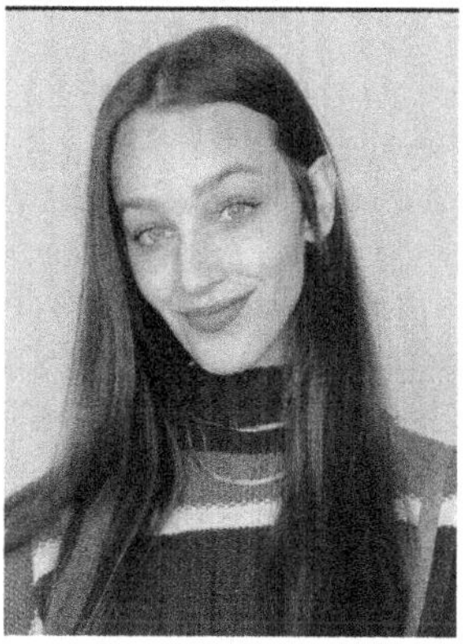

Rebecca J. Neisler is a student at the University of Florida majoring in psychology with an emphasis on neuroscience. She is interested in clinical psychology, neuropharmacology, and psychotherapy. Particular interests center around psychedelic-assisted therapy and the research of entheogens to improve the lives of patients struggling with mental health.
rjoan.neisler@gmail.com

A Journey Into Psychedelic Realms

In the endeavor to share my encounters with psychedelics through writing and anecdotal reports, initial doubts arose concerning the relevance of a 30-year-old female student's perspective without (yet) the scholarly imprimatur of a PhD. However, what I hope to achieve in this personal essay is to show the intrinsic value embedded in my tapestry of erotically spiritual and occasionally challenging voyages with psychedelics. By sharing my experience, I hope to shed light on the potential benefits of these potent substances and on the utmost importance of their study and research to attain a world where psychedelics are used safely and effectively in clinical practice.

Reflecting on my life's trajectory, marked by a search for healing, audacious escapades, and experimentation with psychoactive compounds during adolescence, I cannot but acknowledge the transformative potential of psychedelic medicines. After being sent away to an all-girls home at the age of 12, I held resentment towards my parents and struggled with releasing negative emotions. This fueled a yearning for deeper understanding, eventually leading to the exploration of psychedelic realms. Undeterred by the situation that swayed me to embrace LSD and later partake in an ayahuasca ceremony with a Brazilian shaman, these experiences and subsequent reflections on them led toward profound healing, forgiveness, and new beginnings. These verbatim accounts integrate rich descriptive narratives of visions, physiological effects, and perception changes. However, no human-created words or language could ever come close to fully describing the experience of ingesting this holy, spiritual vine.

Unveiling LSD at Thirteen

At the tender age of 13, amidst the background of an unsettling childhood, I embarked on a journey, gulping the overflow of my cup, running like a river streaming alongside its surface. It was 2006, in Valrico, Florida. Despite my impending curfew, I sensed my return home would unveil a markedly altered teenage daughter. The story unfolds with the discovery of an LSD-laden paper sheet. It was painted with dripped acid onto a tree corpse's saturated, bleached skin, moistening the dried yet dead bark shedding, delicately wrapped in foil and concealed in the freezer, reminiscent of Picasso's lost murals—a surreal Christmas list for any teenager. One hundred equally sliced quadrilaterals rest within a larger one, a mise en abyme effect. Saints they genuinely are. The trees, that is.

I was advised to place four of these tiny square-saturated LSD tabs under my tongue and let them marinate. Several hours after the substance hit my bloodstream, I was hysterically laughing until I cried. Vivid, colorful, and precise lines danced to the music playing in the background in perfect concurrence behind my eyelids as if my mind were attuned to each vibrational beat. I was witnessing the harp's divine strings. I had not laughed this hard or witnessed such joy in my life. After admission into an all-girls home the year prior, I was now in a different realm and dimension. What is this place, and how is it possible?

Time ceased to exist. After a year of shock, I was again a toddler, an innocent child enjoying everything. Something shifted inside me that evening. I had a sensational feeling of knowing true freedom and its sweet-savory taste. Finally breaking away from the horrific life I once knew, ridden with trauma and pain, there was hope around the corner, a light at the end of the tunnel, a reason to believe everything would be all right. There was something much more beautiful about life than I had ever realized, and it was worth appreciating in total joy. At this moment, I understood the need to move forward on my path and forgive my parents to begin healing.

Emotions were all over the place when the sun came up, with the main question masking my thoughts: Was this a religion I had only yet discovered? Perhaps when our ancestors prayed, it was for this road to redemption. Luckily, my life was back on God's table for review. We all have something to leave behind, whatever it may be. A legacy would be ideal. As for now, it is how I put together the English alphabet like a soup of symbols, markings, and swirls in hopes of explaining the influences of LSD on the tainted virgin brain of a 13-year-old. I played with the cards at hand—no judgment taken; no remorse given.

Of course, I struck moments of paranoia. My survival instincts lit up to help me navigate the meaning behind what I was going through. Most importantly, my prefrontal cortex was not fully developed yet, making the ability to process my experience even more difficult. Despite these circumstances, it was a life-changing moment that inspired me daily to pursue a career in behavioral cognitive neurosciences. I hope my story, coming from a young woman who statistically should not be where she is today because of unfavorable childhood luck, is accepted positively. I do not owe all my progress to psychedelics, but it would be dishonest if I said it had no impact on my course in life afterward. The circumstances handed to me early in life leading to the exploration of psychedelics at an abnormally early age hold even more value, knowing my once repressed stories can impact a large community and contribute to the tidal wave of peaking interest to understand and analyze their short- and long-term effects on mental health and the role they play in a person's life.

Ingestion of LSD at an early developmental stage was overwhelming, especially without guided support and pre- and post-therapy sessions. I do not advocate for the consumption of these substances or similar ones by any minor or in any illegal context and setting. At the time, I had to navigate these hurdles alone, as exploring the psychedelic realm was highly looked down upon. However, 18 years have passed, and I see the grit, determination, and hope it gave me throughout adolescence and young adulthood to continue life with love, passion, purpose, meaning, and beauty. More than anything, my experience gave me a deep desire to seek a more scientific and evidence-based understanding of these compounds and their effect on the brain. I wish to see a world that advocates for the professional administration of similar compounds and pushes for their approval and proper application within the medical field. My spiritual encounters have been under the influence of psychedelics, resulting in a much more caring, loving, understanding, and accepting person. Psychedelics have influenced my life dramatically and in an exceptionally positive way by instilling a sense of hope, purpose, and contribution to my community.

The Tunnel Down Ayahuasca

Spit it out. Purge it out and throw it up. The cup spills.
Facilitators: On the count of three, say: Purge. 1. 2. 3.
Attendees: PURGE!

Banisteriopsis caapi, also known as yagé, is a South American liana of the Malpighiaceae family. Added to the caapi brew are parts of the *Psychortria viridis* bush. *P. viridis* has a common name of chacruna—a perennial, shrubby, flowering plant in the coffee family of Rubiaceae. The brew is a decoction of the two entheogenic latter plants containing N,N-dimethyltryptamine (DMT), a tryptamine alkaloid (Hamill et al., 2019). The common names of the ayahuasca brew are Vine of the Soul or Rope of Death. These thoughts and feelings of death will make sense later—days, weeks, months, and sometimes years after unfolding the experience through integration tools and sound research. During this death analogy, hell is a concept, a mindset, and this determines if one gets the Vine of the Soul or the Rope of Death. Mind over matter never had such valid reasoning, and there is a fine line between that equation.

Friday, 6:00 PM

Before initiation into the ayahuasca church, the facilitators prayed four prayers in each direction of the wind—north, south, east, and west—placing what members call a sacrament over the heart, giving thanks to God for allowing consummation in his ever-so-beautiful creations. The first participating medicine in the ceremony is *Nicotiana rustica,* known as Rapé/Hapé, shamanic snuff, or mapacho—a sacred tobacco plant predating Incan times (Tushingham, 2013). When turning in line, one meets the traditional healer, who blows Hapé up the nose using a large pipe made from animal bone. Fireworks set off in each brain hemisphere as she blew the snuff into each nostril. I blurted out profanities in response to the painful discomfort and the powdery discharge dripping from my nasal cavities and suddenly felt terrible that this American gesture would offend the traditional healer. However, it did not, for the Brazilian healer embraces all.

The following rite of passage is the introduction and beginning of the sacred ritual, and consuming the potion is the final initiation step into the church. Upon receiving the first ayahuasca sacrament from the Brazilian traditional healer, I drank 2 tablespoons of the dark-grated leaves and roots in the small glass cup. A dark, chocolatey, molasses-honey, bitter taste and scent that lingered for days even after the ceremony—a new olfaction one always remembers. Throughout the weekend, the bitter taste became manageable.

Within 20 minutes, all previous realities shattered behind both of my oculars. Before I could crawl out of my mat to let the facilitator know I would surely die, I already did. The top center of the maloca took a helical inward shape, a logarithmic swirl with many geometric patterns and colors. Symmetrical boxes of around 15 separated each showcase of artwork while focusing on the maloca's ceiling. One cube had a black and white checkerboard; the next was swirling, another was bright pink, and another bright blue. So much art in one moment, but then vertigo took off exceptionally when the colorful circus reached a black hole effect, sucking one in, or so I thought, only briefly. The world appeared animated and cartoon-like.

This moment was unpleasant because of the intensity and anxiety caused by the unknown—in my first ceremony, I admit, I swayed towards the Rope of Death. Soon, the circle spun too fast. Lightheadedness and emesis set in. There was no alleged body coordination to reach the facilitator sitting directly in front of the mat a yard away, nor the strength to push vocals into making the right sounds. At this point, all there is to do is observe. Here comes the beginning of a purge, coming out like black tar, vomiting the water turned to wine. The tar in the purging bucket turned into a soup of alien sludge with speckles of pink and green appearing as my ten fingers grew longer around the white bucket. Weird!

It was as if I had just slightly scraped the surface of tunneling too far down Alice's rabbit hole (Carroll & Hague, 1985), mirroring the many written accounts about near-death experiences. After purging and settling into this new alien skin, I could write my thoughts in my journal, although it came out like a 3rd grader trying to get out all the images, links, and memories. Discombobulated and unorganized, slouched and tilted, because a straight line was unimaginable.

Friday, 8:00 PM

Around 2 hours after the first sacrament, we were due for a second one. One tablespoon would do this time—less is more. Twenty minutes after ingestion, the floor began to wave like a purple, fluorescent ocean, with electrical light arrays gently flashing throughout the maloca's foundation. Soon, the thin electricity lines traced each body, including mine, as if I had just entered Pandora's world, only one more beautiful. Images of an intricate, beautiful woman flashed in the center of each eye with extraordinarily complex and endless fractals.

This fractal dimension felt like I could zoom in and out, microscopically or macroscopically. There was a rush into time and space, where the universe only had majestic purple and pink colors slightly mixed with blue hues. There were two stars, one larger than the other. Both rested diagonally and slept sideways of each other, with the brighter, larger one on the left top corner and the smaller one on the bottom right. Precise and detailed electricity lines emanated from each star portal as the silvery white lights bounced off the faraway planet stars and dripped both horizontally and vertically. The delicate and thin bolts leaked in perfect symmetry, math most people had never witnessed. I sat in awe as the visions continued to the tambourine's beat and the maracas' rattles.

Benevolent tears streamed down my face while observing the most magnificent places I have ever been as my body picked up the droplets of alligator tears filling up like a balloon in each tear duct, releasing the excess gasses into fairy water, a stream forming that trickled alongside the round Earth of my face. Although aware of my altered consciousness, nothing else was visible except these two stars dripping with light energy. It was an experience analogous to God placing his hands on my eyes, leading me to one place and one place only. The stars were so close I felt I could reach out and touch them. In the moments of the ceremony, the decoction of each vein in the leaves of the plant brew seemed to be the gatekeepers to all levels of the universe, God, the infinite, the past, present, and future. The alkaloids in the decoction are a harmonious pairing, orchestrating life into a symphony as if Beethoven and Mozart had a baby. This time, it was the Vine of the Soul.

Saturday, 8:30 AM

One tablespoon was blessed and handed to each member of the church. At that point, even remembering the taste arouses shivers. This ceremony is held outdoors instead of under the maloca structure. Attendees are assigned a woven rug underneath a *Pinus palustris* tree. Less than half an hour after ingestion, the *P. palustris* tree began to wave and topple over with teal colors and beautiful intricacies within the trunk's large bark shards. Ascension into the sky started here, all wrapped in the tree's embrace. The tree swaddled and then swallowed. Vertigo. Emesis. Purge. Alien bucket. Alien fingers. Alien sludge.

Then, there was the carpenter bee that approached me mid-ceremony. He was so large he appeared with sleek black armor covered in obsidian and gold. His wings were large and fierce, clicking like metal brushing against metal while staring into my soul. Naturally, there was a moment of terror with thoughts of getting stung. I began ducking repeatedly and found my oversized jacket to be a security blanket. The inside of the coat layers with fuzzy black cotton rubbed across my arms like silk. Fetal position. What does he want?

A facilitator walked over to my rug with a white blanket, swatting away the bee in slow motion. Glancing at each facilitator and seeing their returning smiles was comforting and assured my safety. This must have been entertaining for them, considering their smirks as I silently wailed my arms around, making a quiet scene. When the bee departed, saltwater tears streamed profusely down my face yet again, on the Earth's face, smiling from ear to ear and giggling in awe. Not tears of fear or fright, tears of immense love and appreciation of the astounding beauty of nature. My hair felt like velvet, and I internally apologized to my body for being so harsh and crude towards it my whole life. I felt my soul could recall what it has known all along—an infinite connection with self, animals, and others. Each encounter felt significant, like an underlying message waiting to be translated.

Saturday, 6:00 PM

The altar has crystals, sound bowls, incense, sage, Florida Water, a palm frond of the Arecaceae, and candles that display neatly over linen cloth. Pillows and blankets awaited on the white mat. After the Rapé/Hapé and ayahuasca sacraments in this last ceremony, Sananga eyedrops are offered by the traditional healer. Sananga is derived from the *Tabernaemontana* species and is a powerful sacred plant medicine among the Amazonian tribes (Feeney et al., 2018). The Sananga eye drops felt like lightning bolts penetrating and sinking into my orifices. However, the fire and heat of the accompanying burning sensation are only temporary, much like everything else.

Soon, I transformed into a snake. Starting at the spine, each vertebra cracked and morphed into my new slithering body, harmonizing synchronously while I moved to the musical tunes. Images of jaguars appeared, and my eyes took the lens of two diamonds. Once light hits the surface of a diamond, three optical effects occur—reflection, refraction, and dispersion. All the women in the maloca rose to their feet and danced so gracefully, majestically, and powerfully. There was a sense of connection, familiarity, and oneness I had not experienced before. I recalled scripture verses from my childhood and thought, "This must be what standing in the presence of God is like."

My ayahuasca ceremony led to complex mystical experiences modulating the sensory, perceptual, and cognitive systems with emotional processes and increased introspection. After that weekend, I felt reborn. I reached out to people in estranged relationships with me, wanting to pour endless love towards them and rekindle them. My mind felt sharp, and I could communicate positively and efficiently on tough conversation topics. I felt incredibly thankful that the traditional healer and her people were willing to share their botanical knowledge with me and all their guests to undergo such a transformative and spiritual experience.

Conclusions

Consuming psychedelic medicines invariably induces a range of experiences, including mystical feelings, ego dissolution, altered body perception, synesthesia, visions, and a sense of connection to the world and others. The actual dividends of these substances manifest in the aftermath of the psychedelic sessions when individuals undergo profound internal changes and transformation of their life perspectives. The transient nature of psychedelics and their otherworldly visions can be challenging to describe with ordinary language. A trustworthy individual who validates the complexity of these descriptions is paramount. This highlights the importance of integration for prolonging mental health improvements.

Metaphor is a powerful tool for understanding the unusual core of psychedelic realms and has been my most valuable integration strategy. Understanding a vision as a metaphor has helped me reframe my interpretation and describe the otherwise indescribable aspects of psychedelics. When writing down the imagery in detail, metaphors are often inevitable because of the ineffable characteristics of entheogens. By analyzing the connection between psychedelic use, storytelling, and metaphor, we can gain a deeper understanding of both traditional and clinical practices. Developing a literacy of metaphor can be beneficial for both therapists and those who use psychedelics. Just as narrative medicine helps healthcare providers understand patient stories, metaphor can enhance a therapist's ability to understand and respond to a patient's psychedelic experience. This skill is not only beneficial to patients but can also enrich the lives of those who use psychedelics in a non-clinical setting.

Through personal odysseys with psychedelic medicines, I acquired the capacity to navigate and transcend enduring childhood traumas and lingering psychological distress. My story is a testament demonstrating the transformative potential inherent in botanical and synthesized psychedelic medicines. These substances can be pivotal in dismantling entrenched false beliefs and surmounting life obstacles. It is essential to acknowledge that psychedelics are not universally suitable, necessitating ongoing research to delineate their potential therapeutic benefits within a professional and controlled setting—a cause I ardently champion and hope to continue contributing to.

I hope to see the day when this metamorphosis will occur through dedicated practices of controlled integration, therapy, and various support mechanisms. My experiences show me the transformative potential of psychedelic medicines within the psychoanalytic and psychological fields. These substances serve as catalysts for therapeutic breakthroughs, demanding a meticulous understanding of their effects, ongoing research, and incorporation of their benefits into professional therapeutic frameworks. I remain committed to advocating for continued exploration of these therapeutic modalities, recognizing their potential to effect enduring positive change in people's lives and communities.

References

Carroll, L., & Hague, M. (1985). *Alice's adventures in Wonderland.* New York: Holt, Rinehart, and Winston.

Feeney, K., Labate, B. C., & Hudson, J. H. (2018). Bubbling with controversy: Legal challenges for ceremonial ayahuasca circles in the United States. *Plant Medicines, Healing and Psychedelic Science,* 87–111. https://doi.org/10.1007/978-3-319-76720-8_6

Hamill, J., Hallak, J., Dursun, S. M., & Baker, G. (2019). Ayahuasca: Psychological and physiologic effects, pharmacology and potential uses in addiction and mental illness. *Current Neuropharmacology, 17*(2), 108–128. https://doi.org/10.2174/1570159X16666180125095902

Tushingham, S., Ardura, D., Eerkens, J. W., Palazoglu, M., Shahbaz, S., & Fiehn, O. (2013). Hunter-gatherer tobacco smoking: Earliest evidence from the Pacific Northwest Coast of North America. *Journal of Archaeological Science, 40*(2), 1397–1407. https://doi.org/10.1016/j.jas.2012.09.019

The mind, unfettered by the constraints of the ego, dances with the cosmos in ecstatic union.

—J. R. Damon

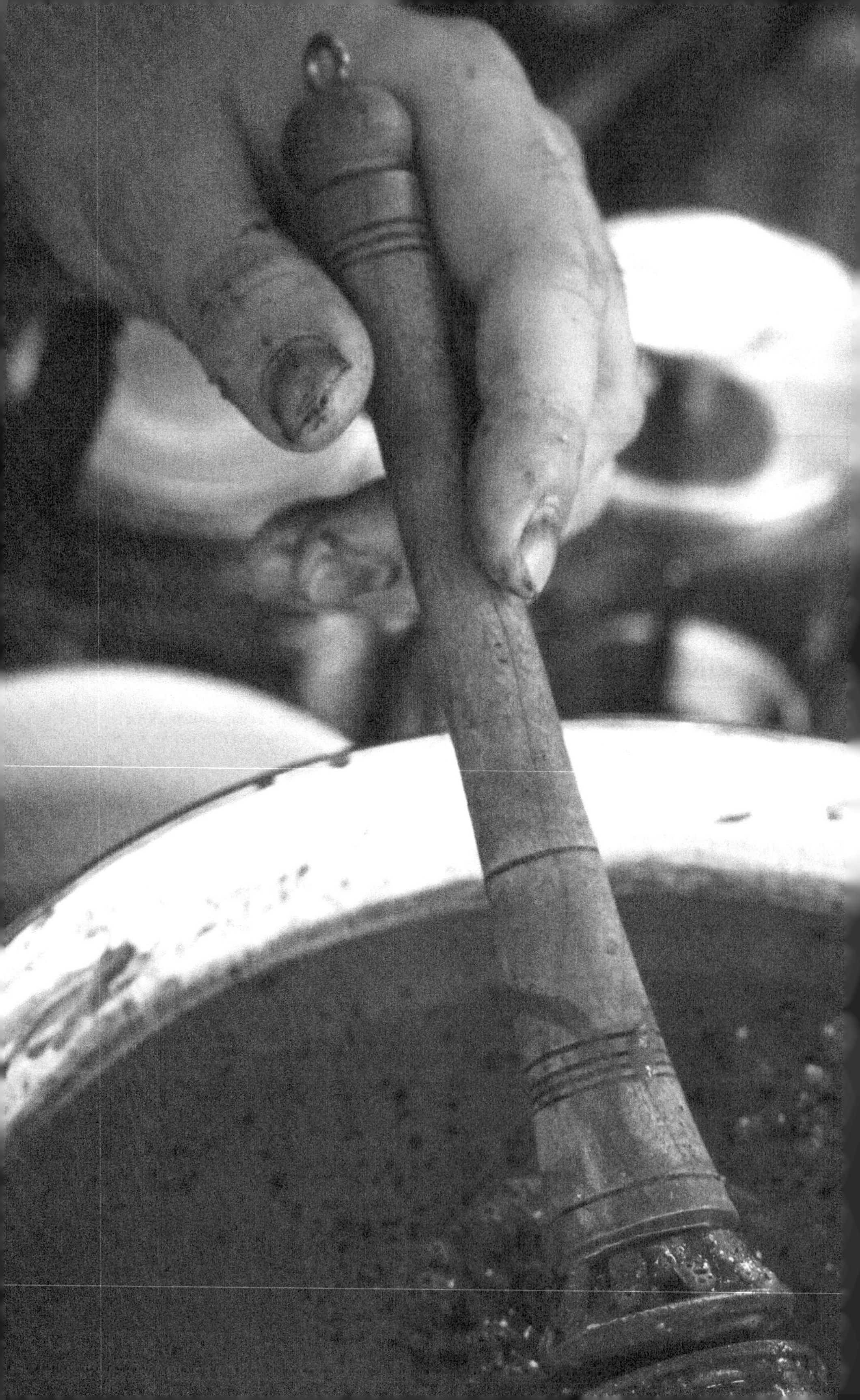

Vanessa Nguyen

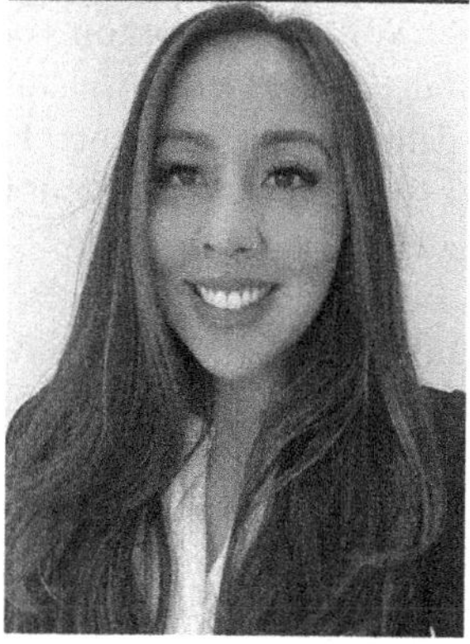

Vanessa Nguyen is a therapist, doctoral student, freelance writer, and advocate for psychedelic-assisted therapy. She earned her master's in clinical psychology at Meridian University. Vanessa has experience in higher levels of care with clients who struggle with mental health challenges and addiction. Her therapeutic approach combines DBT, ACT, Internal Family Systems, Eastern philosophies, and a mindfulness-based holistic approach to navigating difficult life experiences. A second-generation Vietnamese-American, Vanessa is particularly interested in exploring the effects of intergenerational and cultural trauma on immigrants and children of immigrants.
nguyenvanessa0502@gmail.com

Indigenous Plant Medicine Ceremonies: Healing Generations of Pain

If you asked me a few years ago where my journey of healing and grieving would take me, I would never have imagined I would be traveling all the way to a beautiful jungle in Chemuyil, Quintana Roo, Mexico, and right into the heart of a plant medicine retreat. After a few years of being in a doctoral program and working as a therapist, I felt a growing urge to deepen my therapeutic practice, improve my relationship with myself, and heal the parts of me that continued to feel fragmented. The weight of my identity as a second-generation Vietnamese American and daughter of hardworking and loving migrant parents, and the pain from unexpectedly losing my father in 2015, were the catalysts for my decision to embark on a deeply transformative journey with the unconventional.

Throughout my entire life, I have tied so much of my self-worth to these culturally and socially constructed identities, and I had lost sight of who I truly was underneath these layers of labels. When I lost my father, it felt as if any remainders of my most authentic self had died with him. My entire life and the decisions I have made to carve out a safe and predictable path for myself have always been conventional, rooted in adherence to culturally and socially accepted standards and expectations. I wanted the perfect grades, a successful job, and a life that did not attract any negative attention. Being conventional has kept me safe in so many ways. But a strictly conventional life also caused me to fear uncertainty and question my place in the world. What would happen to me once the perfect grades were no longer needed? Once my job no longer gave me meaning? I have spent most of my life trying to repay my parents for the sacrifices they made for me, and in the process, I lost sight of my own purpose.

When my symptoms of anxiety and depression began to worsen during my early 20s, I decided to seek a therapist. At the same time, I was volunteering as an intern at a residential treatment center for individuals struggling with various mental health disorders. I started off as the client in therapy and eventually made it through school to become a therapist myself due to my growing passion for helping others heal from their own mental health challenges. I have had a deep respect and admiration for our current mental health system in the United States, and I have found so much joy and meaning in being a therapist. After years of therapy and antidepressants, my symptoms had reduced enough that I no longer felt as if I didn't want to continue living life anymore. My anxious and ruminating thoughts had reduced enough that I could function and find joy in life again, for the most part. However, I continued to struggle with the pain of losing my father, from the pressure to succeed and be able to provide for my family, and from feelings of guilt and shame that I didn't always understand.

Aside from losing my father in 2015, I've also experienced trauma from being assaulted as a teenager and being emotionally abused in toxic relationships. I had always believed that my trauma helped me empathize with my clients. But if this were the case, shouldn't I deserve to heal with them? I have felt drawn to the healing potential of plant medicine for quite some time now, and I realized that to be fully authentic as a therapist and human being overall, I needed to allow myself to be completely vulnerable. For as long as I can remember, I have had this protective armor up, guarding the parts of myself that I was deeply ashamed of. So much of me felt lost and incomplete, and I was ready to explore a new way of being, a new way of showing up in the world.

I have read up on the studies done by Johns Hopkins Medicine researchers on the efficacy of psilocybin in relieving symptoms of major depression (Davis et al., 2021), in reducing activity in the brain's ego center (Barrett et al., 2020), and decreasing existential anxiety in participants with cancer (Griffiths et al., 2016). My ego had always been my downfall. I remember receiving my first grade of a C in elementary school and crying because I thought I deserved better. As much as I've tried to silence my ego, parts of it have always manifested as a need to prove myself to everyone around me. My fear of failure haunted me, and every rejection felt like a deep wound. Perhaps psilocybin could help me.

I contacted a psychedelic-assisted psychotherapist and medicine woman named Yessica at Mindful You Experiences, who together with her partner, Mac, assist others along their healing journey by facilitating and conducting indigenous plant medicine ceremonies in Mexico. A few weeks after booking my retreat, I would meet with Yessica, Mac, and two shamanic healers from the Indigenous and Original Pueblos of Mexico. The minute I stepped foot into the vast and beautiful jungle where the ceremonies would take place, I felt like it was where I needed to be.

I made the decision to experience psychedelic healing in the context of Indigenous plant-medicine practices and ceremony because I wanted to pay respect to the traditions and roots of these practices. Psychoactive plants have been used by Indigenous people for healing purposes long before they made their way into the modern West. According to Indigenous knowledge, when individuals go through traumatic experiences, they lose parts of their souls that can be accessed through altered states of consciousness. Practices such as the use of psychoactive plants, dance, chanting, and being out in nature can lead to the dissolution of habitual patterns of being and thinking that no longer serve the individual. My own habitual patterns of thinking brought me a life of anxiety and pressure, and I felt stuck in a cycle of self-blame, guilt, and shame.

Many Indigenous cultures believe that altered states of consciousness reveal the parts of our souls that have been lost through intergenerational and present-day trauma (Ringland, 2019). Indigenous cultures also embrace the healing potential of Mother Nature, engaging in practices such as using sage and other plants for energy cleaning. They view the root of illness as a disconnect from the land, from each other, and from our ancestral origins.

I have struggled with anxiety for most of my adolescent and adult life. After both of my parents migrated over to the United States during the Vietnam War, they worked hard to create a comfortable life for my sister and me. Memories of my childhood include feeling loved and supported by an amazing family, yet still experiencing the self-inflicted pressure to succeed and give back to my parents. My self-perception and sense of identity growing up were rooted in achievements and how well I could assimilate into Western culture while still honoring my Vietnamese heritage. The knowledge of the hardships that my parents went through back in Vietnam became my biggest motivator to succeed, while simultaneously contributing to my own descent into anxiety and a deep fear of failure.

In his book, *Trauma and Memory: Brain and Body in Search for a Living Past,* Peter Levine (2015) speaks about the generational transmission of trauma and how symptoms of anxiety and depression can be passed down from generation to generation. Levine reflects on a conversation that he had with a Navajo medicine man, who taught him that the generational transmission of trauma is especially undeniable when parents and ancestors have lived through times of social upheaval and war (Chapter 9). Although indigenous knowledge varies according to the culture, people, and area, there are common approaches to healing that seem to be universal among many Indigenous people. Most Indigenous approaches to healing are holistic in that they focus on the mental, emotional, physical, and spiritual aspects of a person (Robbins & Dewar, 2011). Additionally, Indigenous practices of healing are done communally and focus on collective healing, which explains why the consumption of plant medicine is usually done alongside others as a symbol of inclusivity, respect, and love (Ringland, 2019). Finally, where Western therapeutic approaches tend to focus on the individual experience, Indigenous approaches include healing ourselves, our ancestral and intergenerational trauma, our relationship with the earth, and our relationship to our loved ones and our community.

As much as I am my own person, I am also a combination of my mother, my father, my sister, my ancestors, my loved ones, and my community. I see myself in my clients, and I see their pain within myself. For quite some time now, I've known that to truly feel fulfilled, I needed to heal myself so that I could heal those I cared about. But healing myself was where I felt stuck, and the mind-opening, consciousness-expanding potential of plant medicine was exactly what I needed.

On a warm and moon-lit night in November, I sat in my jungle cabana and began to write down my goals for the plant medicine ceremony. There were so many things that I wanted to happen, including being able to grieve my father and heal from past traumas. But as I began writing down all the things I hoped would be accomplished through my experience, I heard Yessica's voice in my mind: *The medicine gives you what you need, not*

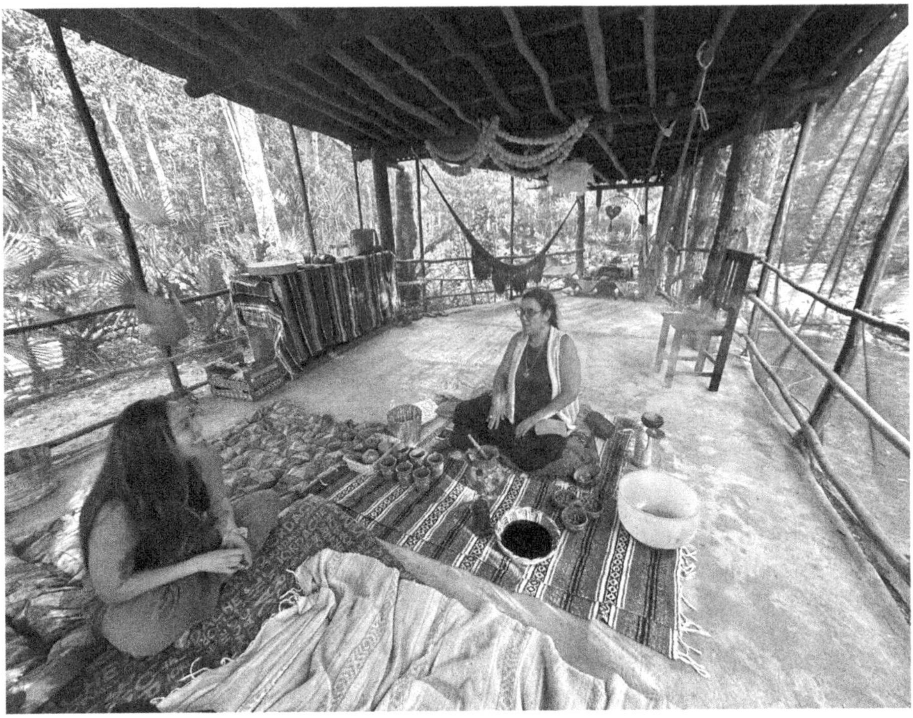

what you want. In the very few minutes remaining before the ceremony would begin, I let go of all the goals I had thought of and focused on an intention instead. *I am going to let go of this need to control my experience, and just allow the mushrooms to guide me. No more goals. No more expectations,* I told myself. Then, I closed my journal and made my way to the ceremony.

It was around 7:00 p.m., and we all sat in a large circle outdoors, surrounded by the various trees and plants in the jungle. As the light from the moon above illuminated the faces of Yessica, Mac, the two shamanic healers, and the fellow travelers who would become like family to me, I suddenly felt a deep sense of love and gratitude for everyone who was present, and for my loved ones back home. I was where I needed to be, but I still felt nervous.

Is it too late to back out? I thought to myself, as my anxiety increased. I had so many reasons for wanting to experience psilocybin in ceremony, but as I sat there completely overwhelmed by my own fears and doubts, my mind went to the one reason I shouldn't: *What if I am never the same again?* What I would come to realize weeks after this experience is that I in fact would never be the same person again. The plant medicine would transform my relationship with myself and my loved ones, how I showed up for my clients in therapy, and how I saw the world. Being the same was what brought me a life of anxiety and a need to control every narrative and outcome. Being the same was what brought me on this very trip and into this plant medicine ceremony.

I had some hesitance about writing this article. As an Asian American female who was brought up on very traditional norms and values, I was aware that writing this article meant coming out to my family about my use of psychoactive plants and coming out to the world as a therapist who supports psychedelic-assisted healing and therapy. The minute I sat down at my desk to begin writing, however, I realized that the fear of being judged was gone. I went through something life-changing, and I was ready to talk about it.

Someone wise once told me that the medicine will call to many, but very few will respond. As I sat there in the middle of the jungle, completely overwhelmed by fear, uncertainty, and anxiety, I realized that this was exactly where I needed to be, at this very moment. The medicine had been calling to me for years now, and I had finally responded.

"Are you scared?" Addy asked me. Addy is a third-generation shamanic healer from the Sacred Children, originating from Oaxaca Mexico. I have so much deep reverence for Addy's knowledge and wisdom, as she made sure to pay respect to the tradition, rituals, and Indigenous practices during each ceremony we participated in. Addy handed me a ceremonial cup of cacao mixed with the psilocybin. As I reflect now on that moment, there has only been one other time that I have ever felt fear and uncertainty so intensely, and that was in 2015, when I was sitting in the hospital, wondering if my dad would make it out alive. "Yes, very." I answered.

"Don't worry, everything that you will see and feel are things you have seen and felt before." She responded. At that time, I did not fully understand what she meant, but looking back now, those words resonated so deeply with what would unfold in the following hours throughout the night.

As I drank the cup of cacao mixed with psilocybin, I felt the resistance begin to surface, and so many thoughts came into my mind. *What if I have a bad trip? Will I get out of this, OK?* "There's still some more left," Addy's voice cut through my thoughts as I set down my cup. I hadn't even noticed it, but my deep fear and anxiety stopped me from finishing the full cup. *Well, here goes. There's no going back now,* I thought to myself, as I finished the concoction.

Ever since my father's sudden passing, I've had an increasing fear of death and uncertainty. I feared death so much that it held me back from taking more risks and living my fullest life. I remember being anxious to even go on my trip, because it meant I would be so far away from my mother and my sister back home. I ended up backing out of an ayahuasca retreat a few months prior to this one. Looking back now, I can only explain it as divine intervention, because the deep connection I had to the shamanic healers and everyone there and the relationship I felt to the mushrooms all felt so personal and intimate, as if every little puzzle piece had to fall into place exactly how it did for me to have the experience I had. My dad's presence and spirit would be with me throughout my entire psilocybin trip, but I wouldn't begin to feel it until I allowed myself to let go of control and surrender.

It took about 45 minutes before I began seeing odd geometrical designs in the trees and on the ground. *Well, it's starting,* I remember thinking. I was terrified, but in that moment, I knew that the only way out would be to go through. There was no going back now, no reverse button.

So much happened in the first hour after the psilocybin started taking effect, but what I can remember vividly is that I was actively trying to control the experience in the beginning. As the effects from the psilocybin continued to increase, I kept rehearsing things inside my mind: *I am safe. I am on a plant medicine retreat. My family is safe back at home. I will come out of this alive. I am safe. I am OK.* The more I rehearsed these words, the more my anxiety grew. Slowly yet gradually, these words stopped making sense to me, as did everything around me. I forgot my name in those moments, and where I was. I remember saying out loud, "I feel lost," before deciding to lie down on my blanket and close my eyes. *I give up,* I remember thinking at one point. And at that moment, it finally happened. I let go of control, and I surrendered.

The moment that the surrender happened, I began to feel so many intense emotions but no thoughts or labels to go along with them. I felt joy, fear, connection, love, grief, and guilt, but it felt as if the guilt was slowly leaving me. The judgmental voice that was always at the back of my mind was suddenly no longer there. I didn't try to make sense of the experience as I usually do. It was chaotic yet liberating, all at once, and none of it needed to make sense. I had no identity, no name, no need to be anywhere except for where I was at that moment. I believe that was the moment my ego dissolution happened. I saw myself not as a therapist or student but as embodied love, joy, and connection to all things. That sense of separateness from others went away, and I felt immense gratitude for my loved ones, my ancestors, for people I haven't even met yet, and for the beautiful earth that I sat on.

I cycled between so many emotions and feelings for quite some time before I felt such an intense feeling of relief that I began crying uncontrollably. In that moment of relief, I grieved my father stronger than I have ever grieved him before. As I cried, I felt years of guilt, shame, and self-blame leave my body.

I still felt weak and disoriented, but I took out my journal and began writing. I didn't want to ever forget everything that I was feeling. My hands felt as if they had a life of their own, and I began writing down every thought that began to finally appear. The next morning, I would finally look at what I wrote down. *Through suffering, there can be joy. We all go back to the earth. We never suffer alone; we all carry each other's pain. Impermanence is beautiful. We are all connected.*

After I journaled the thoughts and insights that came to me, I decided to write my father a letter. I wrote about how much I missed and love him and how grateful I am for everything he has done for me. At the end of the letter, I wrote, *I finally understand you now.*

In his book, *The Power of the Healing Field,* Peter Mark Adams speaks about altered states of consciousness, and how the West has traditionally regarded these states as pathologies and distortions until quite recently. According to Adams (2021), "An 'altered state' designates an extension or expansion of awareness that fulfills some specific purpose... Altered states provide alternative ways of engaging with reality" (p. 17). Adams (2021) quoted Indigenous American author Jane Middleton-Moz, who once replied to the co-founder of transpersonal psychology, Stanislav Grof, by stating, "I don't understand why you use the term nonordinary states. For my people, these experiences are part of the normal spectrum of human experience!" (p. 16). Altered states can allow us to discover alternate realities and information that can lead to profound healing and transformation. Talking about the nuances of altered states and how they impact our brain chemistry would require an entirely separate article, but the purpose here is to touch on my own personal experiences with altered states of consciousness.

My experience of healing during an Indigenous plant medicine ceremony was different from any form of therapy I had ever received back home. The presence of physical touch and embrace, the use of traditional ceremonial practices such as energy cleansing, the beautiful chanting and music, and the communal aspects of the experience all felt so beautifully unconventional and so deeply liberating. In just a few days, I uncovered repressed pain, let go of so much guilt and shame, and healed the parts of me that were underneath that protective shield. All of this was possible through the wisdom, guidance, and love from everyone present during my journey and with the mystical experience created by the mushrooms. The guards and barriers that I have put in place to seemingly keep me safe from the world were destroyed, and with them, my fear and guilt.

I am no longer that same anxious girl who needed to control every narrative, answer, and outcome. I am no longer the girl who was so traumatized after her father's sudden passing that she had a deeply rooted fear of death. Since my plant medicine ceremony, I'm still getting to know this version of myself that isn't trying to become anyone or anything. As a matter of fact, this new version of myself has been all about unbecoming, unlearning, and detaching from all the things that held me back from being my most authentic self. I feel a deep connection to myself and all things around me. Most importantly, however, I've felt more connected to my father than I have ever felt before since his passing. I've begun to view death not as an end to a life but as a continuance into the next. I have reconnected with my Buddhist roots and begun to embrace the beauty of impermanence and interconnectedness. Most importantly, I am now embracing the unconventional, the things that may not always need to be answered by science. My experience helped me realize that continuing to build that bridge between Western therapeutic approaches and Indigenous healing practices may be just what we all need to heal all parts of us, not just the parts that can be measured and seen. The world may benefit from a mix of conventional and unconventional, a combination of ancient wisdom and modern-day knowledge.

References

Adams, P. M. (2021). *The power of the healing field: Energy medicine, psi abilities, and ancestral healing.* Simon and Schuster.

Barrett, F. S., Krimmel, S. R., Griffiths, R. R., Seminowicz, D. A., & Mathur, B. N. (2020). Psilocybin acutely alters the functional connectivity of the claustrum with brain networks that support perception, memory, and attention. *Neuroimage, 218,* 116980.

Davis, A. K., Barrett, F. S., May, D. G., Cosimano, M. P., Sepeda, N. D., Johnson, M. W., ... & Griffiths, R. R. (2021). Effects of psilocybin-assisted therapy on major depressive disorder: a randomized clinical trial. *JAMA Psychiatry, 78*(5), 481-489.

Griffiths, R. R., Johnson, M. W., Carducci, M. A., Umbricht, A., Richards, W. A., Richards, B. D., ... & Klinedinst, M. A. (2016). Psilocybin produces substantial and sustained decreases in depression and anxiety in patients with life-threatening cancer: A randomized double-blind trial. *Journal of psychopharmacology, 30*(12), 1181-1197.

Levine, P. A. (2015). *Trauma and memory: Brain and body in a search for the living past: A practical guide for understanding and working with traumatic memory.* North Atlantic Books.

Ringland, V. C. (2019). Indigenous trauma healing: A modern model. *Australian Counselling Research Journal, 13*(1), 1-7.

Robbins, J. A., & Dewar, J. (2011). Traditional Indigenous approaches to healing and the modern welfare of traditional knowledge, spirituality and lands: A critical reflection on practices and policies taken from the Canadian Indigenous example. *The International Indigenous Policy Journal, 2*(4).

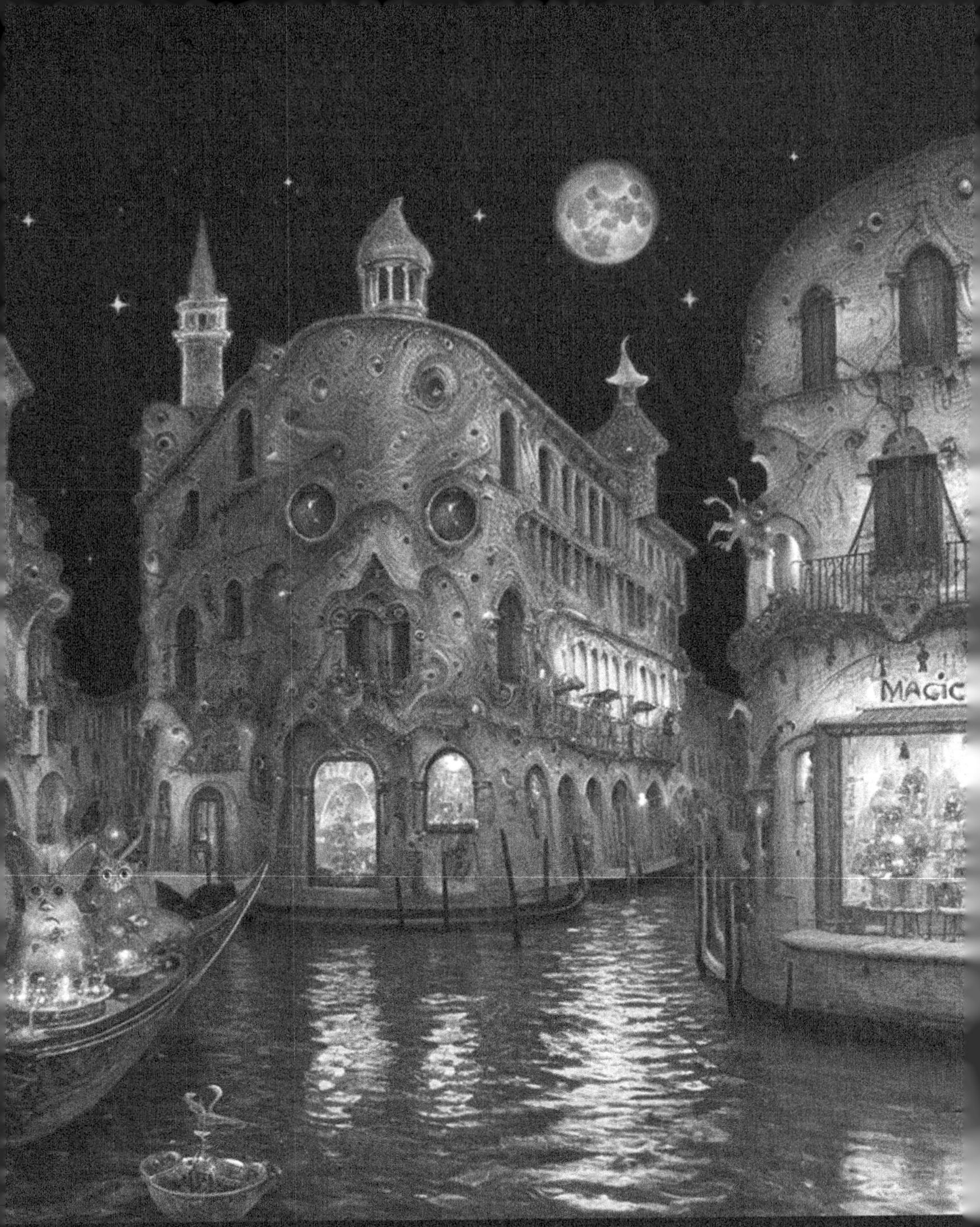
MAGIC

Cathy Roberts

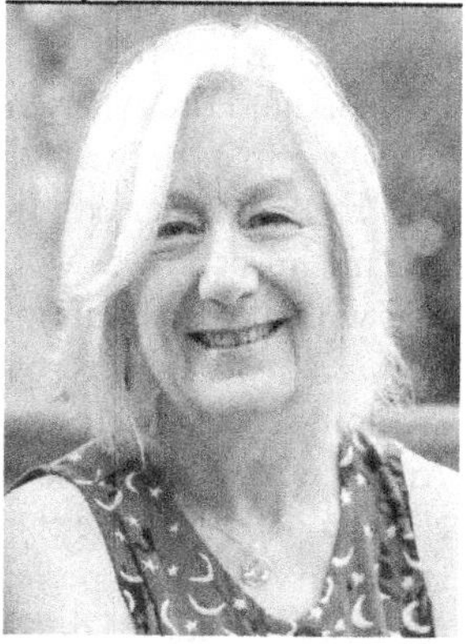

Cathy Roberts, LCPC, lives in Frederick, Maryland, and works virtually with individuals and couples in Maryland, Virginia, and West Virginia. When not counseling clients, you can find her vegetable gardening, writing, and hanging out with one or more of her five grandkids. Her first book, *Fairy Tales for a New Future,* for school-age children and the adults who love them, will be self-published in 2024.
cathy@cathyroberts.net

My Journey Into the Unknown With Ayahuasca

And what we will give you, if you are willing to receive it, is the courage to encounter the unknown.
—Channel Paul Selig, The Book of Alchemy

Good things happen when you go for it.
—Alan Webb (On tea mug, Asheville, NC, April 2021)

Note: Sections in italics are directly from the journal I kept at the time of the ayahuasca ceremony in 2021.

Entering into plant medicine ceremony is encountering the unknown. We may enter into ceremony with intention. We may want a particular outcome. We may expect to feel a certain way or have something specific occur during the journey. But what will actually happen remains unknown. In my first psilocybin journeys, carefully monitored by researchers at Johns Hopkins University, I was seeking a spiritual experience. Period. I wanted to feel something powerful that let me know something about life and meaning. Over the course of four psilocybin journeys and one placebo journey, I received what I wanted. Some experiences were difficult, like when I saw my dead rotting corpse in a grassy, mossy landscape, and some were wonderful, like when I sensed light all around and through everything. Each experience was an entry into the unknown, and I was trained to move towards and dive into whatever was coming up. Great advice for psychedelic journeys and good advice for life.

I like a lot of control, so for me, courage is required to let go and open to the medicine. Courage is not always readily available in my altered state, and while I do my best, releasing myself to whatever it is I am to learn and grow through, I have times of resistance. Then the pain of that resistance becomes so powerful that something else happens, and the experience shifts. In one of my early psilocybin experiences while participating in a study at Johns Hopkins University in 2006, my heart ached as I considered how my older children were working hard in college to become successful adults and my husband was working hard on the job, *all doing what we are supposed to do.* Is that what life is about, my mind on psilocybin wondered? They are doing what we are *supposed to do.* Why is that hurting my heart so much? Would they be doing what they are doing if they were freer to be who they really are? I knew the answer. And it hurt. And I became more free and less controlled by what I am supposed to do. (One of those children later told me they wanted to become homeless for a few months to see if they could survive and experience what it was like. While I didn't want that for them, I liked that they considered doing something that they/we are not supposed to do!)

My interest in mind expansion goes way back to childhood, when I saw my imaginary friends, Mr. and Mrs. Peabody, walking down the hill towards my house. They didn't look human, more like those apple dolls with shriveled faces and gingham clothing you might see at some roadside stand in apple country in autumn. I was told they were imaginary, and I believed that, leaving behind my rich imagination and multidimensional sensory perception. That multidimensional perception never really leaves, though. Participating in the Hopkins study brought thoughts and sensations of what is real for me to the forefront once again. It continues to be clear to me that there is so much more to the world around us than what we see, hear, touch, taste, and smell. I believe in multiple dimensions, mystery, spirit, and soul. Plant medicine encourages my awareness of the unseen, and in that greater awareness, I contact the ways energy and vibration serve me as I move about in the very physical world of matter.

In addition to my imagination and interest in perception beyond the material world, I've been interested in spiritual growth for decades. Reading Annie Dillard's *Pilgrim at Tinker Creek* in late adolescence, I recognized aspects of myself not talked about in my family. The way the leaves on trees waved and whispered to me. The sparkles of sunlight on the waters of Deep Creek Lake after days of rain. These and myriad other experiences touched me deeply, but I had no place to go with my thoughts and sense of awe. The gift of participating in the Hopkins study turned me towards the power of psychedelics to move me along the stream of life towards that divinity, showing up as trees and water, that was always within if I would only slow down enough to realize it.

After my psylocibin experiences under controlled conditions at Hopkins, I longed to try ayahuasca. I'd heard of the mind-opening potentials of the active compound, DMT, and considered traveling to locations where I could experience the plant ceremony. Finally, after over a decade of waiting for the right opportunity, in 2021, friends told me about a shaman closer to home with whom I could experience a community ayahuasca ceremony. I researched the shaman and organization, heard my friends' experiences, and decided to go for it.

In April 2021, I drove 10 hours to Asheville to participate in a sacred ayahuasca plant medicine ceremony. In preparation, I'd had a phone call with the leader and received information about what foods to avoid and how to prepare both physically and spiritually for the weekend. I was excited and a little nervous. I didn't know anyone else in the ceremony, and I was one of the elders in the group of 20 or so who gathered for the 2-night ceremony. My worst-case scenario thinking kicked in. What if something bad happens to me? What if I'm not as healthy as I think and have a negative reaction? Yet I felt a call. A gentle presence nudging me forward. So onward I went, preparing to spend 2 nights on my camping mat with lots of pillows and blankets. I fasted from noon onward, arrived early to get to know other participants, and spent time in silent preparation in the nearby B&B I rented for the occasion.

I've been prepping for this weekend for 10 days. Feeling the call. Aware of my heart connection to ayahuasca. Feeling her pulling me towards her, her roots connecting to my heart. I had deeply painful dreams last night, letting me know how much fear is in my unconscious.

There is so much that goes on during the ceremony. The icaros (medical songs) and sounds of other participants sighing, crying, moving, and vomiting fill the air space around me. The psychedelic visions, nausea, and deep grandmother teachings arise within me. Feeling resistance to the song and medicine dot my interior landscape. Knowing to move towards and dive into whatever comes up helps. And yet I hesitate and hold back. There's a dance of moving towards and moving away from the effects of the medicine. People tell me they feel mother earth's heartbeat and feel at one with everything. Or that they see God and know love. That's not been my experience.

I saw a large wheel-like thing moving. I wanted to make sense of it. What do these turning, colorful wheels mean? Why am I even doing this? Why do people do it again? I was uncomfortable—the nausea, dizziness with the turning wheels. The vision of wheels was expansive. Not located inside my head but outside of it. I opened my eyes for a reference point. I saw narrow lines like a grid in the room. Very straight and orderly. There was a sense of being inside or outside a cage or fence. The lines were floor to ceiling. For some reason the image disturbed me, and I closed my eyes. Eventually I stopped trying to make sense of what I was experiencing and let it move me.

The theme of my first night of aya is expanded consciousness. Consciousness is outside and all around me. I experience it in here, in my mind though. The divide of inside and outside loosened a bit during this experience. It's clear to me now that consciousness exists all around, and I pick up on bits of it and make sense of it in here inside my mind. While seeing the grid, I wondered if I was witnessing the matrix. I'd read enough to believe it possible that we are living in a simulation. My discomfort with something about the grid, that it was something uncomfortable, nauseating to witness, left me wondering if I was indeed looking into a deeper level of the data processing center of the simulation. Is any of what I am writing true? What was true was that I saw something that I didn't want to see, and it was so difficult to see that I began to feel sick looking at it.

After that first night, I thought maybe on the second night I would have one of those amazing, loving, oneness experiences; however, that was not the case.

I wanted the music and singing to stop. It was distorted and annoying in some foreign language. I tried to go with the icaros, move toward it, allow it to move me to a more pleasant place, but I couldn't stay with it. The only thing I knew was to tune it out and go inside my head. What was I doing in my head? Wanting the sounds to stop. Somewhere in here, I noticed my shoulders were hunched and tight as I lay in a fetal position. I could tell the hunching and tightness was a protection from the music and medicine. Somewhere in the midst of this, Grandmother Ayahuasca showed me the mechanisms that I use to keep myself separate from the divine in me and all around me. I avoid what is, because it is uncomfort-

able, and I tighten so that I am unable to open and receive the good all around and within me. Thus, it seems that staying present to what is and relaxing my body to receive what is already here are two of the pathways to my higher, divine spark self.

That sounds so simple. In fact, I work with my clients on these very practices. And yet, it is not easy. I had the sense that I was only capturing a small part of what I was being shown.

While I did not have one of those awesome feeling moments, I did strike gold in this experience: *Somewhere in the midst of this, Grandmother Ayahuasca showed me the mechanisms that I use to keep myself separate from the divine in me and all around me.* My avoidance and tightening around the "what is" that causes that discomfort leads me to retreat from the present. Practicing being open to the what is, working with my body to tolerate the discomfort, and then find the goodness and safety within brings me closer to my highest and best self. As is often the case, that which caused discomfort led to a deeper understanding of how I operate and how I can open to greater love and awareness.

It was weeks or months before the most profound aspect of my ayahuasca journey became evident to me. It garnered only one sentence in my journal: *Sometimes I couldn't contact myself so I focused on my breath for a breath or two, knew I was anchored, and then lost the breath and was in the journey.* When I couldn't contact myself, I had no sense of whether or not I still existed as a living 3-dimensional human! I was in blackness. I was blackness. Endless blackness. Then a thought arose: Am I still in a body? Am I alive or dead? A moment of fear entered, then some part of me told me to breathe, and in the breath, I knew I was in a body. I had to have a body to breathe. That happened a few times. I was in complete blackness—expansive and yet womb-like.

In that blackness, I was in the unknown. I sensed that I was not a being. I felt fear at not being. I heard a message to breathe. I breathed and knew I was still alive. Alive and in the unknown. As I write this paragraph, I am aware of my mother's death just 1 month ago. I was with her for her last 24 hours and with her as she passed. She was going into the unknown. She was scared. I told her that wherever she was going, she would never be alone. I now wonder if that is true. When I said that to her, I believed it. And yet, in that blackness of my ayahuasca journey, I was alone. I had no sense of another presence, no sense of love, no sense of oneness, nothing but my breath. Breath tethers me to my body. Without breath, what happens to soul? What happens to that divine spark of spirit?

As empty as the blackness felt, it was also womb-like. Was it contained? Or was it a vast expanse? It seemed to be both. There was a sense of both finite and infinite. The finite, in the physical, breathing self. The infinite in the limitless spirit, within the body and yet free of embodiment.

There's no way to end this essay, really. While the plant medicine journeys have ended, their effects carry on as I continue to make sense of what I experience.

▼

Brandon Sklar

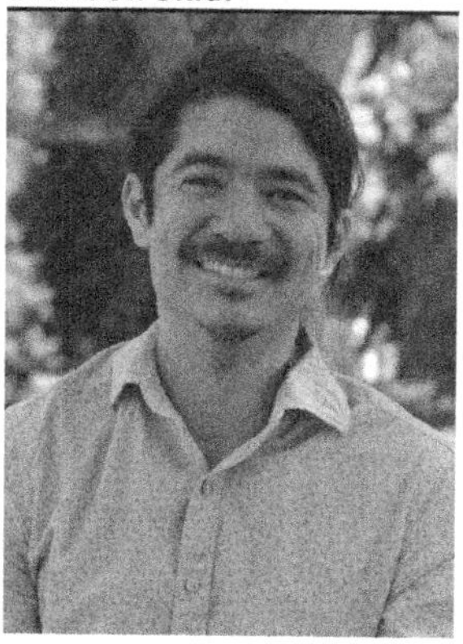

BRANDON SKLAR, MD, is a psychiatrist in Denver, Colorado. He has been in relational psychoanalysis for 4 years and continues to engage in this treatment. He is joining a group practice that will be implementing psychedelic medicines as they become available. He is also planning on opening his own clinic that focuses on helping those who are interested in psychiatric medication tapering.
bsklar1188@gmail.com

My Room

"I DON'T REALLY REMEMBER MY CHILDHOOD."

This is something I would sometimes say when I met new people. I would fumble over myself trying to describe how there seemed to be entire years from my past devoid of any memory. I would feel a mixture of jealousy and fascination with those who could recall their childhoods with a vividness that seemed impossible to me. I would casually shrug this off though. It did not seem to compute with my recollection of my own comfortable, idyllic upbringing that contrasted so heavily with friends who readily told me about deep traumas of being the victims of domestic and sexual violence. I seemed to have a knack for getting others to disclose to me their suffering, something I never thought much about but reveled in.

I had other knacks as well. People used to describe me as unflappable, as possessing a calming temperament that could provide a buffering, harmonic energy to any room I entered. I rarely appeared stressed or anxious or depressed. I surrounded myself with people who were though, and as they leaned on my steadiness for support, I used this role to bolster my self-esteem to such a degree that I gravitated towards becoming a psychiatrist—surrounding myself even further with those who were openly suffering a great deal. "I'm really good at making people feel better," I would tell myself. Probably because I was an expert in making myself feel better. My emotional resilience was unparalleled. I could keep my mood hovering around mild happiness indefinitely. I could weave intellectual narratives that would make me feel good about any situation. I engaged in hobbies that could easily distract me from any discomfort I felt. "I am a beacon of mental health," I would tell myself. "I am nothing like my patients, but I can save them," I would add.

And it was here where psychedelics entered my life.

February 4, 2020, was the first day I took LSD...and the trajectory of my life would be altered forever.

Within that first hour, I began to weep uncontrollably. And much to my horror, that did not stop for several hours following. It felt like the weight of all the suffering in the world was crashing down on me all at once and consuming my entire existence. I entered a living hell that I could not escape as my consciousness was sucked inward by a powerful vortex, into an abyss of agony. At one point, a person I was with remarked, "Wow, Brandon, you are such an...*emotional* person." A comment that shocked me, as it challenged everything I had assumed about myself. Long gone was the Brandon from before, and I left that experience thinking as I was falling asleep, "I will never be the same again." However, much to my dismay, I woke up feeling...basically the same.

But I could not shake the sense that what happened to me meant something. And I kept returning to that psychedelic state again and again, drawn to taking bigger and bigger doses, not really knowing why. I then decided, also for reasons poorly understood, that I should see a therapist. "So I can become a better therapist myself and more effectively help my patients," I rationalized.

As that course of therapy deepened and intensified into psychoanalysis, I started to visualize a walled-off room in my mind, suspended in a black void. It was heavily fortified and had no doors or windows, so its contents were shrouded in mystery and darkness. I started to realize that psychedelics were a tool I was learning how to wield, a hammer and chisel to make small holes into the walls of this inner room so I could peer inside. It took me a while before I could see anything, as small beams of light temporarily illuminated portions of what seemed like just an empty space, until much to my shock, I saw that it was not. In that room...existed a little boy. A boy who looked like me but seemed completely different. He was in immense anguish.

I began to interact with him in psychedelic spaces and in the therapy room. And the more I did, the more horrified I became. He described an existence of severe isolation. One where he was never hungry for food or shelter or material belongings but starved of attention and physical touch. One where he was constantly in the presence of others but left alone. One where he was never yelled at or struck but would go completely unnoticed staring blankly into the wall at dinner every night. Loneliness and abandonment seemed like all this boy ever knew, and his pain was so vast that I struggled to face it. It began to intensify when, together, that boy and I fully felt the gravity of what had been done to me...and why. I then understood why I couldn't remember my childhood, why I was so effective at making myself feel better. Because the depths of underlying suffering could have very well destroyed me, I needed to dissociate from it to survive.

But I started to realize that also came with a cost, because I was not just dissociating from that suffering but from all my feelings. As psychedelics allowed me to peer into the room, they also allowed the boy to peer out and see the world in all of its beauty for the first time. Together, we started to experience realms of awe and love that shattered my entire reality, and indeed, those emotions alongside my grief at never experiencing them before quite literally ripped my life apart, including several dear relationships I had at the time.

While all this was happening, I was also in psychiatry residency, where I had patients coming to me with their own suffering asking me for help. And I started to become deeply confused. I was educated into thinking that I should be tracking people's symptoms of depression and anxiety and using symptom diminishment or absence as a sign of wellness, or at the very least, a job well done. I was taught that feelings such as guilt and hopelessness alongside bodily phenomena such as insomnia and low energy constituted a suffering that should be extinguished rather than an important indicator of a deeper underlying suffering that should be confronted. I watched as my patients who slowly got "better" with chemicals I was giving them reported those symptoms less, but when I thought to ask them other questions not traditionally taught to ask, many of those same patients also began to tell me other things—like how they could not laugh as easily as they used to. I slowly stopped hearing from them about their relationship sorrows or dissatisfaction with their jobs despite nothing changing. And I felt sick. I felt like I was helping patients I grew to care for dissociate...just like me. It felt like I was medicating my patients into submission, helping them create their own rooms where their suffering could be ignored but permitted to fester and spread unconsciously.

I wish I could wrap up this story by stamping my forehead with the word "healed," but that could not be further from the truth. I am still on a healing journey that I'm not convinced even has a destination. My room still exists, that little boy is still frightened to emerge, and I still grapple with my own desire to keep him there, to abuse him in the same way others have. But you find me today not as I was on February 3, 2020. You find me as someone who struggles with depression and anxiety and is stressed all the fucking time. But also as someone who laughs harder, dances longer, and is frolicking through a kaleidoscopic universe meadow. I now recognize that my attempts to save others was really a means of trying to save myself. Psychedelics are helping me do that alongside a few very, very special people. And I am overflowing with a gratitude that I can't wait to express and unleash on the world. ▼

The psilocybin experience can help us access parts of ourselves that are normally hidden from view.

—Paul Stamets

Inner Child

Marcela Bonancio

In the vision, a child—a little girl,
With infectious happiness
And shiny, bright eyes,
Ran through the aisles
Of this antique library.

She played with joy, carefree,
Yet I noticed she was alone.
I took her into my arms, seeking answers
From faces in the library,
Searching for her caretakers.

Until a woman said,
"Caretakers often lose their wards."
Puzzled, I asked, *"What now?"*
She met my gaze and said,
"Perhaps it's time to care for her."
Confused, I hugged the little girl tight.
In the depth of this encounter, I felt wholeness.
A feeling I had forgotten for a while.
Then, the revelation—
The child from the vision was me,
My inner child, whom I had lost in between the battles with myself.

"Little girl, you are no longer lost
In the vastness of time and space.
I found you; together, we'll walk,
Through battles within and without."

Heart Burst Wide Open

Marilise Blignaut

West Coast of Canada
mariliseblignaut@gmail.com

It's 2022. Two weeks before my 34th birthday.

I am nearing the peak of an underground MDMA-assisted psychotherapy session*—and I am reliving a very distressing childhood memory.

In this memory, I am witnessing a younger version of myself cycle through feelings of confusion, rejection, emotional and physical pain, fear, guilt, and shame.

Banished to her room, she sits in the dark alone, hugging her knees close to her body—sobbing aloud and quietly punishing herself more for being so stupid—for upsetting her mom—yet again. She seems to be drowning in her feelings of despair, sorrow, and self-loathing.

The adult me joins her in the room.

I extend an invitation for her to come over to me and squeeze in close under my loving arm. She's reluctant, but she joins me, and we sit together—reconnected. I feel an immense amount of empathy and compassion towards her, and I comfort her.

I tell her I will sit with her for as long as she needs me to. I tell her she will never have to face anything alone ever again. I tell her that our mom's reaction is not her fault. I tell her she did nothing wrong. I tell her what she experienced was awful and unfair, and that she is not to blame. I tell her that all her feelings are okay—all parts of her experience are welcome. I tell her I am not going anywhere.

The visual imagery changes...and I come back to the present moment.

I start to feel a shift happening. An opening.

And suddenly, like pieces of a puzzle, the fragments of my fractured self seem to come together in perfect sequence.

And one by one, message after message is downloaded into my thoughts...

I have never experienced such clarity. Such compassion for myself.

These messages are no longer just affirmations or quotes I read in a book that intellectually resonated... No, I feel these to my core.

At last, my heart and mind...reconnected.

It's exactly what I needed.

The messages?

The trauma you experienced was never your fault.
You did nothing wrong.
You are not inherently bad.
You are not broken.
You have nothing to be ashamed about.
You are a warrior.
You did what you had to do to survive.
You always were enough.
And look at you now: you are no longer only surviving...you have come alive.

This trip with MDMA served as the catalyst of remembering who I am. It allowed me to generate the courage to commit to self-acceptance, self-compassion, and self-love. To establish inner safety (something I seldom had)—and to realize my innate capacity to hold space for my wounded inner child and essentially reparent myself.

MDMA burst my heart wide open.

And then, the real work began...

**At this time MDMA was illegal—being classified as a Schedule I drug in Canada. As of January,2023, it was decriminalized in British Columbia.*

Psychedelics show you what's in and on your mind, those subconscious thoughts and feelings that are hidden, covered up, forgotten, out of sight, maybe even completely unexpected, but nevertheless imminently present.

—Rick Strassma

Marilise Blignaut

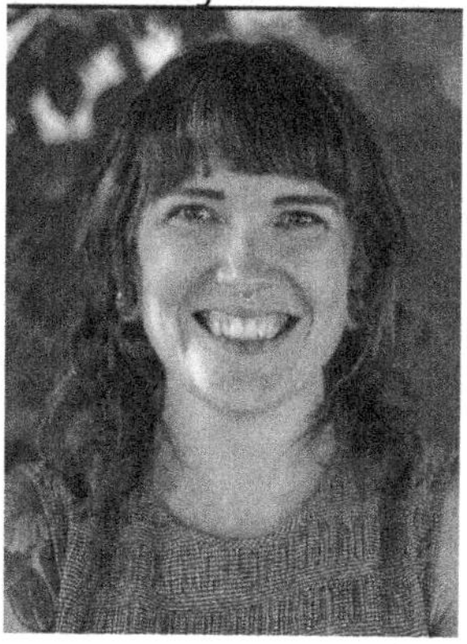

My Psychedelic Journey

I am writing this on World Psychedelics Day (June 20th)—and in honor of this day, I've decided to come out and share how I came to use plant medicine and psychedelics in my healing journey.

My trauma history started in early childhood as I learned from an early age that to survive—to maintain my attachment to my mother, my caregivers, on whom I was dependent—I needed to shut away and exile parts of my self which threatened that attachment. From as young as the age of 8, I can recall feeling a lot of shame, feeling alone with my pain, and having no one to talk to about it. I truly thought that who I was at my core was the issue. My brain rationalized that if my family, the people who are supposed to love and cherish me, could not, it must be a problem with me. I did not dare let anyone know the pain I was in, for fear of punishment and being ostracized further.

It was the fall of 2021, I think, when I watched the documentary *The Wisdom of Trauma* featuring Gabor Maté (Benazzo & Benazzo, 2021). Maté speaks of trauma as the disconnection from our true authentic selves, and healing as the reconnection with that self. He talks about how trauma is not the result of what happened to us but the result of what happens inside of us as a reaction to the experience.

For the first time—after watching that documentary—I felt hope. I felt that I was not alone, that I was not crazy, and that the trauma I had experienced was in fact not my fault. I was one among millions of other people in our society—in the world—who had become so disconnected from themselves. I was one among millions who had experienced and survived childhood trauma and had

Marilise Blignaut is a trauma survivor. She resides on the West Coast of Canada and has been practicing as a critical care registered nurse since 2014. She is pursuing her Master of Science in nursing with a specialization in education. Within the past year, she became a board member of the Okanagan Psychedelic Society. Her passions include writing, painting, reading, and being outside in nature. She is currently working on her first book, a memoir of alchemy.
mariliseblignaut@gmail.com

developed unhealthy adaptations and coping mechanisms as an attempt to fit into the world.

After watching this documentary, I started doing more research: reading books, watching documentaries, listening to podcasts, and hearing others' stories. I was on a mission to seek anything and everything that had helped others and could potentially help me get unstuck from my narrative of suffering as well. By this point, many of the healing modalities I had tried had not been that effective.

I had tried medication from 2017 to 2019—SSRIs (Sertraline/Zoloft) and benzodiazepines (Ativan)—these allowed me to continue to function day to day like a normal person, but I felt completely numb and empty inside. For me, the medication was just another way to numb out the feelings of unease and emotional distress I was having rather than targeting why I was feeling that way in the first place.

I had been to counseling on and off for years trying talk therapy, narrative therapy, cognitive behavioral therapy (CBT), and eye movement desensitization and reprocessing (EMDR). Talk therapy was helpful—but at times would be very challenging as the words to describe my experiences just were not there. EMDR was also helpful, especially in processing the acute trauma and PTSD I struggled with surrounding my dad's fatal motorcycle accident. Still, I needed more.

It felt like there was a major disconnect between my intellectual self and my emotional self. I knew that the trauma was not my fault, but I could not seem to shake these old narratives that were causing my suffering. On a daily basis, I continued to struggle with anxiety and depression, as well as symptoms of developmental trauma, and was having passive thoughts of suicide. I found myself thinking that the world would be better off without me in it—thinking *what's the point?*—that if a life of suffering is what I had signed up for I was no longer interested in playing along. I felt trapped in my reality, and it was evident to me that some radical transformation was needed.

In October of 2021, I emailed a local maestra (Shipibo shaman) to inquire about an ayahuasca (a plant-based psychoactive brew) journey. I had been doing extensive research consuming research publications and books about the healing potential that plant medicine and psychedelics have been shown to have for individuals struggling with anxiety, depression, and PTSD. I was positively intrigued. I did not end up moving forward with the ayahuasca journey at this time due to possible health contraindications—but that did not halt any of my curiosity into psychedelics and plant medicine.

On my own, I began experimenting with recreational micro-dosing and macro-dosing of psilocybin mushrooms. I had a couple of challenging trips as a result—without proper support and integration—and I actually felt a bit derailed from them. Reflecting back on that time, to be perfectly honest, I was feeling pretty desperate at this point... grasping at straws. I felt like my life was on a downward spiral and I needed something to save me from myself. I was under the illusion that I would take the psilocybin mushrooms and then miraculously I just wouldn't have crippling PTSD anymore. Boy, was I wrong! I did not yet understand or truly appreciate the importance of intention, set and setting, safety, and integration. So, psilocybin was off the books.

After my experiences with psilocybin, I decided that if I was to continue exploring psychedelics, I needed to do so in a clinical or controlled setting with a trained guide or clinician; safety was (and still is) paramount to me.

Next, I looked into ketamine-assisted psychotherapy. There was a local clinic opening in April of 2022, and they were offering services for individuals suffering from treatment resistant depression. I decided to go through the intake process and see if this might be the answer I was looking for. Unfortunately, the ketamine-assisted therapy ended up costing more than I was comfortable spending (approximately $6,000)—so, back to the drawing board I went.

Serendipitously, a week or two later, I was in a session with my therapist, and I mentioned to her the research that I had been doing and that I was interested in trying psychedelics as a tool for healing. She chuckled in response and disclosed to me that she was actually part of the underground movement of psychedelic-assisted psychotherapy—and that when she had met me and heard my story, she had immediately thought that plant medicine could be of great benefit for me. To protect herself and her practice, she did not freely offer this modality to her patients unless they brought it up themselves. As many of the plant medicines and psychedelics are still classified as illegal substances under federal law, she was taking a risk—but believed so strongly in their power and had witnessed firsthand the enormous healing potential of these medicines.

Fast forward to July of 2022, and I am attending my first psychedelic-assisted psychotherapy session—MDMA (3-4 methylenedioxymethamphetamine) being the substance of choice. MDMA is known to have powerful effects on getting us out of our default mode network and therefore giving us the ability to allow our hearts to open, release inhibitions, foster connection, and establish safety (Finighan, 2021). Weeks of preparation with my therapist occurred before the session, and together we decided on a comfortable set and setting as well as establishing intentions for the journey beforehand.

The journey took approximately 6 hours, but I was there with my therapist and another sitter for a full 8-hour day. *Hooooooly cow*—what a profound experience it was!

In the span of 6 hours, I was able to establish a sense of safety within myself that I had never felt before in my life. In my journey, I was taken back to a memory of when I was 2 years old, when I was initially excited and proud—seeking approval from my mom for reaching a developmental milestone—and instead received a physical beating and verbal abuse. I was able to sit with this younger version of myself—my wounded inner child—and comfort her, hold space for her, and tell her that I loved her, that she did not do anything wrong, and that I was there to keep her safe. That I would never let anyone do anything to harm her, ever again. The processing of that traumatic memory—along with other things that arose throughout the journey—was truly staggering and life altering.

Above all else, I learned that no one was coming to save me. I had to save myself. Everything I needed was already within me—within my heart and soul. A heart and soul that I had become so disconnected from and had come to hate. After this session, all I felt was love and compassion for myself. I was able to begin the process of reconnecting with my self and breaking down the protective walls I had built around my heart.

Following this, I began integrating this experience and working more closely with my therapist using a therapeutic modality known as internal family systems (IFS) or parts work. Other forms of integration for me have included getting back into my body through yoga, breathwork, and movement (ecstatic dance) and connecting to my soul through sound healing, journaling, singing, allowing myself to play, and meditation...to name a few. I have also been establishing personal spiritual practices, exercising the art of surrender, and letting go of the need for control. I have tapped into and been able to access my creativity again through painting and writing.

Since then, I have also experienced the healing benefits of cannabis, MDMA, and LSD in micro-doses and macro-doses. In August, 2024, I will be attending a women's ayahuasca retreat held locally. The healing effects of these medicines have continued to compound and expand into all areas of my life—and I am so eternally grateful for it. Research has shown that for many individuals, often a single intentional psychedelic journey can yield the same therapeutic results as 10 years of talk therapy. I would have to say that I wholeheartedly agree.

In the last almost 2 years since first feeling a spark of curiosity towards plant medicine and psychedelics, I have grown and changed so much. I no longer identify with the diagnosis of anxiety or depression, and I certainly do not have the same dark thoughts around ending my life anymore. I am continuing to integrate all the journeys I have had—sometimes gaining insight about the meaning around certain parts of a trip a year or more after it has occurred. I am actively working to transmute my trauma into a story of transcendence, strength, and resilience versus one of victimization and suffering. I am creating the life that I desire, day by day—and that is an extraordinarily beautiful thing.

One of the most important lessons that I learned around the use of psychedelics and plant medicine for healing is that it is not some quick fix like we have become accustomed to in this day and age. You have to be prepared and have the courage to put in the work—to surrender control, to integrate the experience, and to lean into challenging experiences and trust. Trust that what the medicine is showing you, albeit difficult and downright terrifying at times, is exactly what you need at that moment. That it will never show you anything that you are not ready for—and the rewards are infinite. Also, set and setting, intentions, support, and integration are essential.

Coincidentally, I am writing this from Denver, Colorado, where I am attending the MAPS Psychedelic Science Conference, the largest conference of this kind in history, bringing in over 11,000 people globally who share the passion for the healing potential of psychedelics and plant medicines. Together we are spearheading the psychedelic renaissance—through education, research, leadership, sharing our stories, building a conscious community. I am so honored and grateful to be here—and to be a part of what's to come.

I realize that these medicines are not for everyone. And that's okay. We all have the right and capacity to choose for ourselves. I do, however, encourage anyone who is even mildly curious to do their own research and make their own decisions based on their comfort levels. Unfortunately, there has been a lot of misinformation and stigma out there around these substances —and I can assure you that the majority of it is false. So, like anything, keep an open mind and decide for yourself. For me, the psychedelic journey has been transformative.

References

Benazzo, Z. (Producer, Director) & Benazzo, M. (Producer, Director). (2021). *The wisdom of trauma (featuring Dr. Gabor Maté)* [Documentary Film]. Retrieved from https://thewisdomoftrauma.com/about-the-film/

Finighan, B. (2021, November 26). Psychedelics and the default mode network. *leafie.* Retrieved from https://www.leafie.co.uk/articles/psychedelics-default-mode-network.

Brodin Anderson

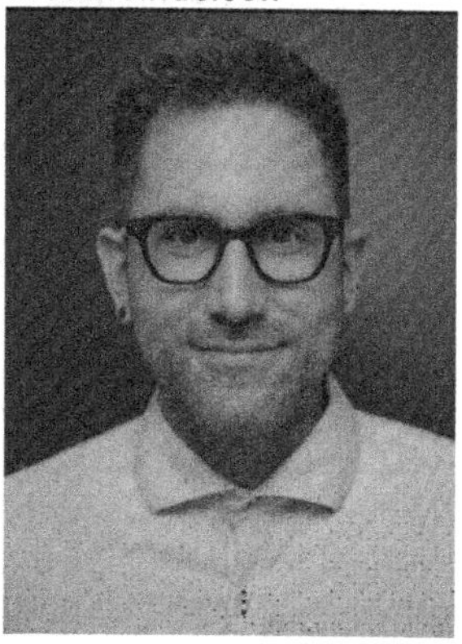

Brodin Anderson, MA, CPC, is a therapist working in private practice in Winnipeg, Manitoba. He and his wife Melissa are excited to open Manitou Psychedelic Clinic whenever legislation allows. It is their dream to work alongside their emerging community of health professionals trained in psychedelic-assisted therapy and share the gifts of psychedelic care with the world. For now, Brodin regifts what the plants teach him through his work as a therapist and writer.
brodinandersoncounselling@gmail.com

What My Grandmothers Taught Me About Pain

Like many who walk in the world of psychedelics as healers, I find it difficult to articulate why I am drawn to such work without telling my own story. Of course, my professional curiosity could not ignore the growing body of research on the subject. I was even more intrigued by contemporary thought leaders I had admired for years beginning to talk openly about the therapeutic potential of these medicines. But there is nothing quite as compelling as pain. And it was my desperation to ease the pain of my own wounds that ultimately pushed me to take my first steps into the emerging world of psychedelic-assisted therapy and plant medicines.

The Wound

I was not initially desperate concerning my own mental health; I was avoidant. Probably less avoidant than the average person on account of my own regular therapy and supervision, but my subconscious found clever ways to conceal the darkest regions of my shadow. That's how my symptoms got so bad so fast. I would still count myself lucky in the sense that panic attack disorder, while an awful thing to experience, is fairly harmless as symptoms go. My first panic attack actually happened in therapy. Though, I was in the wrong chair to be having a breakdown. I was in the midst of administering care to one of my clients.

It will probably forever remain one of the most salient experiences of my life. It certainly helped to know that it was, almost certainly, just a panic attack even as my body screamed that it was dying. My mind kept urging me to stumble into the hall, clenching my chest and screaming for an ambulance. But I assured myself, "You feel like you are dying, but you are not. Even if this is a heart attack, then you will collapse and the client will get you help. This will end." I was right. After what felt like a vast expanse of time the electrical storm inside me began to dissipate. I could detect more milliseconds between my heartbeats. Then I could comprehend my client's speech again. Then I glanced at the clock and realized it had barely been more than a minute!

In hindsight, this terrifying experience was excellent preparation for the psychedelic work that awaited me. I consider myself fortunate to have had access to many legal and well supported journeys. In the pursuit of my own healing, I have had many complex, ineffable experiences within the psychedelic landscape: I have been immersed in unconditional love. I have died; I have re-experienced my own birth. I have been one with all things. I have been fully asleep and fully awake simultaneously. I have perceived myself to be in the presence of God. I have seen my childhood through the eyes of my family members. All of these phenomena and many more, multiple times each in most cases.

It is difficult to articulate how such experiences have reshaped the way I see myself, others, and the natural world or the ways in which they have inspired me. I could fill pages just by focusing on any one of the psychedelic trips I have had along the way. However, what I find most revelatory about my own contact thus far with psychedelics is not what has happened but what has not happened: I have not resolved my deepest wound, the pain that compelled me to seek out psychedelics in the first place.

As far as I can tell, I had met criteria for complex PTSD (C-PTSD) before the first time I ingested a psychedelic substance even though I was unaware of my disorder (our biggest blind spots truly are inside of ourselves). If I go several months without consuming such medicine, I still re-acquire enough symptoms of C-PTSD for a diagnosis even to this day. This is not to say that I have not made progress with my mental health. I had more or less absolved myself of the panic attack disorder which nearly cost me my career even before working with psychedelics. And, as a result of my psychedelic journeys, I do feel I have grown exponentially in many important ways. I have also never again returned to the dark, double-edged shelter of self-harm since my earliest experiences. Indeed, in the weeks following a plant medicine experience, even my C-PTSD symptoms are completely erased. However, no matter how much discipline and focus I dedicate to my self-care and integration practices afterwards, my pathology inevitably resurfaces.

This cycle has repeated dozens of times. It is frustrating to say the least. Especially when I talk to clients who, after taking a few mushrooms at a music festival, report that their own psychopathologies are brought within a manageable range or even completely absolved! I will admit that when I hear of social anxiety and depression being overcome by accident while my malady remains after dozens of highly intentional, guided experiences, it is hard not to resent my position. Having said that, one bit of progress I am grateful for is my cultivation of a deep trust in the process of healing. Specifically, its narrative nature and the immense scope thereof; spanning lifetimes and generations. My journeys, reflection, and research, all motivated by this wound of C-PTSD, have transformed my view of the human experience and the practice of therapy in ways for which I can't help but be grateful.

The Depth

Since the early days of my training, many instructors have cautioned me that I have a strong tendency to lead with my left brain. One supervisor specifically urged me to find another way to engage my own mental health with serious words: "I've seen this play out before, and if you don't find a way out from under it, give it enough time, it will kill you." I had read enough of Gabor Mate's books to know this even before hearing this, but I took in his seriousness. However, I do think that all my overthinking on this matter has produced an intriguing theory as to why the psychological architecture that produces my C-PTSD is so rigid and resilient.

Epigenetic research has uncovered credible mechanisms by which some individuals become vulnerable to traumatization (van Zuiden et al., 2012; Rodgers et al., 2013; Dias & Ressler, 2014; Yehuda et al., 2016, 2018). Based on what I know about my parents' and most recent ancestors' lives, I am a prime candidate for such vulnerability. This was important to me for two reasons. First, without some kind of mechanistic explanation being at least plausible, I would have endlessly blamed myself for the cyclical re-emergence of my C-PTSD symptoms. I also would have judged myself for my own suffering by comparing myself to those of my colleagues who are less affected by vicarious trauma. In light of this research, I have come to believe my wound's roots are on my genome. While my psychedelic experiences reorient me to reality and confound the codependent patterns of my psyche, my genetic vulnerability remains beneath the surface, and eventually my mind and my nervous system succumb once again to hypervigilance.

There are some caveats here. I cannot know for certain that these genes are signaled on for me without medical tests I am unaware of how to access. It should also be made clear that we do have evidence that intergenerational changes in our genes can be reversed (Dias & Ressler, 2014; Yehuda, 2022). Even cognitive behavioral therapy has been shown to accomplish this with combat veterans. So, while I have nothing to offer for why my C-PTSD is so very treatment resistant, my theory is in alignment with some recent research on MDMA and epigenetics that revealed a connection between long-term symptom reduction and the methylation of the glucocorticoid receptor gene (Lewis et al., 2023). I believe this highlights one of the most profound truths that epigenetic and psychedelic research has revealed to the field of psychotherapy: We have a profoundly limited understanding of how we work and the intricate ways in which we can be broken.

My experience may also be a cautionary example for people whose mental illnesses resist even this promising new modality. If trained professionals with ample support resist treatment, then clients with similar struggles need not blame themselves. We just don't have everything figured out yet. As my mentors always told me: your left brain will only get you so far! Thank God the most precious gift that I have received from my psychedelic work resides in my right brain.

The Purpose

My favorite stories from the world of psychedelics are not about the trips themselves but the inexplicable synchronous events that surround some of them. These moments have a profound impact on the individual because it seems impossible to deny that there is some kind of guiding force within their world and within themselves that is fully active before, during, and after their experience. My relationship with my trauma and the work of psychotherapy was reshaped after one such experience of my own. But to understand this, you need to know a little bit about my paternal grandmother.

I visited my grandparents for a couple weeks every summer. Their country home on the shore of Lake Manitoba is one of the most vibrantly alive homesteads contained in my memories. Hummingbirds danced and chased each other through the forests of flowers, set against the splashing waves. I joined the chase one summer and got a nasty splinter from a wooden fence in the palm of my dominant hand. I guess I had gotten one too many splinters that year because I swore I would tell no one lest they decide to remove it with a sewing needle like my mother always did, a poor choice on my part. Within a few days I knew I was in trouble as by then the splinter was floating in pus, my hand pulsating in pain. I covered my face and wept as I reluctantly showed it to my grandma, begging her not to use a needle.

"Oh, my boy. I'm an old Indian woman. I don't use needles! Come, let Grandma see it..."

She sat me down in front of some cartoons and had me soak my hand in warm salt water. I ate a bit of bannock as I waited a little over 10 minutes for her to come back. She gently drew my hand out of the water and said it looked ready. She roughly brushed my palm with a towel, and the splinter was out! Just a brief sting from the friction, and I had nothing to worry about. My grandmother taught me a lesson about healing that day which I will never forget: No matter how good your reasons are for keeping your wounds in the dark, you will only net yourself more pain. And opening them up can be both more simple and more beneficial than you anticipate.

I got a tattoo on that hand to commemorate this experience. I wanted to see this memory every time I looked down to take notes or shake hands with a client. The tattoo is my grandma's name, Louise, adjacent to a hummingbird that is breaking into pieces. The hummingbird holds a thread and suture needle in its tiny feet. For me, this tattoo symbolizes the wounded healer and reminds me of two great teachers: my grandmother and the splinter. Like any tattoo from a reputable artist, it was booked about half a year in advance of the day I received it. So, I had no way of knowing that it would not even be fully healed before the first time I sat with another great teacher: ayahuasca.

It was Daime to be specific; a type of ayahuasca served only in Santo Daime churches. These churches have exemptions to legally serve this brew as their sacrament, and they do so all over the world. I understood immediately why they call her Grandmother Ayahuasca. Without contest, it was the most intimate medicine I had ever had. The ancient maternal energy of the Daime did not leave my mind or my body for several days, which is a difficult thing to explain. I was not high but experienced light differently. All aspects of life contained some subtle novelty I could not put my finger on. Throughout the days that I was within this strange, resonant energy, I was constantly reading all that I could find about the Santo Daime. Amidst this research I stumbled into a realization of the profundity of the timing of my first ingestion of this medicine of medicines.

Naturally, I had taken the Daime with my dominant hand. The hand on which my healer grandmother's name had been inscribed only days before. This alone was incredibly meaningful to me. I could have gotten that tattoo any other time in my life! There was such a warmth to feel that my grandmother had been so close to me in my first experience with ayahuasca. But it was when I was reading through the hymn books of Santo Daime that my jaw dropped. Their hymns contain constant references to hummingbirds! As I delved deeper I learned that the beija-flor (hummingbird) has a totemic significance within the religion. It was even on the cover of some of the books about Santo Daime I sought out and is prominently featured in the decorations of some churches.

This synchronicity was the most impactful I have ever had. Yet, this anomaly was just the capstone atop a collection of others that swirled around it in the months before and after my introduction to Daime. Months earlier, at my previous psychedelic experience (a Grof Breathwork) I was begging to be free from the pain of my C-PTSD. The message I got irritated me: *"Say the word and my servant will be healed."*

This is a quote from the Bible (Matthew 8:8). It is a message sent to Jesus by a Roman Centurion, an outcast among Jewish communities. Jesus is so impressed that this centurion has the faith to trust his servant will be healed without Jesus touching the man that he grants the Roman this miracle.

I resented this message. My complex relationship with the Bible aside, I didn't really know what I was supposed to have such faith in. It was believable to me that I would remain within my cycle of being rebuilt and eroded until I died. If I were ever to lose access to plant medicine, I assumed I might have to forfeit my career as a therapist or work very few hours. This changed after that first time I drank Daime. That ceremony was also the first time I felt I had entered the presence of God. Cognitively speaking, I could dismiss this easily from a physicalist perspective. I could disregard what I felt as a pharmacological event. But somehow, I just know deeply within myself that I was in the company of the divine singularity; call it what you will.

The feeling was so profound and unmistakable that I automatically began to rebuild my relationship with a higher power, something so critical to many successful healing journeys. In fact, in light of Dr. Lisa Miller's work demonstrating the brains of spiritual people to be more resilient against mental illness compared to non-spiritual people, the seeking of a higher power may even be considered evidence-based self-care (Miller & Weigand, 2021). This reconnection to God is just one of the many gifts ayahuasca has given me. I am grateful to have felt this connection many times since. The Daime's message that came with that first ceremony was most welcome: *"You have found what you have been looking for."*

I had found a community where I could be cared for, where I could be held. I believe this container is as much a part of what restores me as the ayahuasca. It was so easy for me to have faith in this plant and in these people who took such good care of me, so easy to see God in it all. With all my heart, I aspire to cultivate a comparable connection between my clients and the therapeutic container of my approach.

Along the way in my healing, I had tried to find relief in many other communities. In my early life this was mostly churches. They meant well, but I found they often missed the mark and delved into the pathologizing of self rather than the healing of trauma. More recently, I had reached out to a Cree elder for help, and he welcomed me into his community that led sweat lodge ceremonies regularly. I have a high regard for this elder and that precious lodge, but I'm afraid after several tries I found no symptom relief from it. Unfortunately, it was another notch in my treatment resistant belt. Also, the dynamic was tricky for me as a White-passing Metis (partly Indigenous) person.

As welcoming as the lodge community was, I constantly questioned my right to be there. I am sure no one there wanted me to feel self-conscious, but it was impossible for me to forget I was an outsider as I observed their profound approach to healing. It was truly beautiful, nothing short of instructive. I believe watching them create the healing container of a sweat was a part of overwriting the negative aspects of some Christian ceremonies hidden in my memories. I was grateful of course, but I was also conflicted and still suffering. In all honesty, if I were to summarize my relationship with my blood into one word, conflict would be that word. It is complex to see yourself reflected in both colonizer and victim.

This played an important role in my journeys the subsequent times I attended Santo Daime. I eagerly returned to the shelter of their ceremony after my first experience. I had discussed the effects of my first visit with the group leader, and he said it sounded as if I may need more. To be sure, whatever my dose was, it did not impede my inner work. Apparently, it was enough to get the visuals moving. The first time I opened my eyes in the ceremony they were immediately filled with tears.

As I looked at my skin, aboriginal artwork danced within it. It was as distinct as a fingerprint, but the art was in constant motion like an immaculate animation. Ancient stylizations of eagles and whales swayed across my body to the tune of the ceremonial hymns. The message came through clearly: *"Your grandmother was a healer. You are a healer. There is medicine in your very blood, but you are not meant to do your work without us."*

The days that followed that ceremony were heavy. With such a complex aspect of my identity having just been operated on, it took time to absorb this truth, but it moved me ahead in my relationship with my ethnicity in a profound way. I now feel a sense of connection to my heritage as a healer through my practice of therapy. I also feel no shame to call on plant medicines to support me. In fact, I believe both are my birthright; though I acknowledge that ayahuasca specifically visits me from a faraway land where it has been stewarded by its own people for millennia. I am forever in their debt and will be watchful for ways to act out my gratitude throughout my lifetime. Especially with the very real threat ayahuasca tourism poses to some communities in South America.

Months later, my intentions for another ceremony were centered on connecting more deeply with God. While my relationship with the intention was complex, the ayahuasca's message was actually very simple and, in fact, aligned with the message I had resented from my breathwork experience:

> *You will be healed when it is time to be healed. Your desire to end your pain has acted as your north star, guiding you to places you are supposed to be. If you are still in pain, the purpose of your pain is not yet complete.*

My grandma took on the care of more than 100 foster children over the course of her lifetime. She died from organ failure attributed to diabetes. I cannot look at the story of her life without thinking of Dr. Gabor Mate's work and his seminal text, *When the Body Says No* (2003). I take the ayahuasca's comparing me to my grandmother to be as much a warning as it is a blessing. I take my supervisor's cautions seriously. I believe that, if I do not manage it carefully, my generational wound will wear down my body and slowly kill me. More specifically, if I had never found psychedelics within my lifetime, it would have killed me like whatever inner wound it was that contributed to the death of my grandmother.

In another experience with Daime, I remember feeling as if it was looking deeply within me, scanning across every part of me from my mind to my spine and organs. The message: *"There is something very much the matter with you. It is not simple to heal, but I will heal this. For now, take your medicine. It is okay to need medicine."*

I believe in the ayahuasca's promise, and I have adhered to this guidance ever since. What psychedelics have given me is truly a profound gift. I am certain I could not maintain a full-time career without them or even a full life. Yet, I know that I am drawn to this work because of the nature of my own trauma which causes me to need to be needed. It also drives me to blame myself harshly for any suffering in the life of another that my craft does not repair. I am as wounded as I am passionate, truly a gift and a curse. However, I can honestly say I would change nothing.

I have faith that my life no longer hangs in the balance because I have been given access to medicine. Psychedelics have done so very much for me, primarily by helping me to see myself more clearly. In my view of what it means to be human, the only possible result of seeing oneself more clearly is accepting and loving oneself more deeply. This is therapy's primary function: for the clients to see and love themselves the same way their therapist is able to. Plant medicines also give me hope, which is all anyone who is suffering truly needs to succeed in their fight for freedom. It is my hope that, in good time and through due process, many more people will be given access to the same gifts that have been afforded to me. Especially my fellow healers in need. For just as we do not yet fully understand the intricate ways in which we can be broken, we are yet to behold the profound ways in which we are to be repaired.

References

Dias, B. G., & Ressler, K. J. (2014). Parental olfactory experience influences behavior and neural structure in subsequent generations. *Nature Neuroscience, 17*(1), 89-96. https://doi.org/10.1038/nn.3594

Lewis, C. R., Tafur, J., Spencer, S., Green, J. M., Harrison, C., Kelmendi, B., Rabin, D. M., Yehuda, R., Yazar-Klosinski, B., & Cahn, B. R. (2023). Pilot study suggests DNA methylation of the glucocorticoid receptor gene (NR3C1) is associated with MDMA-assisted therapy treatment response for severe PTSD. *Frontiers in Psychiatry, 14,* 959590. https://doi.org/10.3389/fpsyt.2023.959590

Maté, G. (2003). *When the body says no: The cost of hidden stress* (1st ed.). A.A. Knopf Canada.

Miller, L., & Weigand, E. S. (2021). *The awakened brain: The new science of spirituality and our quest for an inspired life.* New York: Random House.

Rodgers, A. B., Morgan, C. P., Bronson, S. L., Revello, S., & Bale, T. L. (2013). Paternal stress exposure alters sperm microRNA content and reprograms offspring HPA stress axis regulation. *Journal of Neuroscience, 33*(21), 9003-9012. https://doi.org/10.1523/JNEUROSCI.0914-13.2013

van Zuiden, M., Geuze, E., Willemen, H. L., Vermetten, E., Maas, M., Amarouchi, K., Kavelaars, A., & Heijnen, C.J. (2012). Glucocorticoid receptor pathway components predict posttraumatic stress disorder symptom development: a prospective study. *Biological Psychiatry, 71*(4), 309-316. https://doi.org/10.1016/j.biopsych.2011.10.026

Yehuda, R., Daskalakis, N. P., Bierer, L. M., Bader, H.N., Klengel, T., Holsboer, F., & Binder, E. B. (2016). Holocaust exposure induced intergenerational effects on FKBP5 Methylation. *Biological Psychiatry, 80*(5):372-380. https://doi.org/10.1016/j.biopsych.2015.08.005

Yehuda, R., & Lehrner, A. (2018). Intergenerational transmission of trauma effects: Putative role of epigenetic mechanisms. *World Psychiatry, 17*(3):243-257. https://doi.org/10.1002/wps.20568

Yehuda, R. (2022, February 22). How parents' trauma leaves biological traces in children. *Scientific American.* https://www.scientificamerican.com/article/how-parents-rsquo-trauma-leaves-biological-traces-in-children/

Every Healer Needs a Healer

Brodin Anderson

Whatever it is
that some therapists have
that allows them to leave the stuff that comes up at work

at work,

I don't have it.

I just don't.

I carry it.
And sometimes it hurts me.

I could be a martyr about it.
I could say I care too much.

But honestly,
it's just how I am.

Trauma colliding with nature and nurture.

There's nothing glorious about it.
There's nothing pitiful about it.

It doesn't make me a hero.
It doesn't make me a victim.

It just makes me...

me.

I guess I've learned to live with it,

and I'll tell you how:

The only way
I can do my work
and not fall apart

is by consuming plants,

sacred plants.

They,
along with ritual and community,
have shown me over time that all healers

need a healer,

and that there's more than one way to do it.

Friends can be a healer.

Church can be a healer.

Music can be a healer.

But my healer,
the healer I was designed to align with,

is psychedelic plants.

I'm not entitled.
I'm careful about it.

These plants are powerful.
They deserve respect
and caution.

I don't isolate myself with these experiences.
I involve people in my healing.

But for me,
once these criteria are met,
and I am at peace at the moment of ingestion...

I get somewhere
I am otherwise unable to go.

I love myself
because I see myself clearly.

I can set my burdens down
because I see reality more clearly.

It's beautiful.
It's challenging.
It's transformational.

But...
It doesn't last forever.

There isn't a feeling or state of mind
that ever does.

That's why it's a relationship.

It's partly educational,
partly parental,

and entirely love.

Lauren Parente

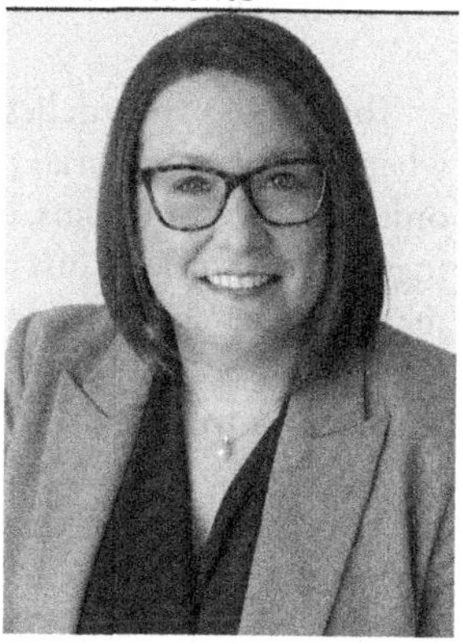

LAUREN PARENTE is a licensed clinical social worker and certified alcohol and drug counselor working at an outpatient trauma treatment center in Illinois. Lauren is most passionate about guiding others in their own healing journeys and is looking forward to becoming a psychedelic-assisted therapist in the future. In her free time, Lauren enjoys creating mixed media art, writing poetry, and spending time in nature.
lparentelcsw@gmail.com

Becoming All of Me:
My Healing Journey With Ketamine-Assisted Psychotherapy (KAP)

HOW COULD IT BE THAT THE VERY THING I PRIDED MYSELF ON FOR MOST OF MY LIFE WAS THE VERY THING THAT ALMOST KILLED ME? Whether you call it a type A personality or, from an RO-DBT perspective, having an overcontrolled personality style—whatever you call it, it's safe to say that I like rules and order. I find great safety in the containment of my self-imposed structure and rules...but I created too many rules. Riddled with constant obsessive thoughts, rigid rules, overthinking, rumination, perfectionism, and constantly falling short of my unrealistic expectations for myself, these rules kept my true self hidden from the world. They convinced me that I was better off dead, that my life was not worth living, and (as I learned in my work with psychedelics) that I was not living my truth.

Here, I share a glimpse of how psychedelics have rocked my world and express my personal and professional opinion on the future of psychedelics in treating mental health conditions. As a cisgender gay White woman, a psychotherapist for over 15 years, and a long-time seeker of personal healing, I'd be remiss if I didn't say that there is some hesitation in outing myself as a psychedelic therapy client. This article is written through the lens of myself as a psychedelic therapy client first and a clinician second. While I mention some barriers to increasing access to psychedelic-assisted psychotherapy, resolution of such barriers remains outside the scope of this article. This writing is deeply personal and raw, perhaps a literal manifestation of what's at stake here—the fragility of human lives and the healing potential of psychedelics.

My Journey

The use of psychedelics in my own healing journey was first recommended in 2021, when I was in residential treatment due to exacerbation of my obsessive-compulsive disorder (OCD) symptoms, depression, and whether I like to admit it or not, a long-standing eating disorder. I just about laughed in the attending physician's face when he asked me if I'd ever considered the use of ketamine to treat my symptoms. How could I, as a licensed clinical social worker and certified alcohol and drug counselor, even consider the use of a drug that some people use recreationally to treat my symptoms? Ultimately, my ego and lack of knowledge of the potential benefits of psychedelics lead me to proceed instead with transcranial magnetic stimulation (TMS) and the current curriculum at the residential facility.

Fast forward less than a year later, around spring of 2022, when I fell into another depressive episode that was almost my last—almost life ending. My best friend had just told me she was moving across the country in June, and my sister, my "person" in the world, decided to move out of state indefinitely at the exact same time. It felt like the perfect opportunity to kill myself.

I was honest with my therapist, who responded by saying, "So what am I supposed to do? Sit here for the next 2 months and sit by as you prepare to end your life?" While I do love her directness, at that moment I was terrified. I thought, "What if she sends me to residential?" followed by immense panic and thoughts like, "I cannot go through that again! I cannot!" My response to her in that moment was "No. I need you to hold me accountable for not writing my goodbyes, not organizing my finances, and not cleaning out my house. And if I do those things, I need you to hold a boundary with me, and there needs to be consequences," to which she nodded and stated, "a higher level of care."

Panic was an understatement. Even if I wanted to go into a higher level of care, I had just started a new job at a start-up company and thus had no short-term disability, and I had already practically drained my finances in seeking a higher level of care the year before. Even if I had the resources, my ego was certainly not going to let me enter a higher level of care less than a year after I had just done the whole residential-partial hospitalization-inpatient (RES-PHP-IOP) cycle.

I felt trapped, like I had tried almost every possible intervention out there in my 21years of battling for my mental health without success. When I say every possible intervention, I mean 21 years of psychotherapy, countless psychotropic medications, outpatient groups, inpatient treatment stays, residential, partial hospitalization (PHP), intensive outpatient (IOP), exposure and response prevention (ERP), somatic experiencing (SE) therapy, electroconvulsive therapy (ECT), and transcranial magnetic simulation (TMS). What was going to be different this time? I thought about my time in residential, trying to glean the most important elements, as if I could recreate them at home and save myself from having to seek a higher level of care again. I thought about the attending I met with in my first 24 hours in residential, who recommended ketamine infusions. My perception of this physician was that he was brilliant, but I wasn't privy to the extent of his brilliance until over a year later, when I followed through on his recommendation. I remember not fully grasping the truth of his words at the time as he looked at me, while motioning his hands as if he was tracing my silhouette, and said, "You see this? This is not you. There's a you somewhere in there, but this is not her."

At the time, I thought he was referencing my high functioning nature, or my ability to present substantially incongruently externally versus internally. As I progressed on my ketamine journey, I came to understand that he was right about a lot of things that day.

Infusions Gone Wrong?

I did not know that ketamine-assisted therapy (KAP) was a thing—or did not fully understand the magnitude of ketamine as catalyst versus ketamine as the medicine—so like many seeking this novel treatment in desperation, I entered the psychedelic space by way of six ketamine infusions over 2 weeks at a standard medical model infusion clinic, where no therapeutic preparation, support, or integration is offered. After the 3rd session, I started to experience a lifting of my depressive symptoms and a lessening of my anxiety...but then it happened—what I now know is referred to as a *ketamine death.* I perceived myself to have died during my 5th infusion. I thought the doctor overdosed me, and I thought he left my body there overnight and was going to come back in the morning to dispose of it. As I perceived my soul to be exiting my cold and stiff body, I pleaded with the universe, "Take me back; take me back! I'm not ready to leave (die)." After 21 years of intermittent suicidal ideation, I was deeply perplexed by my spontaneous declaration. I shared this experience with the doctor, an anesthesiologist, who looked blankly back at me and said, "Huh." Those moments of fear and perplexity made it very clear that I needed someone more experienced to process these experiences with. I needed more than just the medicine. I finished up my prescribed six sessions and worked on connecting to an agency that does KAP for maintenance sessions. This was the best decision I could have ever made for myself in my healing journey.

I knew from my very first appointment with the KAP provider that the process was going to be much different, and while I had some continued skepticism, intuitively I felt like I was where I needed to be. At the most basic level, we spent two sessions with the therapist getting to know me, my history, my needs, and my goals for treatment. I wasn't just handed the standard personal health questionnaire 9-item depression scale (PHQ-9) and generalized anxiety disorder scale (GAD-7), as if my whole life and current struggles could be captured in a series of standardized questions. I felt seen and heard. I am often bewildered by the power of human connection and validation. How did I know after just an intake session or two that this was exactly where I needed to be? Maybe I put a little too much blind faith in others, maybe I'm too trusting of therapy providers, or maybe I was just so desperate to process the ketamine death and prevent any future depressive episodes, like the one I had just gotten out of. Regardless, I continued on, with what I now know to be life-altering work.

The Uncovering

To say that I've learned a lot about myself in my work with KAP is a gross understatement. One of the most profound outcomes has been uncovering my sexuality. Growing up with significant religious trauma as well as my own rigid personality structure, it was never safe to consider that I could be anything other than a cisgender heterosexual female. Certain beliefs about sex before marriage and homosexuality were seemingly burned into my brain. I have always felt a certain pull toward women, but I wrote it off as me being jealous of other thinner, more beautiful women, as I have always been in a bigger body. It wasn't safe for it to be more than that. I also really struggled with dating men, especially with high contamination fears, but I didn't think much of it, again because it wasn't safe to be gay and I just assumed it was my contamination OCD.

I can remember at the end of a KAP session dropping the comment, "We need to talk about my sexuality next session." Thankfully this comment was met with ultimate compassion and noted to be brought up next session. I was and still am so grateful for my bravery in that moment, because it unleashed an avalanche of processing and exploration that ultimately led me to coming out as a gay woman.

At the time, I was training for my 9th marathon, and increased physical activity increased my sex drive. And there was something in me that knew "I just cannot have sex with another man." Was it the ketamine shaking things up in my brain, removing the screens and filters of my usual existence, allowing me to explore who I am and what satisfies me? I'd like to think so. The therapeutic relationship I had with the KAP therapist also contributed to me feeling safe enough to explore my sexuality, and for this I will be eternally grateful.

I did not go into ketamine work thinking, "I must explore my sexuality." It surfaced organically, along with other topics that needed exploration and resolution. For me, this is one of the many beautiful things about psychedelic work—it brings forth what needs to be healed or resolved, and this may or may not be what you think you need to work on. I wasn't exactly privy to this before KAP work, but this was an arena that needed attention. I say needed because at the time, as a single 37-year-old woman with no children who had felt her whole life like she was meant to bring life into this world, this was an important factor in family planning! Not only looking forward with this newfound information, but there was also an opportunity for healing for my adolescent self who felt so othered by not doing what other girls her age were doing at the time. I grieve for my adolescent self who didn't get to explore her sexuality, who was forced into or believed she must only date men. I grieve for the young girl who engaged in sexual behaviors with the opposite gender because that's what she thought she was supposed to do. I have so much compassion for this younger version of myself.

Reconnection To Life

Another example of a profound shift in my life trajectory relates to my relationship with suicidal ideation (SI). My first experience of SI occurred during my first major depressive episode at age 16. At the time I had no plan and no intent, although I contemplated what it would be like to die and there were a lot of nights I spent hoping, maybe even praying, to not wake up in the morning. Throughout the years, my SI has gone up and down in intensity. There were some periods of time when it wasn't there, but those were few and far between. I could never really shake the desire or the belief/fear that I would die prematurely by suicide. In my work with ketamine-assisted psychotherapy, I was able to explore my relationship with SI. I learned the function of it: why it showed up in the first place and why it has been so hard to let go of. More importantly though, I was able to start living my truth, or who I am, and stop living in accordance with who I thought I was supposed to be. I tapped into my own courageous self and started taking action toward family planning. I cannot believe that I had begun forcing myself to start grieving my lifelong value of having a child of my own, of feeling life grow inside me. I believed I was too much for others, thus preventing me from dating, and I assumed that I was on the brink of being too old to carry a child, all of which reinforced this desire in me to die.

It was in this living of my truth and aligning my actions with my values that I started to notice larger gaps of time without thinking about suicide, and I noticed that I was starting to grow an attachment to my future. Never in my 21-year struggle with depression and other diagnoses did I really believe that there was something worth sticking around for in my future. In my previous years of therapy as a client, I had yet to reach anywhere near the level of progress that I've made in my work with psychedelic-assisted therapy. While talk therapy may have kept me safe, or kept me from acting on my SI, the relationship I had with SI remained stagnant. Perhaps I was unwilling to let it go. Regardless, it took stepping into my truth, an outcome inaccessible to me prior to psychedelics, for me to truly comprehend that I don't actually want to die.

Catalyst Versus Magic

It is both my personal and professional opinion that the use of psychedelics for healing has the most impact (intensity and duration) with accompanying supportive therapy. I am aware of Indigenous and other models of psychedelics, but I have not experienced them and cannot speak to them. Psychedelic-assisted psychotherapy capitalizes on the changes in neuroplasticity that occur with ketamine and other yet to become legal psychedelics. It is not just about the initial relief after the psychedelic journey—it's about so much more. As one of the KAP group therapists says, "It's about walking the insights/learnings from the experience into your life." Things like intention setting before the psychedelic journey, the presence of a trusted therapist in the room while the client is undergoing the psychedelic journey, and the integration that occurs in the days, weeks, and months after a given session all help reinforce the changes occurring in the client's life. The client benefits from all components of the therapeutic model. The psychedelic is the catalyst for change and not just the magic pill that promotes feeling better.

My ketamine therapist, also trained as an art therapist, offers expressive directives like artmaking or writing in the preparation or integration phases, which can deepen the therapeutic process and processing that occurs. One does not have to consider oneself creative to benefit from this element. It's about the willingness to explore one's inner world with an alternative medium, one that transcends the limits of human language. Yes, the art gets processed using language, but the movement that occurs, the interaction between the individual, their internal world, and the medium they are using—well that's pure magic. For example, I've done scribble drawings in which I set an intention, scribble with my eyes closed using my non-dominant hand for one minute, and then go back into the drawing with eyes open and color in what appears to me, followed by a few reflection questions such as "What is this image here to tell me?" or "What is true from this image's point of view?" This process has helped me clarify intentions for psychedelic journeys and has helped me shift my relationship with things I've struggled with for many years.

In addition to utilizing scribble drawings in the preparation process for KAP sessions, I have found myself drawn to other forms of artistic expression, such as poetry,

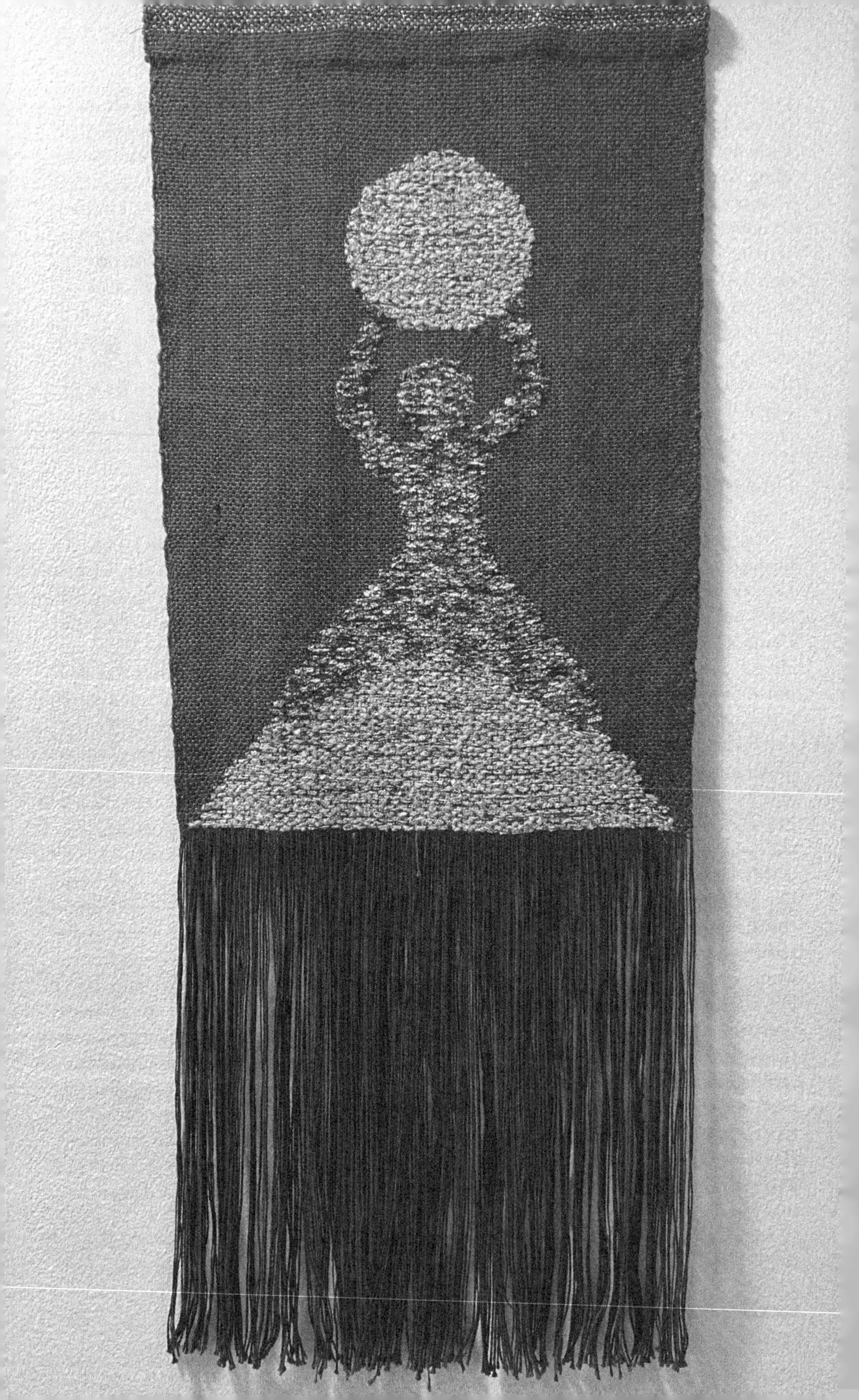

textile weaving, mixed media art, etc. While I have a craft studio in my house, I was only creating things that could achieve some level of perfection or symmetry prior to my experience with psychedelics. My theory is that the work I did, in addition to the unwavering support and encouragement from my KAP art therapist, helped challenge some of the rules and perfectionism I had around my creativity. It stopped being so much about evaluative praise or "Will people like this?" and more a deeply personal expression of my emotional landscape, of my own journey and transformation. I've found that I really enjoy creating a work of art and then writing poetry about the art.

For example, I share here a wall hanging designed and hand-woven by me, and the poem below that I wrote in response to the piece. Her title is "Unbecoming."

The world has shaped me into the being I am today,
but how do I know if that's really who I'm called to be?
Perhaps it can't be.
Force, shape, restrict, deny, avoid, suppress...
all actions I've taken to try to be the "me" I thought the world wanted me to be.
After slowing down and going inward, I'm learning there's much more joy to be had by
unbecoming everything I thought I was supposed to be
and embracing everything that I am.
Oh, what freedom there is in letting go of the expectations of the world
and tuning into me!
Expansion, exploration, curiosity, fluidity...all are celebrated here!
Today I choose courage over fear, aliveness over stuckness, curiosity over judgment.
Today, I choose me!

Implications

As part of the professional community and someone who has greatly benefited from psychedelic-assisted psychotherapy, I believe we have an obligation to educate the public on the pros and cons of the medical versus psychotherapeutic models of psychedelic therapy. We are on the precipice of an explosion in popularity and availability of the use of psychedelics to treat mental health conditions. With the chronicity of the disorders being targeted by psychedelics, the lens must be zoomed out enough to focus not only on ameliorating current symptoms but on preventing or reducing intensity, frequency, and duration of future relapses. Thus, the best way to reinforce lasting changes is involving therapy as part of the process.

I am aware of some of the barriers that exist in promoting such a model, including limited numbers of providers trained, cost (psychedelic medicine sessions plus the cost of therapy), lack of access for underfunded uninsured/underserved populations, lags in insurance support of psychedelics, societal stigma, etc. This is a future worth fighting for, though, and I would like to be part of the solution. It is my hope in the next 5 years or so to engage in formal training to become a psychedelic-assisted therapist to pay it forward. I truly believe I wouldn't still be here on Earth if it wasn't for the introduction of ketamine-assisted therapy into my treatment plan. ▼

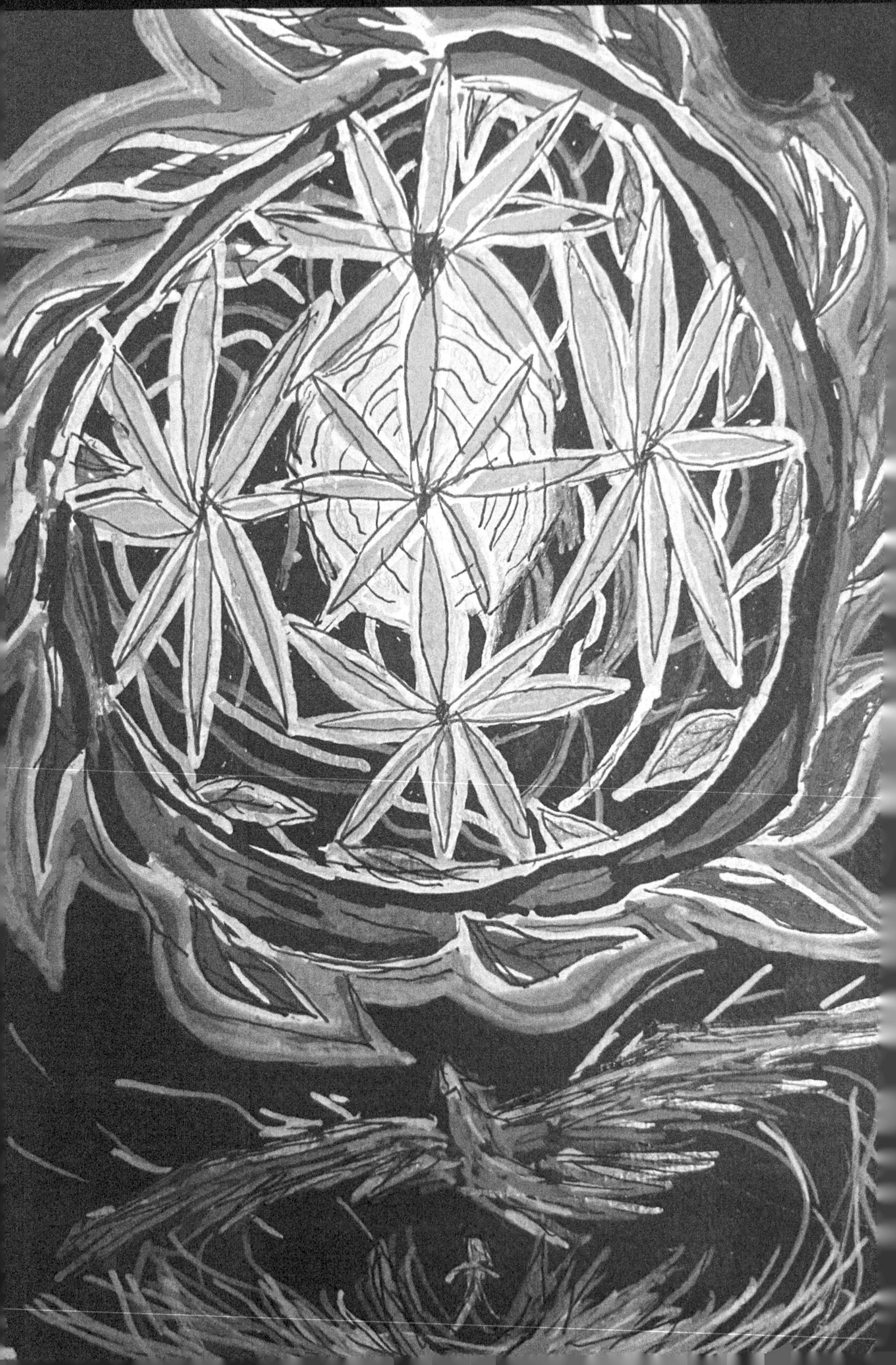

Lisa Noeth

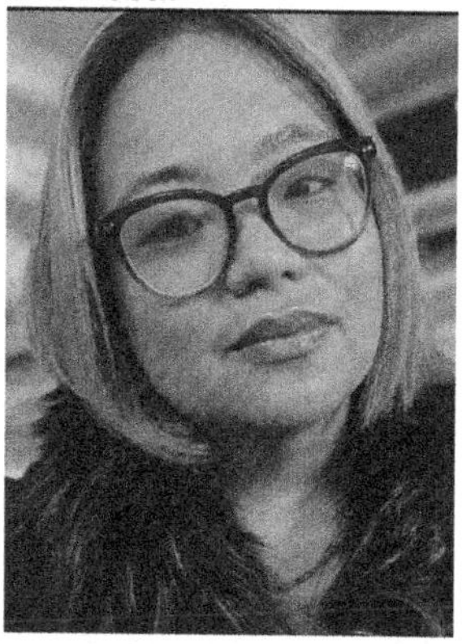

LISA NOETH is a tenacious grassroots leader, entrepreneur, political commentator, and artist. With her master's degree from NYU, she champions drug policy reform by publishing her master's thesis, "Trending High: The Call for Drug Policy Reform." She remains a lifelong advocate for destigmatizing cannabis and psychedelics for therapeutic uses and healing trauma. Lisa enjoys cheering on the Vegas Golden Knights, traveling, painting, and cooking.
lisanoethnv@gmail.com

Reborn from Ashes' Breath:
An Introspective Look at Healing Trauma Through Ceremonial Ayahuasca and Psychedelic Therapy

MY PERSONAL EXPERIENCE WITH AYAHUASCA encompasses the desire to be seen and heard by working through bouts of depression, emotional eating, and intergenerational trauma. I argue that the key to combatting the pervasive issues of trauma, addiction, and mental health crises, exacerbated by the aftermath of the COVID-19 pandemic, lies in the adoption of psychedelic therapy within a controlled and safe setting. I have witnessed transformative personal experiences as well as derived societal observations by participating in ayahuasca ceremonies and using psychedelics. Such alternative treatments have the potential to initiate deep healing and to fundamentally change our societal approach to mental wellness and spirituality in search of a deeper meaning in life. They have certainly changed mine.

After graduating with my master's degree in international relations from New York University in 2016, I settled for a life without meaning in the corporate world. Long before the corporate world swallowed my living soul, my master's thesis, titled "Trending High: The Call for Drug Policy Reform," was about drug policy reform, the historical implications of the War on Drugs in the minority community, and a case study of the positive impact of the decriminalization of all drugs in Portugal (Noeth, 2017). Eight years later, having become an advocate in the interim, educating the general public and promoting the recreational legalization of cannabis in Nevada, my final conclusion supports the larger implications of mirroring Portugal to decriminalize all drugs instead of strict criminal prosecution, in order to tackle the biggest issues facing humanity—trauma, addiction, and the mental health crisis in our post-COVID pandemic world—with alternative treatment options including the use of psychedelics in a safe ceremonial setting or therapeutic session.

The use of psychedelic therapy is becoming increasingly accepted as an alternative option in addressing a wide array of mental illnesses and trauma such as major depressive disorder, anxiety, complex post-traumatic stress disorder, and substance abuse. Examples of psychedelic substances used for therapeutic purposes include psilocybin mushrooms, ayahuasca, MDMA, LSD, and ketamine. Psychedelic therapy allows one to fully immerse in a deeply spiritual and personal experience embedded in embracing oneself through surrender and vulnerability in the moment of using psychedelics.

Many of us have become so lost in our monotonous lives that we forget that deep down we all crave the feeling of being seen and understood by being our true authentic selves around one another. As we grow older, we become trapped in never-ending cycles of self-destructive behavioral patterns of escapism, including distracting and numbing ourselves with substances and food.

Our internalized trauma and coping mechanisms, systemically stemming from childhood, carry on into adulthood. For example, growing up as a first-generation Filipino American in a strict Catholic household, I could not truly express my emotions directly.

I had to show no emotions because whenever I tried to communicate my needs, I was immediately shut down. Standing up for myself was perceived as complaining or being ungrateful, and my feelings were always invalidated. I was taught at a young age that love is conditional and based on transactional relationships. I was expected to follow the cultural norm of going to nursing school in return for familial sacrifice, also known in Tagalog as "utang na loob," which is the opposite of the American westernized ideology of family dynamics.

In addition, we were taught at a young age to be the "good girl" by meeting everyone else's needs and not taking up space. We were expected to manage our older relatives' emotions by not being too loud and by walking on eggshells all the time. Being the good girl, people pleaser, and empath came at a cost. Prioritizing everyone else's needs led me to emotional eating, ultimately binge eating, as I stuffed my emotions with food, the only thing that made me happy. I held on to these repressed emotions of childhood trauma deep inside of me that led me to weigh almost 300 lbs. I dealt with constant body shaming from older relatives, especially in the Philippines, hearing comments about my weight and how I dressed throughout my childhood into my adulthood.

Surrounded by toxic positivity coupled with intergenerational trauma and indescribable forces of family and cultural pressure that weighed heavily on my heart, I dealt with enormous amounts of shame, self-deprivation, and self-loathing, as I put on a mask in a corporate environment and faced disappointments as I followed my own path for my life after graduating.

Little did I know that ayahuasca would reopen the doors to these repressed memories and negative emotions bottled up inside me for so long. There are moments that define our lives, healing our past trauma for us to move forward. I experienced such a moment in a profound spiritual experience of self-discovery by practicing psychedelic medicine in a safe and ceremonial space.

Originating from the Amazonian rainforest in South America, ayahuasca, also known as the vine of the soul, is a psychoactive brewed drink that contains two main ingredients: Banisteriopsis caapi, a bark containing monoamine oxidase inhibitors (MAOIs), brewed with the leaves of Psychotria viridis, or another plant, which contains N,N-dimethyltryptamine (DMT). The effects of ayahuasca induce hallucinations. For thousands of years, ayahuasca ceremonies have been prevalent for religious and spiritual rituals in Peru and throughout South America, practiced by Indigenous tribes as an ancient plant medicine to address health issues and for the religious experience of connecting deeply with one's spirit.

A long time ago, during my thesis research in Washington, DC, about drug policy reform, I learned about psychedelics such as magic mushrooms and LSD. Then I stumbled upon Michelle Rodriguez's (2016) documentary about her ayahuasca experience, *The Reality of Truth,* on YouTube. Years later, I would be called to experience an ayahuasca ceremony with my close friend. Sitting with ayahuasca exposes multiple facets of who you really are by confronting your trauma, inner demons, fears, and true spirit.

On my first ayahuasca retreat, organized by Hummingbird Church and led by Pedro Tiata, I was transported into multiple dimensions beyond my understanding of the physical realm and spiritual universe. My friend and I were greeted with warmth once we arrived at the retreat grounds. As we settled down in the ceremony room, I couldn't know that my life would change forever during this first night of the retreat weekend. I was introduced into the spiritual community with open arms, and then I was introduced to the sacred power of breathwork for the first time.

The guided holotropic breathwork, breathing through your mouth and nose with fast-paced breathing patterns, is a guided exercise to teach each participant to ground themselves with the breath through a meditative exercise. Doing the breathwork exercises for the first time, I experienced an out-of-body experience with a sensation of unblocking the negative energy and repressed memories I had been holding onto by releasing with each breath the stress, anxiety, overthinking, and depression. I felt my mind opening up to a higher state of consciousness and relaxation by controlling each inhale as oxygen flowed through the brain after the tension within my body was released.

Before we were given our first cup of ayahuasca, we were told to come up with an intention. My intention was not to get high or to have an out-of-this-world visual trippy experience; I wanted to face myself in order to heal the parts of my life where I felt trapped and empty, especially my negative body image and intergenerational trauma, growing up as a first-generation Filipino American. I had all these intentions in mind as I stood up and walked in front of the altar to drink my first cup. Pedro Tiata stared straight into my soul by looking me in the eyes as if he could see all my pain, intergenerational trauma, addiction, attachment to material possessions, attunement to the mainstream news and issues, and the physical world of my past and present.

I have always described my first ayahuasca retreat as profound, expanding my mind beyond the conditional understanding of the world learned from society at a young age into adulthood. With ayahuasca, you embark on a spiritual quest to the darkest memories of your mind, as you take a break from the stress of modern society, disconnecting from phones and social media, in order to reconnect with yourself.

I was deeply anxious, not knowing what to expect, as I witnessed every single participant expressing extraretinal emotions triggered by ayahuasca's psychoactive effects, in sync with the indigenous chants, Pedro Tiata playing the harmonica, and the prayers throughout the 3-day ceremony. It was a frightening experience for the first time as the room transformed into geometrical patterns around me. The fire became vibrant, and there were translucent colors even with my eyes closed. Everyone around me slowly started freaking out, including me. Every participant was going through their own personal hell after ingesting the ayahuasca brew. The ceremony room was filled with many emotions, such as anger, moaning, yelling, and cursing, which encouraged us to release the negative energy and repressed memories. Looking back, we were able to navigate these personal tribulations by emotionally releasing the heaviness deep inside our souls as we learned to trust and surrender ourselves to the medicine with the support of Pedro Tiata. It takes an immeasurable amount of courage for each participant to face their worst fears into the night by sitting with ayahuasca.

As ayahuasca begins to break down your ego, you begin to confront yourself on a deeper spiritual level of understanding. It felt like I was dying, falling into the deep dark abyss as I was losing my own mind. I became separated from my physical body as I met my inner subconsciousness. I saw different paths around me being depicted as roots.

The very essence of near-death experience in an ayahuasca ceremony transforms into a sense of relief once you sit down with your inner spirit and subconsciousness. Then, I had an honest conversation with my inner child and my spiritual subconsciousness. In the end, I forgave the different versions of myself—my child, teenager, young adult, present, and future selves—in my own personal experience of internal conflict during the first night ceremony. Ayahuasca assists you in taking off your mask, allowing you to see yourself without any judgment and the distractions from the outside world. It allows you to see past the suffering from traumatic upbringing and bad decisions made from it. For those from a traumatic childhood, we perpetuate the trauma to the next generation. Under the plant medicine, we either end up relieving the trauma or confronting facets of our life that are not working. After I finally surrendered to ayahuasca by allowing my heart to guide me rather than my logical mind, I felt at peace with myself. As a result, sitting with ayahuasca for one weekend overshadowed Western medicine and years of therapy in my personal experience. The isolation and separateness from my inner spirit slipped away in the aftermath of each ceremony. What I witnessed from this experience from each participant was that the world is full of pain in this crazy chaotic life, but once we really set aside our differences, humanity as a whole is hurting from trauma.

On the other hand, I witnessed each participant's eyes light up with pure bliss of white light. I was in awe of seeing the pure joy of everyone dancing with a huge smile after going through their own pit of despair and personal hell by the end of the 3-day retreat weekend. I recognized a collective consciousness of individual and shared pain as we each sought to heal ourselves by doing inner shadow work and then becoming our most authentic selves. The interactions with one another after each ceremony made me realize that we each wanted to participate in an ayahuasca ceremony to heal and breathe in a judgment-free and safe environment by being transparent and vulnerable with our own selves. In all the agony and despair we experienced throughout the retreat weekend, many of us found ourselves, as we are all itching to be heard and see one another for who we are in all of our flaws.

As my friend and I shared reflections upon our first ayahuasca ceremony, it became clear that it had been a profound journey for both of us, a complex tapestry of transformative emotions, visions, and insights.

It was the morning after the first night ceremony. The sun had barely kissed the mountains, but the two of us were already awake, seated on the porch of our tent, a recorder between us. The birds were just starting to chirp, perhaps sharing their own stories, as we began to recount ours.

"Healing," I began, the word hanging in the misty air. "That's how it felt, despite the chaos, the fear...it was healing."

"You're right," my friend added, "it was scary, but it was like there was this dichotomy. Fear mixed with light, visions you want to run from, but then...a surrender to joy."

We recalled the chaotic experience in the room after every participant had received the first cup of ayahuasca. The room had been filled with cries and screams that gave rise to anxiety so intense that a facilitator had to call for the spirit lady, a guide who helped us navigate the turbulent waters of our psyches.

"She sat with me, and just...being told I was loved and safe, it helped me let go," we recounted.

My visions had been intense—a tree of roots that represented the different paths of life converging, dictating a journey others wanted for me. "But I'm following my own path," I said with a newfound conviction.

My friend shared her part, speaking of how the ceremony had heightened her senses, the auditory experience merging with colorful glimpses into a realm beyond: "But it wasn't just sights and sounds; it was emotion—raw and unfiltered. People's pain, their purging...it was like a chorus of suffering, and I felt trapped in it."

Our shaman's songs, also known as icaros in Spanish, the language of his ancestors of past shamans before him, became a bridge to understanding between the spiritual realm and our own personal journey. I saw my mother, her life, her pain, and her strength. It was overwhelming, a torrent of generational trauma and love.

"And then," my friend interjected, "it wasn't just our pain. It was everyone's—the whole room, the whole family lineage. It's like the ayahuasca was showing us the roots of our pain."

This was a testament to a shared experience that was deeply personal yet universally human amongst all the participants in the ceremony room. We spoke of ancestors, of the medicine of the sky, and of the profound realization that our parents were more than just caregivers—they were individuals with their own stories and struggles.

The conversation shifted as we explored the many aspects of the ceremony—the people around us, the contrast in reactions, the guidance of the shaman, and the profound shifts in perspective. Laughter mixed with tears, moments of fear interspersed with revelations of love and forgiveness. We spoke of our personal experiences and the realization that the path we were on was our own to shape. The visions had been clear, guiding us through past and potential futures, urging us to understand, to forgive, and to embrace our inner strength.

As our conversation neared its end, we acknowledged the difficulty of the experience, the moments we swore we'd never return to another ceremony, and yet, the undeniable pull of the ayahuasca's call to heal. "We'll see how tonight goes," my friend mused, "maybe a half cup this time." We both captured a final thought, a profound understanding of the interconnectedness of our pains and joys, before we agreed it was time to rest, to process, and to prepare for the ceremony to come. Afterwards, there was silence once more, just for the whispers of the wind through the trees, perhaps carrying our story to ears unknown.

My personal story is one of discovery, of facing inner demons, and of finding a path through the pain to a place of healing and understanding with ayahuasca. This is a snapshot of a spiritual journey that is both deeply personal and universally resonant, as a testament to the power of ancient practices and the resilience of the human spirit. I hope to go into it with more depth in my screenplay pitch for a limited television series about healing our intergenerational trauma as psychedelic use continues to become no longer a taboo as a sacred medicine.

After two ayahuasca retreat weekends, I desire to become more in touch with what truly brings me joy—tapping into my creative side again after being in the dark for so long and trapped in the corporate world. My inner child wants me to become a writer, storyteller, researcher, policy advocate and leader, chef, artist, and a healer by becoming a future breathwork instructor or facilitator in my post integration life. I still struggle with slips of depression post weight loss surgery, but I had to be ready to do the work as a part of the integration process post ceremony. I felt a stronger connection to taking care of myself and my health by protecting my boundaries. In a world where I felt like I didn't belong, growing up as a first generation Filipino American, I now desire to be my authentic self by creating meaningful connections to walk the path of figuring out my true purpose on this earth. Moreover, I learned in my first retreat that I have to forgive both my parents and accept them for their own faults; my grandma and older half-brother who passed away a long time ago were my ancestorial guides throughout each ceremony. I want to continue to write this entire profound experience. I embarked on undergoing the weight loss surgery approval process right after my first retreat weekend with ayahuasca, a step in this new journey to self-love and self-acceptance. Will I ever attend another ayahuasca ceremony again? I am not sure what the future holds, but I know that I will continue to shine a light as an advocate and storyteller to help each and every one of us save our own selves with psychedelics.

Notwithstanding this positive personal transformation, looking back at our first ayahuasca encounter 2 years ago, there are moments when I have regrets about taking the plant medicine because I am now awake to the failed constructs of society. Our modern way of living destroyed our natural human form of living in nature, hugging trees, taking in the sunlight every day, and dancing in the moonlight together under the stars, not inside an office cubicle. Secondly, I learned that worldly material possessions do not matter to me anymore, nor does the chase to climb the corporate ladder. Ayahuasca made me more aware of living life in the present. There is a quote from the TV show *Six Feet Under* that made me reflect on my ayahuasca experience: "You hang onto your pain like it means something, like it's worth something—well let me tell ya, it's not worth shit. Let it go. Infinite possibilities and all he can do is whine" (Ball, A., & Oliver, N., 2015). This holds true as our bodies remember the trauma all the way back from childhood. Ayahuasca brings the past to the present, to teach us to let go of the pain. Lastly, I now feel more deeply connected to God after ayahuasca by seeing God all around me in nature, in fire, in the earth, in water, and most importantly in each other, not just in a church building.

My story is one of many accounts of life transformation through psychedelics. I can only imagine how many more stories there would be if psychedelics were more accessible as a therapy modality. As a result, I advocate for policy changes to be able to further conduct research for the therapeutic effects of psychedelics for public health, including ayahuasca. Research to date shows promise for the efficacy of psychedelic-assisted therapy (Maia et al., 2023; Jimenez-Garrido et al., 2020), but more groundbreaking research on a larger scale needs to be done to evaluate the long-term effectiveness of the improvements of physical, emotional, and mental health after using psychedelics, in order to assess the risks and potential benefits.

Where do we go from here, considering that psychedelics are still illegal under the Drug Enforcement Agency's regulations? We need to lift the barriers imposed by Schedule I status to create a safer environment for comprehensive clinical research. This will innovate the future landscape of psychedelic research and development. Advocating for change at a legislative level is crucial, and we can do this by openly sharing a wide array of personal stories about profound breakthroughs for medicinal use, as I have shared mine here. The legalization and decriminalization of psychedelics should be promoted by engaging and educating the general population and stakeholders.

References

Ball, A., & Oliver, N. (Writers). (2005). Nathaniel Fisher. In *Six Feet Under*. Season 4, Episode 12, [Untitled]. HBO.

Jiménez-Garrido, D.F., Gómez-Sousa, M., Ona, G., Dos Santos, R.G., Hallak, J.E.C., Alcázar-Córcoles, M.Á., & Bouso, J.C. (2020). Effects of ayahuasca on mental health and quality of life in naïve users: A longitudinal and cross-sectional study combination. *Scientific Reports, 10,* 4075. https://doi.org/10.1038/s41598-020-61169-x

Maia, L.O., Daldegan-Bueno, D., Wiessner, I., Araujo, D. B., & Tofoli, L. F. (2023). Ayahuasca's therapeutic potential: What we know—and what not. *European neuropsychopharmacology, 66,* 45-61. https://doi.org/10.1016/j.euroneuro.2022.10.008

Noeth, L. (2017). *Trending high: The call for drug policy reform* [Master's Thesis]. CreateSpace Independent Publishing Platform.

Rodriguez, M. (2016). *Reality of truth* [Documentary Film]. Mike "Zappy" Zapolin & Laurent Levy (Directors).

We're all just walking each other home.

—Ram Dass

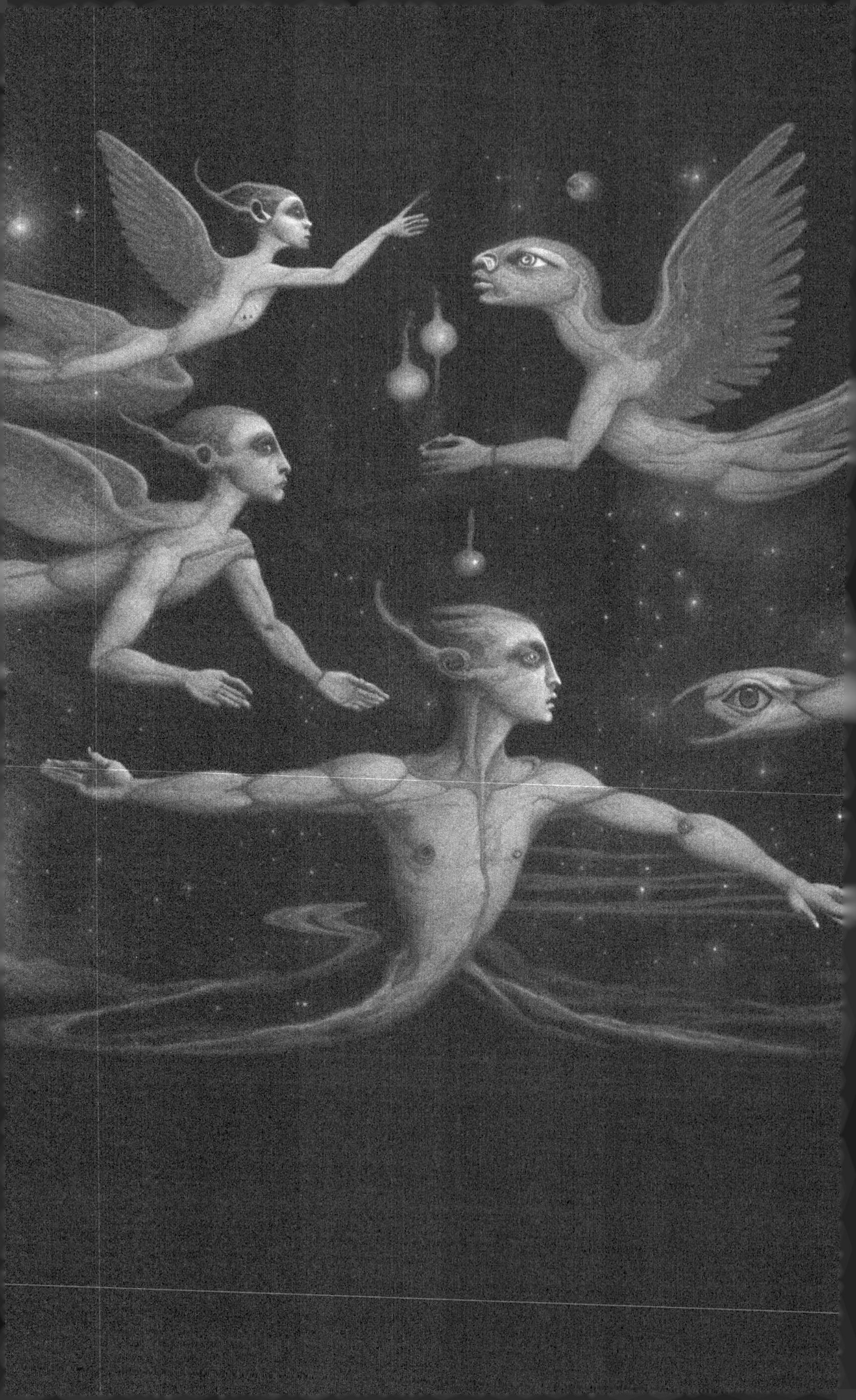

Michael Conti

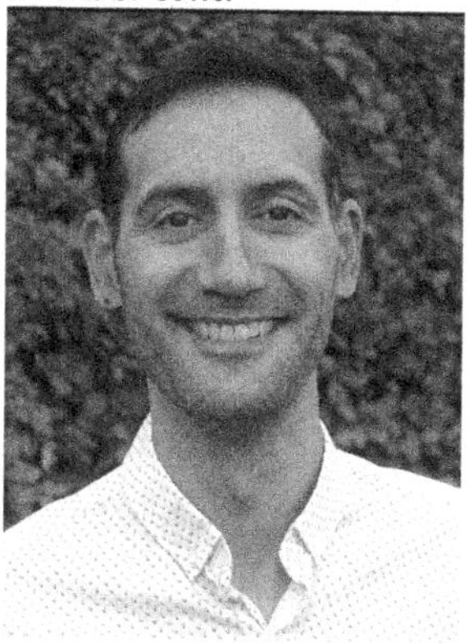

Michael Conti, MA, MSc, ECP, is a consultant psychotherapist, coach, and clinical supervisor working from an integrative somatic perspective. Trained in EMDR therapy, ketamine-assisted psychotherapy (KAP), and somatic sexuality, he specializes in working with altered states of consciousness, trauma, and gender and sexuality with a particular focus on the LGBTQIA+ population. He is the author of *Living Better with Yourself—A Practical Guide to Embodied Growth* and runs workshops internationally.
info@michaelconti.net

I'm Not F*cked up!—Healing Shame Through Erotic Transference While Using MDMA

This article is a reflection on my experience of erotic transference during a couple of MDMA experiences with a friend and how they furthered my development of freedom from shame and changed the associated compulsive self-regulating behaviors that I had in place.

Having done previous research in erotic transference and countertransference, I am quite aware of the attention the term has received in literature and the complexity of defining the erotic. In this article, the aim is not to elaborate a highly refined definition of erotic transference. Instead, I will approach erotic transference from a space that integrates its physical, sexual, emotional, intellectual, and spiritual dimensions.

I would describe erotic transference as a person's experience of desire for intimate connection that presents itself in an embodied, physically-intimate, and potentially sexual way. This experience does not accurately reflect the relationship that exists between the people involved but is an altered relationality generated primarily by the core psychological processes of one person (the client's, in the case of a therapeutic setting) which get projected onto the other person (e.g., the therapist) and the relationship between them. This altered perception of the relationship could be fictitious in nature or it could have its roots in a dimension of that relationship that already exists, such as a friendship dynamic. Although it occurs in a relational context, the experience of transference has a one-sided dimension to it; consequently, one could say that it is always a partially distorted perception of reality. The two-sided nature of the experience of the erotic comes into play when one also considers countertransference, which I will not be addressing in this article.

After presenting some aspects of my life story as context, I will describe a few important themes that were present in my two MDMA (3,4-methylenedioxymethamphetamine) experiences and explore my understanding of what brought about the personal change I went through. Finally, I will highlight some important points to consider when looking at erotic transference in the practice of psychedelic-assisted therapy.

Splitting Off the Sexual Self

Growing up in a religious, Catholic family in southern Europe in the '80s didn't really provide me with easy access to pornography. My parents' illustrated Bible and the collection of art books they possessed were the only naked bodies I spent considerable time staring at during my first years of puberty. In my family and the culture I grew up in, the erotic was either invisible or primarily looked down upon as embarrassing, shameful, disgusting, or sinful. This led me to develop an internal psychological split between the good boy persona that the adults in my life expected of me and were happy with and my sexual desires, which I was left alone to make sense of. What I wasn't aware of then, and only came to realize at the age of 24 while training to become a Catholic priest, was that I was gay and that my sexual desires and fantasies were primarily of a fetish nature. As if believing that being sexual was something to be ashamed of was not problematic enough, at a young age I unconsciously learned that I also needed to protect myself from being associated with the shameful abomination of homosexuality and, even more so, from the utter disgust of being a boy turned on by kinky eroticism.

By the age of 11 I had developed a completely split-off sexuality, enjoying my erotic body only when I was alone at home and then completely denying that experience from my consciousness the moment I sat down at my desk to continue studying and being the good boy the people around me wanted me to be. Masturbation happened regularly but was never labelled as such. My sexual body lived a life of its own in a completely different realm of consciousness: a very restricted one! During those formative years, I learned and came to believe what would become the basis of how I fundamentally saw myself and my sexuality for the many years to follow: My erotic desires should never be manifested to others because they are a fundamental flaw that makes me an intrinsically thwarted and disgusting person—a pervert.

Around the time I turned 17, our home got connected to the world wide web, and my pornography resources expanded considerably. I was no longer limited to the books lining the shelves in the living room, so I started exploring other bodies and scenarios—always male and in fetish situations. The split-off nature of my sexuality, however, perpetuated the denial of my identity and desires, and my sexual life continued being completely bracketed out of my awareness.

In the many years that followed, I came out as a gay man, attended many therapy sessions, quit my studies to become a priest, was in a few very significant romantic relationships, received a lot of support from my friends and family, and started incorporating a more embodied perspective to my personal development. All of this brought me a considerable level of healing and enabled me to start seeing myself as a more loveable person than I ever believed I was. I came to a better acceptance of my sexual desires. A part of myself, however, still held on to this inner shaming voice that believed I was intrinsically and fundamentally fucked up, and no relational or self-awareness experiences managed to convince me otherwise because only my deepest psyche knew the extent of my desires.

Looking back, I now realize how pornography and the compulsive sexual behavior that accompanied it had become my primary mode of regulating my emotions when confronted with the intense and horrific shame of looking at my sexual identity and erotic desires. It allowed me to enter into my own secret space, thus ensuring that I was the only one exposed to my shameful and flawed self. It also trapped me in a cycle I could never step out of. On one hand, pornography became my primary access to the inner sanctuary of erotic desire and allowed me to embody my emotional experience and link it to pleasure. On the other hand, this enjoyable erotic experience was precisely that which generated my shame and inner judgement. My way of coping with this dysfunctional dynamic was to progressively dissociate from my body and sexuality, something that endured for a long part of my life.

Ecstasy

I had my first experience with psychedelics at the age of 43. Half a year after having attended an ayahuasca ceremony, I shared an experience using MDMA with a close friend who was also a therapist and very much experienced in the therapeutic use of psychedelics. The aim was to use MDMA for personal growth rather than to have a psychedelic-assisted therapy session.

It was during that first experience that I definitely understood why MDMA was called "ecstasy"! It was the first time in my life where I had the most profound awareness that I am fundamentally OK as a person. This was also accompanied by a lot of trauma-releasing body movements that continued in the subsequent days. It was an experience of complete alignment of my cognitive, emotional, embodied, and spiritual dimensions, and this led me to start seeing myself in a completely new light. I was primarily loveable in all my totality without the internal splitting that had been a constant in the previous 3 decades.

One moment that particularly stood out for me during that experience was when my friend touched me on the shoulder to check on how I was doing. It was the first experience of human touch as this loveable version of myself. That moment of touch became the crystallized, embodied experience of release from the shame of being myself and provided me with a new body memory: I am not flawed, disgusting, and repulsive but fundamentally loveable; I am not someone to be shunned and despised but someone who can be lovingly touched.

This experience was followed by many months of integration during which I continued developing a less judgmental approach to my sexual desires. I became more accepting of myself as a gay man and of my kinky eroticism. Overall, I felt less ashamed of being myself. And yet, the secretive side of sexual shame started to slowly creep back in, and pornography and compulsive sexual behavior continued serving the function of emotional regulation as they always had. I could see myself in a different light, but I still had an ingrained inner belief that I was inherently damaged and still had not acquired new tools to manage my emotions in a different way.

"I'm Not Fucked Up!"

Ten months later I decided to repeat the experience using MDMA with the same friend. This being my second time using the substance, I was very open to whatever came up during the experience and only went into it with the intention of continuing my personal journey of inner freedom. Three themes were significantly present for me during the experience, and the relational component turned out to be a very salient one throughout.

At one point during the experience, I was placed in front of the 11-year-old version of myself. I wasn't him. I was the adult who held him, loved him, and protected him. As I write these words I feel the futility of trying to describe in words the intensity of such an experience. It was a quantum leap forward from the previous ways in which I had tried to relate to my inner child. Prior to that evening, I had tried to get my adult self to interact with my inner child. I knew what the adult wanted to say. I knew what he wanted to do. But the child remained out of reach. During that MDMA experience, however, I felt myself become the adult, and I could intimately connect to that boy.

Before this second MDMA experience, whenever my shame came up, especially in relation to my sexuality, my inner voice unequivocally repeated the following phrase over and over with a deep conviction: "I am fucked up!" After my MDMA experience, however, something has radically shifted in me, and I find myself unable to use that phrase about myself anymore. There have been many opportunities for that internal script to be played out again, and my life is definitely far from perfect, and yet, whenever the thought of it comes up, I experience a strong inner counter-voice that actively resists that statement and deeply believes that, although some things in my life could be fucked up, *I* am not.

I also find that I have stopped using pornography, that the compulsive dynamics in my sexual life have significantly decreased, and that there is, on the whole, a stronger desire to connect to the other person on more than just a physical level. It's not that I'm actively trying to avoid pornography or control my sexual behaviors. I don't find in myself an inner judgement, as such, in relation to these behaviors—my training as a somatic sexuality practitioner radically widened my perspective on the different facets of sexual behaviors and desires! Instead, I believe that what has happened is that I have found a more direct route to what I actually desire in the moment rather than regularly displacing my emotions onto my sexuality. Because of my new experience of being the adult holding the child and the deep belief that I'm not intrinsically and fundamentally flawed, I am now able to sit with and connect to my actual emotions without the usual shame being activated. The emotional-regulatory function that pornography and compulsive sexual behavior served seems to no longer be necessary because I—including all my desires and sexuality—am not someone to be ashamed of.

Erotic Transference

This change was so significant for me that it left me with great curiosity as to what it was during my MDMA experiences that had made this shift possible. There is no precise way of knowing how such change occurs, so I will offer the best understanding I have come to, namely that erotic transference was the fundamental force involved.

During the second MDMA experience I reconnected with the sense of being fundamentally OK as a person. At the same time, I also perceived a strong desire for physical intimacy with my friend. The desire wasn't primarily for explicit sexual contact but more for physical intimacy and closeness that could not be separated from an erotic charge that I was feeling in my whole body. This desire would, previously, have been precisely one of the strongest triggers of my internalized shame and the compulsive need to regulate it. Under the influence of MDMA, however, I could see myself as being fundamentally OK while at the same time perceiving, with stark clarity, my desire for embodied intimacy with another man. What ensued was that my desire became integrated into the loving perspective I had acquired of myself, helping me shed another layer of shame, this time specifically related to my erotic and physical desire for intimacy. I came to see myself as fundamentally OK as a person and with my desires—all of them!

The change that happened in me during the second MDMA experience was to such an extent that, instead of only becoming aware of my desires, during the experience itself I actively shifted my behavior away from the usual pattern of closing myself in, in the shadow where shame festers. At different points during the MDMA experience, I consciously decided to physically reach out to my friend with simple gestures of physical affection. Instead of this triggering the usual shame spiral that would inevitably ensue, the physical connection gave me the opportunity to relive the experience of being fundamentally OK in an embodied, relational context. This time, however, it was not just about the embodiment of being touchable by the other but also that of being able to step out and touch the other. My desires were permitted. They didn't turn me into a disgusting and repulsive monster, but they became an experience of strong connection that flowed from this loved and loving self that I saw myself as being. Hence, through this erotic transference I experienced a deeper integration of myself (Luca, 2014). Because my experience of my desires didn't trigger the usual feelings of rejection and shame and the subsequent emotional dysregulation, the need for my typical coping mechanism fell apart.

I now realize that the experience of erotic transference with my friend gave me the opportunity to experience my desires in a real manner rather than in the typical deformed way that my shame had turned them into. The term reality here does not refer to the form of the relationship itself, as this was a very particular context that entailed me being under the influence of a substance that produces feelings of empathy, sociability, and interpersonal closeness (Bravo, 2001). Instead, the reality lies in that I could connect to my desires without them being suffocated and distorted by shame. The transferential dimension of the relationship with my friend was not separate from the real one and become a place of transformation, generating a more mature relationship of a person-to-person nature (Mann, 1997).

Applying This to Psychedelic-Assisted Therapy

What is the relevance of this account for psychotherapy involving the use of psychedelics, namely MDMA? I am well aware that the setup I am describing is different from the context of psychedelic-assisted therapy. I do believe, however, that there are a number of things that are very relevant to the practice of such therapy.

First, it would be helpful to consider that not only is erotic transference not something to be afraid of in therapy but its foreclosure could easily constitute harm to our clients. This applies to all therapeutic settings but all the more so when psychedelics are being used due to the client's heightened ability to pick up what is happening on the therapist's side in such contexts (Feldmar, 2021; Grof, 2008). If, as therapists, we approach erotic transference with our unconscious judgement or fear, it is more likely that we contribute to further entrenching our clients' internalized shame around the experience and expression of erotic desire. If, on the other hand, we allow it to be ethically present even in situations where our clients are in a highly-perceptive state, while we are being compassionate and non-judgmental, we would be offering a deeply corrective relational experience that could have a profoundly transformative effect in our clients (Phelps et al., 2017).

Because of the depth of experience that erotic transference entails, especially when psychoactive substances are being used, and the importance of keeping it within an ethical framework without foreclosing it, it is of paramount importance to explicitly and appropriately bring up the topic of erotic transference during integration sessions by inquiring about it and allowing enough space to talk about it over the course of a number of sessions. This gives clients explicit permission to acknowledge what they felt during the session and articulate the experience of the relational space in its full entirety. By doing so, as therapists we would be helping to reinforce our client's freedom from internalized shame. At the same time, it is equally important that this is done in the most appropriate way possible where it is crystal clear that such an exchange is explicitly being done for the client's benefit and not for that of the therapist. As therapists we need to always hold in mind the power differential that exists in such conversations and have our intentions and actions aligned in the pure interest of our clients, while doing our own personal work in a separate context.

Touch is a tricky subject in psychotherapy and all the more so in psychedelic-assisted therapy. Out of our concern for our clients, we might lean towards avoiding touch, seeing this as being potentially harmful due to matters related to power, exploitation, or boundary violations (Hunter & Struve, 1998; Pinson, 2002). While bearing in mind the relevant professional guidelines in relation to the use of touch, especially when it comes to consent and sexual contact, it is also helpful to examine our own fears of engaging in touch. It helps to check in with ourselves about how much of our hesitation actually stems from our ethical obligation not to cause harm and how much of it comes out of the cultural and social scripts that we have internalized. These scripts have generated highly individualist notions in our societies where physical contact is often seen as suspicious and dangerous, and this has led to societies made up of individuals with embodied isolation. It is, thus, precisely in the spirit of not harming our clients that it is vital to question how much withholding touch can be harmful to our clients, reinforcing the disconnection that has been generated within our societies with all the resultant mental and physical health consequences (Kumar & Salinas, 2021).

All of what's mentioned above needs to be situated within the context of an ethical therapist-client relationship. That is why boundaries, clarity, and consent are of paramount importance, especially when working with psychedelic substances. This implies that we always need to consider our clients' histories—particularly when trauma is involved—when deciding how to be present in situations where erotic transference comes up. It is also undeniable that, as therapists involved in psychedelic-assisted therapy, we actively and constantly examine our own countertransference (Grof, 1985) because this is always present given the relational nature of therapy (Mitchell, 1988; Stolorow, 1994). As therapists we need to do our own work on our countertransference, both personally and in a supervisory context (Conti, 2016), to ensure that erotic countertransference dynamics do not negatively impact our clients.

Conclusion

Erotic transference can be seen as a minefield in psychotherapy and potentially more so when psychedelic substances are involved. One could, however, see the use of psychedelics as a way of allowing for the experience of erotic transference in such a way that it profoundly transforms and heals clients' internalized relational or erotic shame, together with any associated self-regulating compulsive behaviors. To work ethically with clients in psychedelic-assisted therapy settings, as therapists we need to do more than our utmost to work within the boundaries of a professional relationship, while also ensuring that we do not foreclose the experience of the erotic, thus further reinforcing our clients' internalized shame.

References

Bravo, G. L. (2001). What does MDMA feel like? In J. Holland (Ed.), *Ecstasy: The complete guide. A comprehensive look at the risks and benefits of MDMA.* Park Street Press.

Conti, M. (2016). *Supervisors' experience of the erotic in supervision: An interpretative phenomenological analysis* [Unpublished master's thesis]. Middlesex University.

Feldmar. A. (2021). On the therapeutic stance during psychedelic psychotherapy. In T. Read & M. Papaspyrou (Eds.), *Psychedelics and psychotherapy: The healing potential of expanded states* (pp. 7-17). Park Street Press.

Grof, S. (1985). *Beyond the brain: Birth, death, and transcendence in psychotherapy.* State University of New York Press.

Grof, S. (2008). *LSD psychotherapy: The healing potential of psychedelic medicine* (4th ed.). Multidisciplinary Association for Psychedelic Studies.

Hunter, M., & Struve, J. (1998). *The ethical use of touch in psychotherapy.* Sage. https://doi.org/10.4135/9781483328102

Kumar, A., & Salinas, J. (2021). The long-term public health impact of social distancing on brain health: Topical review. *International Journal of Environmental Research and Public Health, 18*(14):7307. https://doi.org/10.3390/ijerph18147307

Luca, M. (2014). Editorial introduction: An encounter with erotic desire in therapy. In M. Luca (Ed.), *Sexual attraction in therapy: Clinical perspectives on moving beyond the taboo—A guide for training and practice* (pp. xvii-xxiii). John Wiley.

Mann, D. (1997). *Psychotherapy: An erotic relationship. Transference and countertransference passions.* Routledge.

Mitchell, S. A. (1988). *Relational concepts in psychoanalysis: An integration.* Harvard University Press.

Phelps, J., Anthony P., & Grob, C. (2017). Developing guidelines and competencies for the training of psychedelic therapists. *The Journal of Humanistic Psychology, 57*(5), 450–487. https://doi.org/10.1177/0022167817711304

Pinson, B. (2002). Touch in therapy: An effort to make the unknown known. *Journal of Contemporary Psychotherapy: On the Cutting Edge of Modern Developments in Psychotherapy, 32*(2-3), 179–196. https://doi.org/10.1023/A:1020545010081

Stolorow. R. D. (1994). The intersubjective context of intrapsychic experience. In R. D. Stolorow, G. E. Atwood, & B. Branchaft (Eds.), *The intersubjective perspective* (pp. 3-12). Jason Aronson.

To Be Known

Allison M. Hammond

The ache of mine lingers and burns.

This pain lodged in me from the hands of a father, an "uncle," the Priest, an athletic trainer, a boy, and a boyfriend.

My body raw, cold, exposed, without consent.

The feeling of being cooked from the inside. Such pressure and confusion from the heat of those six. Someone else's shame crossed through my skin.

I was tossed aside like the trash from another young girl's birthday party.

Time did not stop.

The stiff, stuck walls of icy bricks built within me. Boulders dammed my water's flow.

My nervous system froze.

Wounds then scars formed like jagged icicles.

My flame of hope unsupported, alone, flickering.

Survival unsure.

Repression necessary.

Escape welcomed.

Trapped. Inside. This. Frozen. Tundra.

Three. Decades. Pass.

The budding thaw of frozen pain and trauma.

How?

A temperature change with psychedelics and warm guidance. An opening to my own internal medicine.

A safety to feel and move through my freeze.

A homecoming. A coming home to self—myself.

Welcoming all parts of me home.

Death became a less sought escape.

Compassion. To know myself. My story.

Seeing power in my own nurturing darkness.

A choice—the cycle of abuse stops with me.

A choice—to root into Mother Earth.

To birth my creation. My truth.

A remembering of self within the ache.

A new ache born—a worthy desire to discern my own voice.

Ah, yes, my pen as an IV for the pain.

A message roared, "I matter."

Acceptance.

My own fire.

Courage to be known.

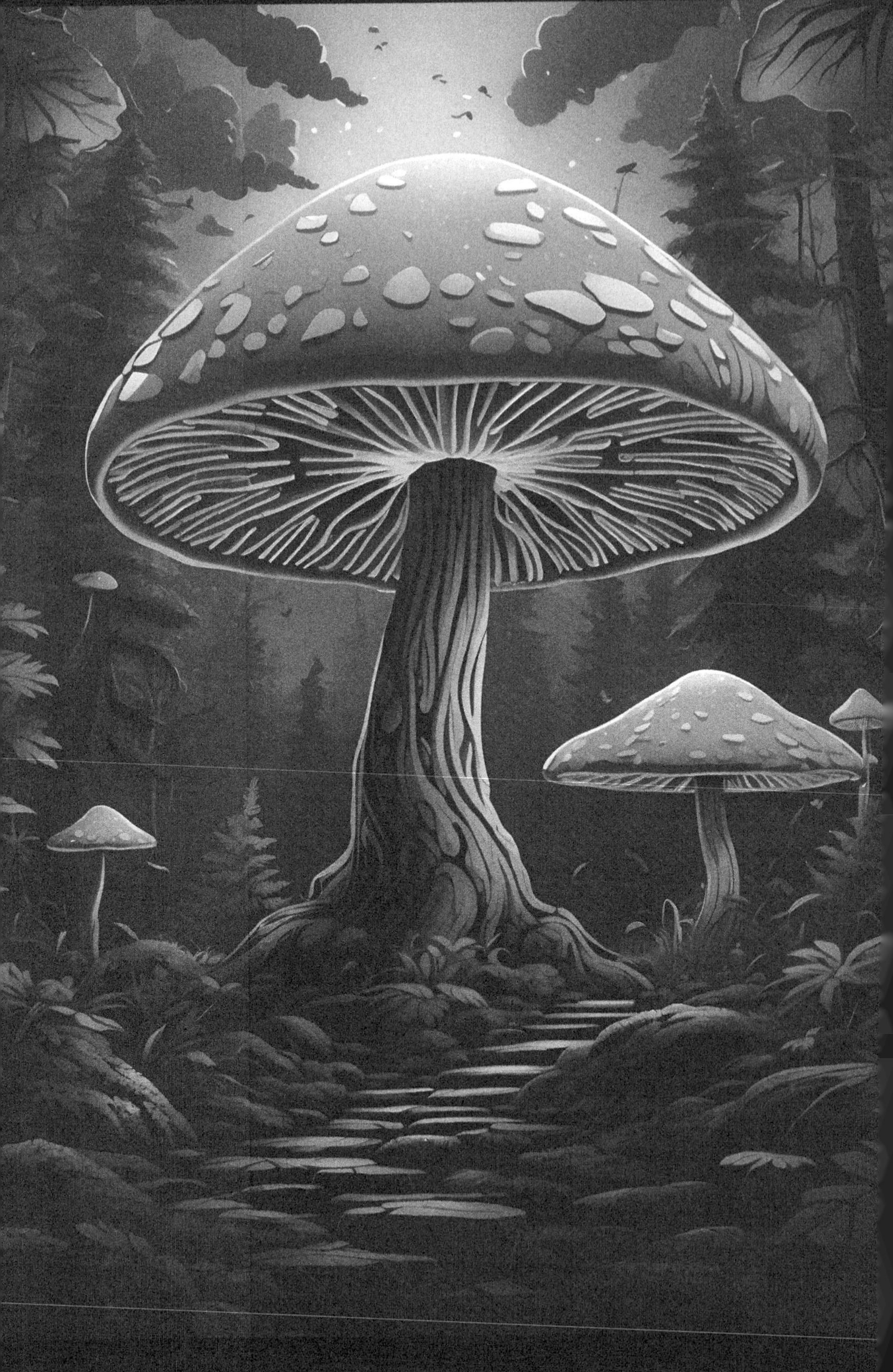

Denise Rue

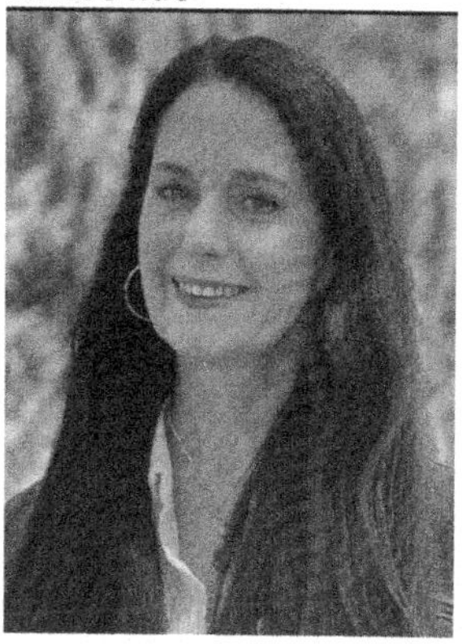

DENISE RUE is a licensed clinical social worker and hypnotherapist. For over 3 years, Denise worked as retreat leader and lead therapist at a legal psilocybin retreat center in Jamaica. Denise has had the privilege of overseeing over 1,500 psilocybin sessions and as many group integration sessions. She has a profound respect for the healing potential of this medicine, as well as a deep sense of the responsibility practitioners hold in shepherding people on their journeys. Denise has a private practice in New Jersey, specializing in complex trauma. Denise is the founder of the New Jersey Psychedelic Therapy Association.
deniserue59@gmail.com

How Magic Mushrooms Made Me a Better Therapist

I LIKE TO THINK THAT BEFORE I TOOK MAGIC MUSHROOMS, I WAS A GOOD THERAPIST: compassionate, committed, and continuously striving to improve my skills. But my experiences with magic mushrooms over several nights in July of 2018 contributed more to how I conceptualize my work as a healer than any amount of education, reading, or workshops ever could.

I was a latecomer to the psychedelic world. Like many of my Catholic school peers, I'd fallen prey to the Nixon-era propaganda that demonized all recreational drugs. So, what compelled me to try psilocybin so late in life? As a psychotherapist working with individuals with complex trauma, particularly adult survivors of childhood sexual abuse, I became frustrated with the slow pace of healing afforded by conventional therapy and psychiatric medications, as they did little more than take the edge off. Was this really the only option for my clients? After reading the studies with psilocybin coming out of New York University and Johns Hopkins, I became motivated to experience first-hand this medicine that had shown such promise in helping individuals with end-of-life anxiety, treatment-resistant depression, and addictions. So, soon after my 58th birthday I took a leap of faith and booked a 10-day, four-dose psilocybin retreat in Jamaica.

> *(now the ears of my ears awake and/now the eyes of my eyes are opened)*
>
> —E. E. Cummings

In the hundreds of psychedelic integration circles I've now had the privilege of leading, it's not uncommon to hear from a client that one session with the medicine is like years of traditional therapy. That was certainly true for me.

And while I went to the retreat wearing my therapist's hat, I also sought healing for myself. I especially wanted to address the deep grief I'd been experiencing following the deaths of my husband, father, and brother, as well as my anguish over my mother's recent descent into dementia. The first morning's preparation session with the retreat leader, facilitators, and the other 14 participants extended into the warm afternoon. As evening approached, I journaled and set down my hopes for the session. At sunset the group gathered, and with very little ceremony each swallowed our allotted dose of psilocybin capsules (3 grams for me). I found a vacant corner in the open-air pavilion, unfurled my yoga mat, donned my headphones, closed my eyes—and waited.

After about a half hour, I began to experience classic psychedelic visuals—colorful fractals and sinuous paisleys, morphing into minarets, turrets, and Corinthian columns. It was all very beautiful, straight out of *Alice in Wonderland.* Then I began to descend into the earth. There were jewels in the mud, and I thought, "I'm going to have to dig for the treasures here." And then I began to cough. And cough. No amount of water would soothe my throat. My body was trying to release some pent-up energy, trauma stored in the deepest recesses of my being.

One of the facilitators gently suggested I might want to scream. At first, I demurred, not wanting to upset other members of the group, but I finally allowed her to lead me out into a nearby field. Light rain began to fall, and I could feel the ground pitch and heave. I dropped to my knees wailing, "This earth has swallowed everyone I love!" I keened for what seemed like hours, great rivers of mucus coursing down my face. My lovely guide, Sidi, steady by my side, offered tissues and a hand on my shoulder. What a blessed catharsis. The mushroom brought me face to face with the grief I'd been holding for years, perhaps at a cellular level, and with the aid of a kind and nonjudgmental guide, I was gifted release.

But the night was far from over. For some reason, I intuitively felt I needed a male facilitator for the next part of my journey. I asked specifically for Dan, a young midwestern man in his 20s who sported a killer tattoo of a praying mantis and an extraterrestrial on his right arm. As we walked under the Jamaican sky, I told him my story of loss. When I spoke of my grief, the ground turned to mud and threatened to swallow me; the gnarled branches of the almond trees clawed out to engulf me. But when I uttered words of gratitude—for the love of these wonderful men and for my own courage—that very tree burst into blossom. In that moment, I experienced the power of my thoughts, how they could rob me of strength and keep me sunk in despair, or fortify me. It was a night of searing pain and absolution: years of therapy in a single evening.

The atmosphere of this retreat was a far cry from the structured settings typically followed in clinical trials and many other retreats. While there were several experienced guides present, the guests were not required to direct their attention inward while wearing a mask and listening to music. I felt completely safe and cared for and always had a guide with me. It was helpful for me to move, to feel grounded by the earth, to engage with the stars and trees. Most importantly, I needed to tell my story to a compassionate listener. Since the deaths of my father and husband, 4 months apart, I had never been able to tell my story beginning to end. My guide, Dan, sat like a Buddha and simply listened. What a gift it was that night to be met without judgment and with infinite patience. Telling my story was what I needed, and while it was not technically evidence based, it was profoundly transformational.

The Big Night

By the second psilocybin session 2 nights later (my 5-gram dose) it was clear that I was tapping into the experiences of the other group members, a frequently observed phenomenon with psychedelics, which tend to erode our false sense of separateness from others. These substances dissolve, as Alan Watts put it, the notion that we are "isolated 'egos' inside bags of skin." (Watts, 1989, p.9). Grof (1980) observed repeatedly that his LSD subjects were able to tune into the feelings of their sitters with great accuracy. So, it made sense to me that my intuitive nature was heightened while under the influence of psilocybin.

The great challenge was that once I soaked in another guest's energy, I didn't know how to release it. The retreat leader showed me how to work energetically, taking in and releasing, a breathing practice I had utilized while working in hospice. There in Jamaica, I was instructed to release energies to the ground, the ocean, or the air, releasing through my breath but also through my hands and feet. I got the message from Mother Earth that she could handle it all. Just as Dan had received my pain and gratitude on that first night, I was learning how to receive the experience of another with deep presence and compassion and release it so I wouldn't go down with the ship. It was a crash course, to be sure, and while I in no way felt ready, I was inspired to offer up whatever I could on the third dose.

That night, with the aid of 10 grams (a dose arguably too high for my delicate constitution), I settled onto my mat on a sand dune at the edge of the Caribbean Sea. I had befriended several women on the retreat, three of whom were survivors of childhood sexual abuse and, as the oldest woman there, felt a sense of protection towards them. Donning my eye shades, I sent up my intention that if the mushroom wanted my help, I would offer up what meager skills I had. The ensuing visuals brought a procession of shamans, medicine women, and alien entities. Each filed past assessing me, shining lanterns, prodding me with scopes, sizing me up as if to say, "Who is this woman who says she wants to help?" Finally, a very serious angel hovered above, regarding me, then silently released me into the night.

Thus began the most terrifying hours of my life. The mushroom catapulted me into the bodies and psyches of my new-found friends. I was transported into the body of the girl who was kidnapped, chloroformed, and raped on a cold warehouse floor. Parts of my psyche splintered and fled in order to endure the ordeal, and the parts of me that remained morphed into a cold-blooded, green-scaled reptile. How else could I survive? I went numb and silent like the little girl whose father crept into her room each night, repaid her in Barbie dolls, and swore her to secrecy. I writhed with the guilt and despair of the soldier who watched her friend walk into an ambush in Iraq. I crawled on the beach for hours that night descending into deeply hellish realms. Yes, it most certainly could be classified as a bad trip. But like many who ascend from those demonic depths, I consider this to be one of the most personally transformative and meaningful experiences of my life (Carbonaro et al., 2016).

Increased Empathy

The capacity for empathic listening is a hallmark of a good therapist and a skill I feel came naturally to me. But since that paradigm-shattering night, my client's trials are less abstract. Symptoms such as flashbacks, hypervigilance, or dissociation are no longer simply diagnostic criteria. Having experienced, survived, and subsequently processed the intense emotional states of my bad trip, I'm better able to maintain an empathetic embodied presence with my clients (Phelps, 2017). I noticed this immediately upon returning to work after my retreat. I was able to cultivate an evenly suspended attention, retain greater equanimity, listen deeply, and truly connect with my clients' emotional states. In my therapeutic training I heard countless times that a therapist can take her client only so far as she's taken herself. I consider the experience of that hellish July night to be one of the greatest gifts I've ever received from the mushroom. While I would never have signed on for the experience, it has immensely enhanced my therapeutic skills and greatly expanded my capacity to be a fully present and empathetic human being.

The Importance of Silence

On my retreat the immense therapeutic value of silence was communicated to me through an unexpected source—lizards. In Jamaica, they were everywhere: eyeing me from the branches of the ackee tree, basking on a near-by rock, observing me in the outdoor shower. They possessed a kind of preternatural stillness, a necessary patience. While on mushrooms, I was struck by the power of their silence and intuited that the lizards were there as teachers. I asked a local craftsman, Errol, to carve a lizard for me. Back home in New Jersey, I placed it on my office desk to remind me of the importance of silence and stillness in therapeutic work.

Too often in therapy sessions, I'd found myself eyeing the clock anxiously, focusing on tackling treatment plan goals and getting the work done. I had forgotten the power of silence—how suppressed feelings can bubble up when given the space and how healing it can be for the client to weep or rage while the therapist simply allows the necessary emotions to flow without need to explain or make it better. A comfortable silence can provide what psychoanalyst D. W. Winnicott referred to as a "holding environment," in which the client feels safe and is given time to reflect (Applegate, 1997). This pause also allows me to better tap into my own healing wisdom and intuition. My wooden lizard reminds me to pause, to observe, to let the client's process unfold in that rare oasis of silence.

Faith That All Is Unfolding as It Should

One of the challenges many therapists face is compassion fatigue, also known as secondary stress reaction. Listening to heartbreaking stories of trauma all day can take a mental, physical, and spiritual toll. Although I was rigorous in my self-care routine, too often my heart was weary from trying to comprehend why some individuals carry such heavy loads. How do we remain buoyant when the scope of human suffering threatens to capsize us?

One of the greatest lessons I have learned through the mushroom is that the world is unfolding precisely as it should be. On my second trip, I simply asked the mushroom how to retain a healthy sense of compassion. The mushroom answered that the world is immeasurably more complicated than our brains can grasp. "Just stay in your corner and weave," I heard a voice say. There is an undeniable wisdom, intelligence, and cohesiveness in the web of existence, in which we all play a part. And in each moment, we have a choice—will we contribute to the healing of the world, or will we create suffering? This sentiment may sound like a Hallmark confection, but when experienced in the context of a psilocybin trip, it holds a noetic quality that surpasses any feel-good greeting card bromide.

There is peace in this for me. I don't have to beat my fists against the heavens, demanding *How?* and *Why?* Pema Chodron (2000) wrote that when she doubts she has what it takes to stay present with suffering, she takes heart from Buddhist master Trungpa Rinpoche's reminder that there is no cure for hot or cold. Things simply are. The mushroom has allowed me to accept that an innate wisdom is in charge. That allows me to better maintain equanimity, roll up my sleeves, and with as much grace and good humor as I can muster, get on with the work.

Healing My Own Wounds

It is essential that therapists tend to their own healing. The experience of having been in therapy allows us to empathize with our clients' struggles and to understand how challenging it can be to lay oneself bare to a stranger. Therapy helps us to heal childhood wounds, examine our blind spots, and learn how to accept feedback. I have been diligent over decades in tending to my garden, as it were, but the healing I have received through the mushroom has exceeded my wildest expectations.

With each successive psilocybin journey, I have learned to relax into the experience, no matter how painful, confusing, or downright weird. I've trusted that the mushroom has a higher wisdom, and all is unfolding as it should. I no longer feel I need to cure or overcome my challenges, but can embrace their teleological value. Psilocybin has allowed me to greet my wounds with acceptance and kindness, to travel the distance, and emerge transformed.

Conclusion

At the retreat's closing integration circle, I remarked to the others that, while I felt excited to return to my work at the mental health agency, I mourned that I would be unable to utilize psychedelic medicines with my clients. As luck would have it, a year later I was asked to return to the retreat as their lead therapist. In the 3 years at the retreat, I had the privilege of working with hundreds of guests having their own transformative psilocybin experiences. Witnessing over 1,500 psilocybin sessions, and leading as many group integration sessions, has been the greatest privilege, and responsibility, of my career. I am often humbled by the trust my clients place in me, and I am honored to create space for their pain and their triumphs. And I'm forever grateful to magic mushrooms which have allowed me to meet my clients with greater compassion, patience, and humanity than I ever imagined was possible.

References

Applegate, J. S. (1997). The holding environment: An organizing metaphor for social work theory and practice. *Smith College Studies in Social Work, 68*(1), 7–29. https://doi.org/10.1080/00377319709517514

Carbonaro, T. M., Bradstreet, M. P., Barrett, F. S., MacLean, K. A., Jesse, R., Johnson, M. W., & Griffiths, R. R. (2016). Survey study of challenging experiences after ingesting psilocybin mushrooms: Acute and enduring positive and negative consequences. *Journal of psychopharmacology, 30*(12), 1268-1278.

Chodron, P. (2000). *When things fall apart: Heart advice for difficult times.* Shambhala.

Cummings, E. E. (n.d.). i thank You God for most this amazing [poem].Retrieved from https://www.americanpoems.com/poets/eecummings/i-thank-you-god-for-most-this-amazing/

Grof, S. (1980). *LSD psychotherapy.* Alameda, CA: Hunter House.

Phelps, J. (2017). Developing guidelines and competencies for the training of psychedelic therapists. *Journal of Humanistic Psychology, 57*(5), 450-487. https://doi.org/10.1177/0022167817711304

Watts, A. (1989). *The book: On the taboo against knowing who you are.* New York, NY: Vintage Books.

> There are aspects to those two particular drugs [psilocybin and LSD] that the places you can go in your brain are much deeper and more healing than anything else.
>
> —Kristen Bell

Rachael O'Donnell

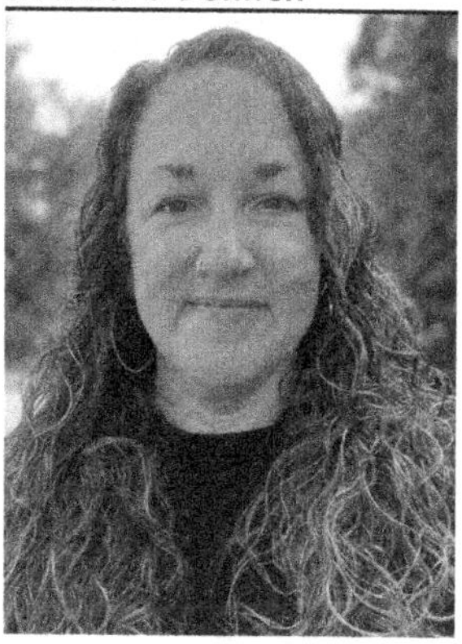

Rachael O'Donnell is an LCSW and licensed alcohol and drug counselor (LADC), with a certificate in psychedelic-assisted therapy from Naropa University. She has maintained a private practice in Maine for 13 years. She specializes in ketamine-assisted psychotherapy and formal consulting services for psychedelic therapists. Rachael's personal transformation with psychedelics has led to her truest work, educating others and bringing these life-saving treatments to those who need them.
rachael@therapyuntethered.com

Healing with Psychedelics:
A Therapist's Journey

My discovery of psychedelics as a tool for mental health treatment happened in 2021, when a friend and fellow healer asked me if I had heard of psychedelic therapy. I had experienced a significant loss during the pandemic, which triggered a depressive episode that I couldn't seem to find my way out of with traditional methods. I was struggling, and she thought this might be a tool for my healing. "No," I replied in shock. "They do therapy with psychedelics?" I was both surprised and frankly embarrassed that this was my field and I had no idea this was even happening.

She proceeded to tell me more about it, specifically ketamine-assisted therapy and suggested I look into it, so I did. Over the next few weeks, I took a deep dive into the psychedelics and mental health world, consuming all the information I could about the current landscape of treatment, and I was intrigued. After reading Michael Pollan's (2018) *How to Change Your Mind,* I decided that I was going to explore it for myself.

I was no stranger to psychedelics. Having been a teenager and young adult in the '90s when all-night music festivals called raves were all the rage, I had done my share of psychedelics recreationally. It had been more than 2 decades since those adventures though, and I had never used them in the context of healing. Because of these experiences I was familiar with their power and could see how they might serve as an incredible tool for healing. I decided to reach out to the local clinic doing ketamine-assisted therapy and began a long 6-month wait for treatment.

After completing a comprehensive history and assessment form online, the day arrived for my 2-hour intake with two providers. As a therapist, being in a room with two other therapists for treatment is a little overwhelming. I felt safe enough to be open and let my defenses down, but I think there is always a little fear of being entirely vulnerable as a patient when you are also a clinician. I did my best to keep those fears quiet, not let them run the show, and to be as vulnerable and authentic as I could.

There are two things I remember distinctly from that appointment. The first is when Matt, the doctor and facilitator who would work directly with me, said, "First off, Rachael, I just want to take a moment and acknowledge what an incredible amount of trauma you have survived and just take a moment to honor that." *What?* I thought. *Trauma?...OK.* I mean, I knew I had been through a number of challenges in my life, but trauma? That really isn't a label I have used in regards to my own life experiences. But something inside of me cracked open when he said that. For the first time, someone saw something deep inside of me that I hadn't been able to access, and at the same time, I had doubts that it was actually true.

The second thing I remember was during a conversation about why I sought out this treatment. I shared my grief around closing the business I had worked so hard to build for 3 years, because of the pandemic. As I became more and more emotional telling the story of that loss, the other clinician suggested I pause to take a couple of breaths and be in my body. Then he looked at me and said, "You know, it sounds like you worked so hard and were able to show yourself that you can do all this hard work to be successful and make sure you are OK. And then here comes this pandemic, and no matter how hard you worked, you just couldn't change the outcome, which was to lose everything you had worked for. That sounds a lot like other times in your life, where even though you worked really hard, you couldn't always control the things that came in and took those things away."

I stared at him and blinked. *Um, What?* I thought.... Did I just find out that my entire personality is a trauma response? Has everything I have ever done in my life just been driven by this desperation to prove that I can survive and take care of myself because I never felt safe? *No wonder I can't get over this loss,* I thought. Maybe I wasn't grieving this loss at all but had a whole lifetime of hurt get opened up by it and had no conscious idea of what I was really processing. How did a clinician who has never met me before just see such a deep truth about me? And how did I—a therapist—not know any of this about myself? I was stunned. The intense emotions I felt when he said that confirmed the truth behind it.

I left that appointment and just sat in my car for a while thinking, *my god this is going to be hard.* I mean the reality of the work I was being asked to do just hit me like a freight train. There are things I was not aware of that needed to come to the surface so I could heal, and it hadn't even occurred to me. Until this moment, I hadn't really connected with the work I was signing up for, but now it was clear, and I was ready.

At my second ketamine session, which was a high dose intra-muscular injection, the effects of the medicine came on quickly, and I was deeply immersed in another world. The most profound piece of this journey came well after the peak effects of the medicine. The music I was listening to was soft and ethereal with a harmonica gently playing and leading the tune. In the journey, I was looking at my old house, one my husband and I built together and lived in for 10 years. The sunlight was dappling the front porch and yard as it set, and a man sat on my porch swing playing the harmonica. I watched the tall grass in the side yard blow in the gentle breeze and just took the scene in. My heart swelled from the beauty of it all, and I began to cry. I then experienced what can only be described as a complete and total immersion into my husband's experience of deep loss around selling that house. I felt everything that he went through during that difficult time in our lives, that I couldn't see or make room for at the time because I was so immersed in my own experience. I took my blindfold off and sat up on the floor cushion so I could blow my nose, and I continued to cry. Matt, a doctor and trained psychedelic facilitator, sat on the floor next to me supported by a back jack. "My god," I said, "I thought I had done all of this work. I thought I had moved through this grief." "Yes," he said, "you probably did, and here are some deeper layers that need attention." He provided witness, support, and a safe space for me to do my own healing work. He wasn't analyzing, suggesting, directing, or teaching. He was simply holding space for me—for my inner healing intelligence to show up for the work I needed to do.

This was one of the most profound, emotionally intimate, and supportive experiences I had ever had. The way that Matt created such a safe space for the deep expression of grief and so fully trusted the process that was unfolding was astonishing. Even his physical proximity, just sitting next to me on the floor instead of across from me in a chair, made me feel like he was truly there with me, that I was not alone. *This is what therapy is supposed to be,* I thought. This is what actually helping people heal looks like.

I knew, in that moment, that I had been missing something so deeply profound in my work as a therapist. I had been missing the tools I needed to help people actually heal. I finally understood that the burnout and frustration that led to me stepping away from my practice in 2017 wasn't about not wanting to be a therapist but not wanting to be a therapist who couldn't seem to help people get as far in their healing as they needed to. Perhaps I had just been missing out on having the right tools to create deep and meaningful change for my patients.

After 18 months of my own healing work with ketamine, and eventually other plant medicines, I decided to pursue formal training to be able to do this work in my practice. I was accepted to the Naropa University Psychedelic-Assisted Therapy program and began my training. The feeling that I had throughout my education with them echoed my experience in the room during my second ketamine session: that so much of what I had been doing as a therapist was missing something. That this work—the work of supporting humans in healing with psychedelics and plant medicine—allows space for deeper human connection. It also invites the spiritual into the healing room and creates space to honor indigenous practices, wisdom, and knowledge alongside the traditional therapy process. That the real work of therapy is getting to and healing the root causes of anxiety and depression, not just improving a person's ability to manage the symptoms.

At one point in my healing work with ketamine, I saw the friend who introduced me to it, and I remember saying to her, "I had no idea how traumatized I am." Ketamine brought all of my past to the surface, showing me the places that needed acknowledgement and providing me the opportunity to do just that with an open heart and mind. If you imagine that your emotional health is like a large house with many rooms, some of whose doors are locked, psychedelics unlock the doors of those rooms. You still have to open them and walk in, but it makes it possible to do so with less fear and more courage. You learn how to heal yourself, and you build confidence in your ability to do so.

As a therapist, providing psychedelic-assisted therapy requires you to do less and trust the process that unfolds uniquely for each patient. It is a challenge to much of what we have learned about being a therapist and creates a rich opportunity for personal and professional growth. It allows us to help clients heal instead of just cope better and change the trajectory of their lives with the depth of awareness and healing that it provides. It asks us to get more comfortable with silence and to invite our clients to learn how to be their own healers so that they can continue to show up for themselves through their lives.

As a patient, psychedelic-assisted therapy asks you to do the hard work of healing. It asks you to move toward that which is painful and scary and move through it and challenges you to stop hiding, running, and numbing from discomfort and fear. It invites you into deep healing work and challenges you to show up for yourself and your life in a whole new way.

Psychedelic-assisted therapy seeks to use altered states of consciousness as a tool for exploring the subconscious with our defenses quieted. It takes the experiences and insights that a person has during a medicine journey and helps them translate those into real actionable changes in their life. It develops the skills needed to interrupt avoidance patterns and build confidence in one's ability to handle discomfort. This work is not for those who are seeking a quick and painless fix to their suffering. It is work that is designed for those who want to transform their suffering into meaningful change and growth.

Psychedelic-assisted therapy has made me believe in my profession again and has renewed the hopeful spirit that drew me into being a therapist in the first place. It has shown me that deep healing is indeed possible, and significant personal transformation can be the norm rather than the exception in the therapy world. It has also shown me that this can be accomplished in less time than traditional talk therapy, reducing how long a person has to suffer before finding relief.

On a personal level, psychedelics have given me the very best version of myself, freed me from the emotional response to triggers that have kept me trapped in unhealthy patterns for much of my adult life, and renewed my compassion for the world and my connection to and reverence for nature. They have helped me break bad habits and create and stick with new ones. They have changed the way I show up for my life and interrupted my desires to escape from it so frequently.

Most importantly, my personal work with psychedelics has transformed me as a therapist. I show up for my patients with more presence, deeper compassion, renewed hope and excitement about this work, and personal experiences of healing with psychedelics that allow me to meet them deeply in the work and be present for the challenges and gifts it brings.

I am forever indebted to the friend who started me on this path and for all of the healers that have supported me in my personal journey, as well as to all the patients that so deeply trust me to guide them in this work. I believe that psychedelics will transform the way that we conceptualize and treat mental health in the coming decade, and I am grateful to be a part of that.

References

Pollan, M. (2018). *How to change your mind.* New York: Penguin Publishing Group.

Mary Gresham

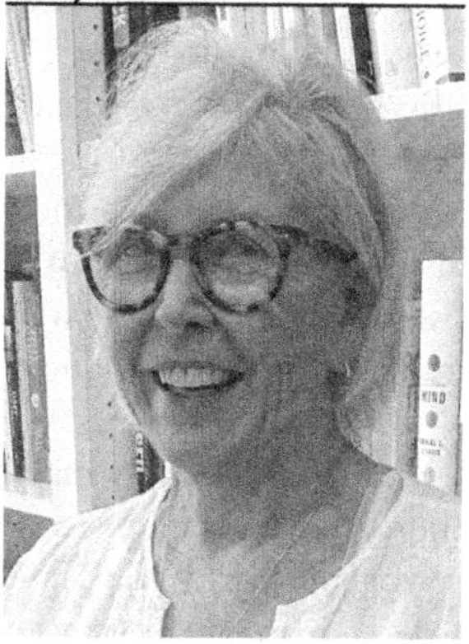

MARY GRESHAM, PHD, loved her studies at Tulane, Emory, and Georgia State in clinical psychology and set a record for years spent in school. She has practiced clinical psychology in Atlanta for 40 years and is still learning how to be a therapist. In 2019, she was drawn to the certificate program in psychedelic therapy at the California Institute of Integral Studies and currently works in research trials studying psilocybin at Emory University. Her recent interests include ketamine-assisted psychotherapy and internal family systems. She typically stands out as the oldest person in the workshop.
docgresh1@gmail.com

My Year of Living as a Seeker

IN 2018, AT THE AGE OF 70, I ASKED MY HUSBAND OF 17 YEARS FOR A SEPARATION. This was a courageous act on my part since I was afraid of living alone as an older woman. I found a therapist to help me navigate my fears but also had been googling terms like "existential anxiety," "older women alone," and "gray divorce" for many months. In one of my searches, up came the phrase "psychedelic therapy" as a treatment for existential anxiety associated with cancer. As I followed that thread, I discovered a training program in California that could teach me how to become a psychedelic therapist. I felt hopeful and excited for the first time in many months and waited for the application process to begin. The practicalities of commuting to San Francisco, paying the tuition, and studying seemed unimportant compared to the benefits of the new energy I felt.

I began the program at the California Institute of Integral Studies (CIIS) in 2019 and now feel very lucky that I was in the last group to meet in person, to have a smaller cohort of 80, and to accept students from Georgia. The challenges of balancing my private practice with my school schedule, where to stay, and how to navigate San Francisco were both anxiety inducing and exciting. My hope was to find some kind of spiritual connection that would ameliorate my loneliness and fears. During my program, I read about the mystical experience and the bliss of oneness with the universe and heard about it personally from luminaries in the field, big names like Bill Richards and Tony Bossis (Richards, 2015). I was also hoping to find access to a skilled psychotherapist who could lead me on a psilocybin journey. I began to realize that as one of the oldest students in the group, from

Georgia and not in a big psychedelic center like DC, San Francisco, or Santa Cruz, this would be harder than I thought. I made friends with the other older women, and we discussed how to make this happen. In general, I heard that when it is right to happen, it will just appear. One of my friends grew her own mushrooms and took them alone. Another found a connection via her daughter. Another woman had been part of an ayahuasca circle in another state. The thought of traveling there and doing that seemed way ahead of my psychonautic skill set. I settled into just working through the program and asking here and there, but nothing really came my way.

Our training week with the Multidisciplinary Association for Psychedelic Studies (MAPS) was deeply inspiring, with meaningful and touching videos of veterans receiving MDMA therapy for PTSD. I thought often of my parents, undiagnosed PTSD survivors of World War II, who became alcoholics as their way of dealing with war trauma. My training group stayed in a wonderful state park in Marin County, with fresh air, beautiful scenery, group meals, and great conversations. I had thought that we might get to experience MDMA therapy ourselves, but that has not yet been part of the MAPS protocol.

Realizing that I had to take matters more into my own hands, I was finally able to secure some MDMA from a much younger friend. Being cautious, I sent it off to a lab for testing to see if it was pure. I was fortunate to find a therapist who was willing to help me with a guided experience if I could supply my own. I had a very good first experience with this medicine and was able to see myself in a new light and to see both the beautiful and limiting parts of my recent marriage. Reclaiming my lost identities and declaring what I wanted in life were especially prescient for me. Years later I re-read the notes from this session and realized that what I said I wanted had come true, without my ever recalling having declared it.

I took a river rafting trip down the Grand Canyon during this time, wondering if the natural world would be the key to my search for a deeper spiritual life. I realized on this trip that my spiritual self actually resides in my relationships with other people, not in the natural world or feeling united with everything. I had an experience of finding a kindred spirit in my river raft, and we had a wonderful connection around our mutual appreciation of folk artist Henry Darger and folk art in general. We both walked away saying, "Who would have thought that I would find another like this in the middle of a river raft?" and that was the beginning of my understanding of where spirituality lives for me.

To teach us budding psychedelic therapists more about guiding in non-ordinary states of consciousness, CIIS set up a weekend of holotropic breathwork, a legal method to shift consciousness. Gifted facilitators from the holotropic community led us, and I learned about the perinatal matrices and the psychedelic work of Stanislav Grof. I again set an intention to experience unitive consciousness...or whatever needs to emerge. I was learning by this point that holding intentions lightly and being open to whatever comes up organically helps me more than wishing for a certain kind of experience. This awareness continues to be useful in my life.

Although our program did not teach us about ketamine, I did hear a lot about it from other students who lived in the Bay Area. One of my colleagues arranged a training with ketamine-assisted experiences for those of us commuting from out of town. I knew little about ketamine-assisted psychotherapy (KAP) and studied the book *The Ketamine*

Papers (Wolfson & Hartelius, 2016) to prepare for it. About ten of us signed up and I finally had the group psychedelic experience that I had hoped for. I did feel a closer connection to my fellow students after we went through our 2-day training course. We experienced the use of low dose psycholytic lozenges, taking turns sitting for each other, and a high dose psychedelic intramuscular injection (IM) experience. Since ketamine is a Schedule 3 drug, it was legal and done in the open. My IM experience was an amazing experience of feeling shot into space and then an intense reliving of conceiving my son, going through my pregnancy, and delivering him into the world, ultimately letting him go to live his own life and take care of himself. I still work with the body sensations and meanings of this vivid experience.

As I came to the end of my year of training, my research project was to collect the psychedelic experiences of others over the age of 65. Strangers I found through mutual connections were kind enough to share with me their experiences in their journeys as elders. There was a mix of experiences from "nothing much happened" to "it was profound." There is little research on the use of these medicines for elders, and perhaps that reflects the state of ageism in our world. Many studies have age cutoffs of 55, and those without cutoffs do not break down the results by age group (Dore et al., 2019; Ross et al., 2016). Most elders who wish to experience psychedelics will need to find underground therapists who are willing to take them as clients. Since we elders are closer to the end of life and the major consciousness shift known as death, it seems only natural that we would want to practice with this and gain as much insight as possible.

After my program ended, it took me five journeys and several consultations with experts to realize what needed to happen to create a good psilocybin experience for myself. These did not come just because I was ready. I had to seek them out just as I had to seek out my MDMA and ketamine experiences. The first four journeys were at the hands of people who did not understand my aging body's needs. I had to figure it out and arrange my own protocol. On my 5th attempt, I did have a very meaningful journey where I could feel the evaporation of myself into a vast empty universe, broken into bits of light, joining with other bits of light. It was not blissful, but it felt truthful. Since then, I haven't been afraid of dying...but I continue to fear poor health care in the hands of those who do not understand what is needed.

In December of 2019, my divorce was finalized. I applied and was hired to work in a research trial for psilocybin because I had the certificate from CIIS and was willing to work for the pay that was offered. I benefit from learning about the unpredictability of these experiences in our trials. We are in the infancy of building a knowledge base that can be accessed by the public and hopefully used to their benefit to consider safety as well as other factors in psychedelic therapy. It is meaningful to me to work towards the rescheduling of these substances that do not belong as Schedule 1 drugs. I believe that as Mary Cosimano (2021) says:

> We should learn to live each day with the same attitude as that during a psychedelic experience: that all that happens is welcome, even what is disturbing...ask why certain things are arising and what can be learned from them...you don't have to like it but allow and accept it...when we try to resist what is happening, we get into trouble. (p. 391)

I have been especially grateful for this particular year of so many discoveries and the psychedelic community that I have been building since then. I continue to be fascinated by the topic and wonder what will happen for our patients and ourselves when psychedelic medicines are finally rescheduled, hoping it will be in my lifetime.

References

Cosimano, M. (2021). The role of the guide in psychedelic-assisted therapy. In C. Grob & J. Grigsby (Eds.) *Handbook of medical hallucinogens* (pp.377-394). Guildford Press.

Dore, J., Turnipseed, B., Dwyer, S., Turnipseed, A., Andries, J., Ascani, G., Monnette, C., Huidekoper, A., Strauss, N., & Wolfson, P. (2019). Ketamine Assisted Psychotherapy (KAP): Patient demographics, clinical data and outcomes in three large practices administering ketamine with psychotherapy. *Journal of Psychoactive Drugs, 51*(2), 189–198.

Richards, W. A. (2015). *Sacred knowledge: Psychedelics and religious experiences.* Columbia University Press.

Ross, S., Bossis, A., Guss, J., Agin-Liebes, G., Malone, T., Cohen, B., Mennenga, S. E., Belser, A., Kalliontzi, K., Babb, J., Su, Z., Corby, P., & Schmidt, B. L. (2016). Rapid and sustained symptom reduction following psilocybin treatment for anxiety and depression in patients with life-threatening cancer: A randomized controlled trial. *Journal of psychopharmacology (Oxford, England), 30*(12), 1165–1180. https://doi.org/10.1177/0269881116675512

Wolfson, P., & Hartelius, G. (Eds.). (2016). *The ketamine papers.* Santa Cruz, CA: MAPS.

The purpose of therapy is not to remove suffering but to move through it to an enlarged consciousness that can sustain the polarity of painful opposites.

—James Hollis

Elizabeth Hoke

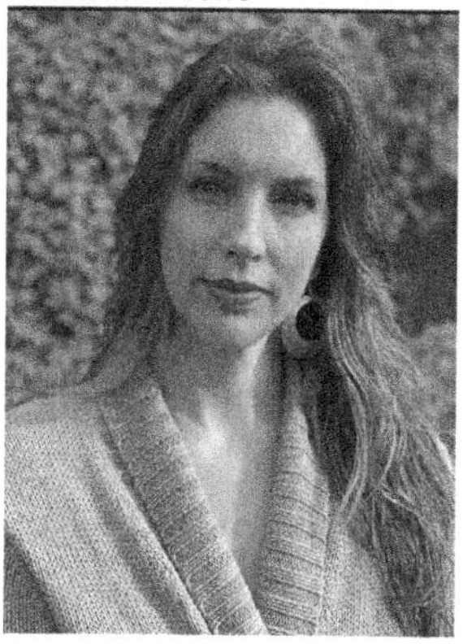

ELIZABETH HOKE is a licensed marriage and family therapist in California and Oregon. She is the clinical director of Liberation Institute, a community mental health clinic that provides therapy for all on a sliding scale. Elizabeth works at Rainfall Medicine, helping individuals explore their unconscious with the support of a medicine called ketamine. Elizabeth lectures on psychedelic- assisted therapy at Lewis and Clark College and facilitates recovery groups for Portland Psychedelic Society.
elizabeth@liberationinstitute.org

Right Relationship, Psychedelics, and Addiction Recovery

IT WAS 7:45 A.M. ON A TUESDAY MORNING, AND I WAS GETTING READY FOR MY 8:00 A.M. KETAMINE-ASSISTED PSYCHOTHERAPY CLIENT. I was watering my plants in the office when Dr. Rosonke walked in. I greeted him with my typical large smile, and he said, "Are you happy all the time?" I told him that I used to live in hell and that every day I'm not living there feels like a gift. I am one of the lucky ones who managed to not die from her addiction, and plant medicines, fungi, psychedelics, and therapy are big reasons why I'm still alive today.

As far back as my memory goes, I always felt out of place and deeply insecure. I didn't sleep at night and spent most of my days tracking everyone's reactions to me so I could figure out how to feel more loved and connected to them. I'm not sure which came first—my lonely feelings of being constantly misunderstood and invisible to my parents, who were too busy either working or fulfilling their obligations with their new families after the divorce, or not trusting that my needs were valuable and that I deserved love even when I wasn't doing anything to earn it. Either way, it was around the same time in early childhood that I also learned that if I was a good girl I would get more attention. So, I tried desperately to be helpful and make everyone around me happy. This worked half of the time, but with undiagnosed ADHD, school was incredibly challenging, and I constantly felt inadequate and unworthy. Because I deeply believed that I had no value unless I was doing something for others, I quickly became overly stressed and chronically uncomfortable in my body.

When I was 12, I spent a lot of time at a friend's house whose single mom was never home. We spent most of our time there, after walking home from junior high school, eating macaroni and cheese, drinking Kool-Aid, and watching Jerry Springer. One day, we decided to drink a beer from the fridge, and the relief it brought me was so instant that my life was changed forever.

My need for numbing quickly progressed to using any drug I could get my hands on by age 15. At 17, I was kicked out of my mom's house for throwing a party that resulted in a childhood friend robbing us while I was passed out. By 20, I was a full-blown alcoholic. I didn't drink every day or alone, but when I did drink, which was three or four times a week, I would black out. I desperately longed for connection and love but felt further and further away from it. Fast forward to 24, I was bartending in San Francisco, and my blackouts were getting worse. I was drinking and using drugs most days and started to wake up in places I didn't know. I would wake up and promise to not do it again, then by 5:00 p.m. be drinking again, and the cycle repeated. I felt so out of control. I was ashamed of my behavior and terrified that I was going to die. My desperation to feel loved and valued paralleled my intense need to take care of everyone around me. The extreme people-pleasing wouldn't allow me to ask for help, and no one in my family knew the truth about my struggle. I was deeply depressed and had suicidal ideation. I also truly believed that I would be alone forever because if anyone knew the truth of who I really was and all the shameful mistakes I'd made, then they'd see that I was too disgusting of a human to ever deserve love.

I was lucky enough to have a friend who took me to a taqueria after work one night to confront me about my destructive behavior. He cried while he ate his tacos and told me that I was killing myself and that he wasn't going to pretend otherwise any longer. He said he loved me and that I deserved better than the current life I was living. I didn't change anything about my behavior that night, but I couldn't get his words out of my head. I wanted to quit drinking, but 12-step programs didn't work for me because I didn't believe in a higher power and couldn't surrender to it or believe that it would help me get past my addiction.

As a child, I was raised Jewish, but only by way of celebrating at Grandma's. There was no connection to traditions, rituals, or ceremonies, only Grandma's matzo ball soup on holidays. My father was Christian and married a woman who was Catholic, which meant that I had to start going to church when I visited them. When they got up for Holy Communion, I was told to stay in the pew because I was Jewish. I felt so much shame sitting there as the rows of people got up and walked to the front of the room, staring at me as they walked by. This experience solidified two beliefs: that religion was a crock and that if it wasn't a crock, I was someone that didn't deserve to be a part of it.

Many years after that night at the taqueria, a different friend offered me some mushroom tea in a country where it was legal. We drank the tea and ended up in the middle of a park around 11:30 p.m., alone with the tall trees and quiet rain. I lay on the wet grass and for the first time in my life felt what it was like to live inside my own body, and had so much gratitude for it. I felt, for the first time in my life, unconditional love for myself. It was also the first night in a long time that I was not blacked out and was not swimming in thoughts of being a disgusting worthless person. I saw myself as part of the earth, realizing that I and the rock in space I was living on were connected and I wasn't separate from it. New thoughts were being formed in my head, saying I was valuable and deserving of love despite the mistakes I had made. I vowed that I would stop trying to destroy myself and would do everything I could to help others get out of the hell they felt stuck in from their addiction.

It didn't happen right away, but over the next few years, I was able to get sober thanks to therapy and my new found belief that I had value and deserved a different life. I went back to school to earn a master's in counseling psychology and found my dream job in 2011, at a community mental health clinic called The Liberation Institute. While my first 8 years of sobriety were focused on abstinence, I was able to find my way back to psychedelics, which helped me deepen my spiritual practice and recovery and became the focus of my career.

I am now working as a ketamine-assisted psychotherapist, specializing in addiction recovery. I also teach psychedelic-focused continuing education workshops and volunteer with psychedelic communities, running recovery groups for people who use psychedelics to aid their recovery. I have sat with hundreds of clients for ketamine-assisted psychotherapy and psychedelic integration, many of them coming to deal with issues of addiction. Some come in speaking directly about their struggle with alcohol, drugs, nicotine, sex, shopping, gambling, etc., while others come in suffering from problematic thinking and challenging behaviors that cause them to over use substances and other dissociative practices. While everyone has a different life story and reaction to addictive substances and pathological behavior, I do see a few common threads between their stories and mine.

The first common thread is the feeling of disconnection and loneliness. It seems that the individual-focused capitalist structure we live in has caused people to forget what it means and feels like to be in *right relationship* with each other and with plants, animals, and our environment. I learned about this term of interdependence in the Multidisciplinary Association for Psychedelic Studies (MAPS) MDMA therapy training program. Kylea Talor (2017) discusses the importance of being in right relationship with ourselves in order to be in right relationship with clients in her book *The Ethics of Caring.* This concept is common in the Buddhist tradition, where Thich Nhat Hanh (2017) describes it as interbeing, and has also been shared through stories by Indigenous communities around the world.

So how do we get in right relationship? I had a client who wanted to quit smoking, but nothing seemed to work. She tried the gum, patches, 12-step programs, and even psychotherapy. One day, she met with an Indigenous healer who encouraged her to buy a nicotiana tabacum plant, which is used to produce smoking tobacco. She found one, planted it in her garden in the spring, and was instructed to love it and nurture it and heal the relationship she had to it so that it was no longer abstract and abusive. Instead of quitting through demonizing the tobacco and telling herself she was powerless over her addiction, she changed her relationship to it.

She and I spent months talking about her original relationship to smoking. We unpacked the story of how she started as a teen, and she shared how smoking tobacco helped her feel calm and less activated when in painful and challenging situations. She started a journaling practice around her relationship to the plant, noting whether she was using and abusing it or enjoying and honoring it. The more time she spent in loving forgiveness of herself and seeing the tobacco as an ally not an enemy, the more she cherished it and didn't want to have an abusive relationship with it any longer. She decided to do six ketamine sessions with me to help with the withdrawals, which were very challenging since she'd started smoking so young. While her desire to smoke was never completely relieved, she slowly quit by continuing her compassionate self-care inquiry and plant tending. She changed her relationship to her cravings, being with them patiently instead of rushing to appease them. This allowed her to gain control over her addiction, and a year later, she's still abstaining from smoking.

The second common thread is people feeling utter hopelessness and a deep distrust in their ability to heal themselves. Most people with addiction issues show up so disconnected from their body that they can't remember the last time they slowed down enough to feel their heartbeat in their chest or witness their breath move in and out of their lungs. Before doing any type of ketamine-assisted psychotherapy or psychedelic integration, I always start by reconnecting the person to their body.

Breathing exercises and guided meditations help clients gain awareness and internal grounding to support them through the psychedelic experience. Somatic exercises and psycho-education also help clients gain awareness of their body armoring and defensive character structure. The body storming in addicts typically shows up as pressure to be in an upright posture while the chest caves in to protect the heart and the neck and shoulders constantly feel sore from being held in a tense up right position. When helping clients feel into this, they start to relax the muscles instead and find themselves opening up more. When the body armoring is deactivated, the defensive character structure shifts to more vulnerable and open. The more a person utilizes their body to feel safe, the less they need to numb or disassociate. The more connected they feel to their body, the more they can use it as a tool for healing. Trust and deep connection with self bring remedies for loneliness, helping clients feel less urgency to numb and disassociate.

Our external living environment and institutions don't always support everyone's inner light and being. The individual-focused consumerism-driven society we've created doesn't feel safe for people who are deeply sensitive, and when they seek professional help, they are often given labels and medication to help them change. This leads to feeling misunderstood and hopeless and creates a deep desire to constantly dissociate or numb these feelings.

From my experience as a ketamine-assisted therapist, I have witnessed and been told by clients that their addiction recovery feels different when the focus is on right relationship and the body. Using ketamine in conjunction with somatic techniques, talk therapy, and a relational framework with a biocentric focus can help people change the story they believe about themselves. Helping clients foster *right relationship* and develop a deep trust in their inner healing intelligence can strengthen their ability to heal from their addictions. Humans are like the flowers found growing through the cracks in the sidewalk. The environment is not conducive for thriving, but with the right amount of support, they can learn to grow and blossom and find strength in their wildness to break through concrete confines. To borrow words and inspiration from Robin Wall Kimmerer:

> Action on behalf of life transforms. Because the relationship between self and the world is reciprocal, it is not a question of first getting enlightened or saved and then acting. As we work to heal the earth, the earth heals us. (Kimmerer, 2015, p. 328)

References

Hanh, T. N. (2017). *The art of living.* San Francisco: HarperOne.

Kimmerer, R. W. (2015). *Braiding sweetgrass.* Minneapolis, MN: Milkweed Editions.

Taylor, K. (2017). *The ethics of caring: Finding right relationship with clients.* Santa Cruz, CA: Hanford Mead Publishers.

Valeria McCarroll

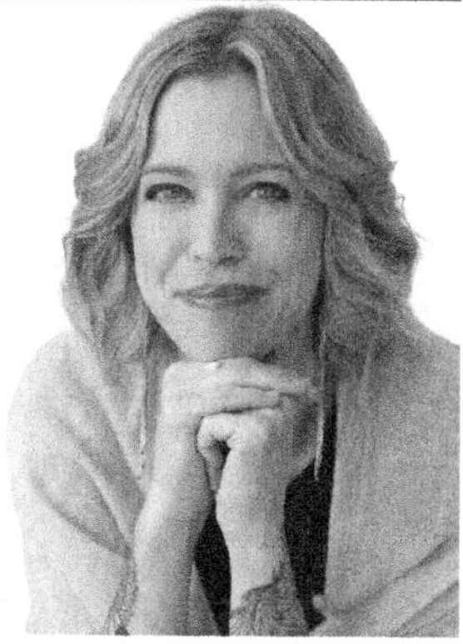

VALERIA MCCARROLL, PHD, LMFT, is a psychedelic educator, writer, and speaker. Formally trained as a guide in expanded states of consciousness, she teaches critical courses on psychedelic humanities to students at the California Institute of Integral Studies. Having been in the field of psychedelic work over a decade, her interests lie at the intersection of nondual wisdom traditions, somatics, psychedelics, and social and transformative justice.
www.valeriamccarroll.com
valeria.mccarroll@gmail.com

Towards the Practice of Soul Midwifery

MANY OF US HOPE, THE FIRST TIME WE USE PSYCHEDELICS WITH INTENTION, that we will have a complete spiritual awakening, achieve enlightenment, and resolve all our trauma. We long for the possibility that psychedelics are the answer. The truth of psychedelic work, however, is rarely so straightforward. Instead, it is more like a series of progressive illuminations, a peeling back of layers of patriarchal wounding, one by one.

If the landscape of psychedelic experience is a mountain range, then my first two ceremonial encounters were molehills. Both were working with *ayahuasca*, a potent psychedelic beverage that tastes something like rotting earth, day-old coffee, and rancid chocolate. Even now, the memory of the flavors causes a slight internal shudder. Aside from the crippling nausea that gripped me from beginning to end, and the one-millisecond vision of a sky filled with stars, both experiences were for the most part uneventful on the visionary front and brutally uncomfortable on the physical. At this point, any logical person would probably throw in the towel and call it a day. But I am a stubborn human being, and my desire to understand why the other people in the room kept showing up for this torture overrode all other feedback. I am a sucker for the promise of a peak experience.

To a certain degree, I was also desperate. I was in the middle of a graduate degree learning how to become a psychotherapist. I felt frustrated by the limitations of traditional talk therapy. While I had been in my own personal therapy for several years by that point, I felt stuck in symptoms of unresolved trauma: depression, anxiety, and disordered eating. I knew what needed to change in my life; I just couldn't seem to actually change it.

The healing potential of psychedelics is poised to revolutionize the way we think, talk, and orient toward health. MDMA-assisted psychotherapy for PTSD (Mitchell et al., 2021), social anxiety (Danforth et al., 2018), and eating disorders (Brewerton et al., 2021). Psilocybin mushrooms for depression (Carhart-Harris, 2021) and end-of-life anxiety (Yu et al., 2021). Ayahuasca for addiction (Thomas et al., 2013). Ketamine for depression (Krystal et al., 2019). After years of embargo on research, the resurgence of psychedelic-assisted therapy is startling. With plenty of interest: Of those Americans who have mental health conditions, 65% said that they would like access to psychedelics (Bartlett, 2022).

Finally, in my third ceremony, desperate and hopeful, something happened: I vomited rainbows. It was utterly glorious. This is an odd thing to say, coming from someone who dislikes losing control and particularly loathes vomiting. But as the hot, thick liquid surged up the back of my throat and into the bucket in front of me, I felt only a profound sense of relief. Visions of rainbow light collided, kaleidoscopically refracting off each other. I was struck by the deep knowing of the holiness of my offering into the bucket. Widespread gratitude and well-being flooded my system. At that moment I was at a loss for articulating exactly what had transpired, but I was clear that something had shifted for the better.

Of the panoply of psychedelic medicines, ayahuasca is well-known for both its visionary and purgative effects. That is, it makes you puke and see things (Domínguez-Clavé et al., 2016). From the perspective of the Indigenous Amazonian peoples who have cultivated and used ayahuasca for thousands of years (Labate & Goldstein, 2009), what I had just experienced was a healing: the *purga* (Mabit, 2007), as the purgative effects of ayahuasca are called, is a form of catharsis, an expulsion and clearing of negative energies from the body (Fotiou & Gearin, 2019). This kind of excavation creates space for the restoration of wellness in a system. I was inclined to agree. Beyond being physically emptied out, I felt expansive, open, and free.

The term *expanded state of consciousness* is often used to describe the vastness of the territory you might encounter during a psychedelic experience. There are other terms: *altered state* or *non-ordinary state*. An expanded state is when your perception of the world (including how you experience yourself and your internal landscape) seems distinctly different from your usual, everyday consciousness. Expanded states are marked by their departure from normative reality. What happened to me was not ordinary. I don't normally see kaleidoscopes of rainbows in my vomit. My perception of consciousness was radically altered. The morning following, an internal quiescence pervaded my being. My somatic experience felt notably softer, less pervaded by the thrum of a low-level anxiety, more grounded in an easeful flow.

Over time and across integration, I have come to understand that psychedelics catalyzed a profound personal belief in somatics. Concepts that were entirely theoretical before my ceremonial encounters were suddenly grounded in the reality of lived experience; my theories of healing were brought into an embodied consciousness. Fast forward the better part of a decade and a half, and I find myself formally trained as a psychedelic guide, teaching critical courses on psychedelic humanities, and forever picking apart the Rubik's cube that lies at the intersection of psychedelics, nondual wisdom traditions, somatics, and social justice.

During that time, here is some of what I have learned about the possibilities of these medicines: Psychedelics can potentiate deep and powerful healing when used with intentionality. Conversely, they can engender great trauma and suffering when weaponized or used to recapitulate systems of oppression. Psychedelics are illuminators of consciousness. They reveal what lies beyond our normative constrictions and limitations. They can support us in releasing the contractions of our small-mindedness and perceiving the fullness of the world as it really is, in its awesome and awful glory. Psychedelics can help us not only to identify where we are wounded, but also to develop the resiliency to be with the parts of ourselves we would normally reject or deny. In this capacity, they are great agents of the healing of trauma and initiators of cycles of rebirth. Psychedelics can develop our interoception, our capacity to perceive our inner experience, giving us a greater sensibility and somatic engagement as we move through the world—the lived experience of our fundamental interdependence with all of life. Expanders of perception and potentiators of awareness, they can awaken us to our own sovereignty, inviting us onto a path of liberation. We can work with psychedelics to cultivate better versions of ourselves as more loving, kind, and compassionate beings. In their integration, psychedelics can create space for us to walk as instruments of peace, as love embodied.

Thanks to the "Michael Pollan effect" (Brooker, 2022), we in the West have anchored into the idea that psychedelics manifest the contents of one's mind. After all, the word *psychedelic* means mind-manifesting, from the Greek *psyche* (meaning mind or soul) and *-delic* (to manifest). But here we've leapt across the Cartesian divide into the bias of materialistic reductionism that pervades so much of the Western world. The belief that psychedelics center the mind reflects an ontological assumption of fundamental separation between mind and body, spirit and matter, man and nature. This assumption underlies and pervades our systems of medicine, governance, justice, and education. It's engrained in the classification and treatment of psychological symptoms as mental disorders without a somatic ground. It underscores the individualistic lean in the practice of psychotherapy today that encourages a therapist to remain opaque to their clients (Freud, 1912/1964), pathologizes trauma as a problem to be solved, and places the burden of healing on the individual rather than situating that person's suffering within the cultural context of a wildly imbalanced world on the verge of global collapse.

You could say that psychedelics radicalized me, both personally and professionally. To be radicalized is to be rooted into the earth, the soma of the body, and into what Indigenous scholar Tyson Yunkaporta calls "the law in the land" (MacKenzie, 2020). Our white-bodied, heteronormative, ableist, capitalist, supremacist, kyriarchal conditioning lies at the root of suffering. Unearthing and transmuting it as it lives in embodied experience and plays out in our systems is my life's work. As such, I understand psychotherapeutic work to be political in nature, and the healing work of dismantling internalized oppression that can occur in psychedelic therapy as an act of social justice. Psychedelic experience has seeded in me an embodied belief in the fundamentally interdependent, co-arising nature of the cosmos. Universal intercorporeality, so to speak.

While I consider myself a cautious optimist about the potential of psychedelics to engender global change, I am also a realist. The shadows of the field of psychedelics are the same aspects of the collective unconscious that play out in Western culture today: exploitation, oppression, and violence. Psychedelics are not a magic pill, nor are they a panacea. Affected intimately by the impact of both set and setting (Noorani, 2021), the potency of psychedelics can be likened to the razor-edged sharpness of a surgeon's blade. It is the same capacity that allows a tool to cut out a cancer and save a life that might slice an artery and take one. The difference lies in the intentionality with which the blade is wielded. Reports over the past several years of sexual misconduct and abuse in psychedelic spaces highlight the need for specific training for psychedelic guides around consent and power dynamics, as well as the installation of rupture and repair processes.

The history of psychedelics is also the history of colonization, exploitation, and oppression of Indigenous stewards of these medicines across time. As psychedelics move from being the primary prerogative of Indigenous and underground practitioners into a medicalized model, they become increasingly vulnerable to the influence of those in power and those looking to capitalize on their potency. As such, the commercialization of psychedelics and what has been termed the "commodification of the sacred" (Posey, 2002, p. 3) is a growing concern alongside issues of cultural appropriation, equity, and reciprocity. I live inside the question of what it means to be in right relationship: with the populations that have stewarded these medicines historically, with the medicines themselves, and with my own privilege and power. This is to say nothing of the issues of accessibility: How are psychedelics to be made available to the populations who might most benefit from them when legal access can have a baseline of several thousand dollars for an experience? What of potentiating mystical experience within a medicalized model that denies the existence of spirit and reduces what would have been historically considered a rite of passage to a medical treatment?

I hold the role of psychedelic guide with reverence for the responsibility it entails, while in the same breath I am perpetually working to deconstruct the lineages of power-over/power-under that are projected onto that epithet. Beyond patriarchy lies possibility, and at the intersection of psychedelics and psychotherapy I see an emergent practice of *soul midwifery*. Consider that the word psyche refers not only to the machinations of the mind but also the concerns of the soul. That is to say: What if psychedelic psychotherapy was not only about the manifestations of one's mind but also might include the birthing of a soul's purpose?

Soul often feels to me to be a bit of a word that we prefer to brush to the side, relegating it to the wheelhouse of religion. To consider the idea that psychedelics might reveal a soul's calling begs the question: What is the nature of soul? The indwelling of spirit in the material? The connection point between the individual and the collective? Geologian Thomas Berry writes that soul is "fundamentally a biological concept, defined as the primary organizing, sustaining, and guiding principle of a living being" (Berry, 2003, p. xiii). Soul is biologically rooted, anchored into a bodied reality. Within this framework emerges my own working definition of *soul*: the living gnosis of self-as-cosmos. Soul is an animated, ever-changing, evolving phenomenon, the personalized expression of the invisible matrix of energy which connects everything and is connected to everything. One's soul is a seed of possibility, the prayerful chorus of one's ancestors, vibrating in a double helix of DNA.

Here, a layer of patriarchal conditioning sloughs off: For those of us raised within a Judeo-Christian culture, the idea that we have a soul evokes images of the afterlife, narratives of good battling evil, and beliefs in immortality and wholeness. We are immediately cast into a stark reality of good battling evil and of the one true God who, for many of us, was probably a bearded old White dude in the sky who promised salvation from the untrustworthy, sinful, and wicked world we lived in, as well as from the terrible actuality of our carnal nature. The castration of the erotic. Save us from ourselves, so long as we do everything we can to be good. How problematic this mindset is and what insidious suffering it causes when the work of ensoulment seems to lie in the acceptance of one's wholeness as a complicated, shadowy human being who makes mistakes and has unconscious aspects to one's nature and violent capacities within one's personality.

We live in a world experiencing a dearth of soul. The soullessness of the world contributes to lives that lack deeper meaning, instability in human relationships, and a fundamental disconnection from nature that perpetuates suffering (Berry, 2003). Yet paradoxically, our own soul's calling has the potential to change the world. In the 1990's, psychologist James Hillman developed what he called "acorn theory": the idea that every person comes into the world with a seed of destiny, a calling unique to their soul (Hillman, 1997). This theory, obviously, is much older than Hillman. It has roots in the Greek concept of the daimon, touches Buddhist beliefs around reincarnation, and the Roman concept of one's genius. According to mythologist Michael Meade, "the original idea of genius refers to the inborn spirit and natural gifts of each person. In that sense, everyone has a genius nature and something essential to give to the world" (Meade, n.d.). If the threads of genius are what connects a person to their soul, expressing their genius into the world results in a more ensouled world.

As I have withdrawn my projections of the all-knowing guru from the role of the psychedelic guide, I understand instead that the midwife of soul is a maieutic calling. Donning one's Socratic robes, the work with a client is a nurturing and bringing forth their innate gifts, accompanying them on the twists and turns of the journey of remembrance as they uncover the hidden knowledge of self that lies within. Disentangling an understanding of power from a hierarchy that demands over versus under, it is my very strong sense that a guide walks alongside a client, rather than leading them along a predetermined path of awakening. Nor does a guide carry an agenda for what a client's healing might look like, beyond their intention to be of service to that person's integrated liberation. The work of the guide lies in holding space for the birth pangs of a person's process as the luminous seed of their soul's calling rends the veils of illusion and the radiant truth of who they are at the center of their being shines forth.

As a midwife of soul my work lies in how skillfully I can bring the light of my awareness into a field such that another person might recognize the threads of their own genius and trace them back to touch their soul's purpose. In this way, I know myself as a potentiator or catalyst, a facilitator of space. As a practice it demands that I develop my own capacity to titrate and weave between and across the sacred and the profane. My training as a psychotherapist has been invaluable in the development of cognitive maps of healing, my capacity to be with a client, and the cultivation of a witnessing presence.

Often, following the soul's calling asks a person to step off the beaten path of culture and onto the road less traveled. To be a midwife of soul asks one to develop a certain level of comfort sitting in the darkness of the unknown, as well as resiliency when exploring shadowy territory in the psyche. This is of course a practice that is lived rather than a lifeless ethical tenet inscribed in a moral code. This capacity stems from a deep knowing that every moment is fresh, new, filled with the possibility for birth and rebirth, that the present moment is the only moment that truly exists. The more deeply one rests in the groundlessness of this truth, the more one can access the innate potential that unfurls within it. A contemporary practice of soul midwifery is a discipline of uncovering, dismantling, and reconsidering the ways in which patriarchal patterning serves a dismembering purpose. To do so means leaning into the practice of the practice: a living container that is deliberately and intentionally shaped in an on-going way, and then refined to reflect how well it operationalizes the core values centered within it.

In this way, the guide's work is the cohesive and creative expression of their being and becoming, as well as it is creating intentional spaces for regenerative transformation. The art of guiding takes seriously the impact of set and setting on psychedelic experience. As such, a guide understands that the relational and psychic containers created around a psychedelic journey are part of the set and serve a containing function for the client. Said containers would naturally be trauma-attuned, and necessarily include explicit agreements around consent, disclosure of ontological assumptions, psycho-spiritual training and skills, and inherently contain an awareness of personal positionality and power differentials.

Soul midwifery is a spiraling journey of remembrance and realization. It is one filled with potholes and pitfalls, psychic discombobulation and somatic confusion. It is not a path of transcendence that bypasses the sufferings and limitations of being embodied. Rather, it celebrates, calls forth, and uses for healing the inherent aliveness of the body. This aliveness can be a source of healing as it is at the same time a vehicle for healing itself. Paradoxically, the felt sense of aliveness is also a hallmark of healing having occurred: the snake bites its own tail in an ouroboric loop of being and becoming.

The initiation into the practice of soul midwifery lies in befriending the power of paradox, in embracing the both/and. At the center of paradox lies the freedom and spontaneous perfection of the present moment. Here, reality's multidimensional nature reveals itself while intention shapes the event horizon. Not only that, but the material of one's personal unconscious, the unconscious of one's clients, and the collective unconscious becomes a source of power that can be yoked in service of liberative change. As such, the midwife of soul sees the initiatory portals that lie within the wounds of trauma. This is not to say that suffering should be romanticized, only that the adamantine jewel of the soul is often revealed via intense pressure, and polishing these facets occurs along a spectrum of being fully human that includes both pain and pleasure.

Psychedelics are known for their capacity to facilitate a sense of connectedness: to oneself, to other beings, and to nature. If they serve a healing function, perhaps it lies in the reconnection to an innate sense of the sacredness of all life. To affirm and raise up the whispers of the soul. We are, after all, radiant matter. Stardust animated. The practice of soul midwifery lives inside the devotion to lifting the light that radiates out from the center of every person, to remembering and recohering the aspects of self that have been dismembered in the face of oppression. A guide who inhabits this dance of consciousness participates in what Joanna Macy (2009) calls "The Great Turning," the transformational leap from a paradigm of power over/power under toward an epoch grounded in belonging with nature, cultures of peace, and universal human rights, seeding a more beautiful world with each breath.

References

Bartlett, L. (2022). Study finds 65% of Americans with mental health conditions want access to psychedelics. *Forbes*. Retrieved January 1, 2024, from https://www.forbes.com/sites/lindseybartlett/2022/01/18/study-finds-65-of-americans-with-mental-health-conditions-want-access-to-psychedelics/?sh=641660c510f4.

Berry, T. (2003). In Plotkin, B. *Soulcraft: Crossing into the mysteries of nature and psyche.* New World Library.

Brewerton, T. D., Lafrance, A., & Mithoefer, M. C. (2021). The potential use of N-methyl-3, 4-methylenedioxyamphetamine (MDMA) assisted psychotherapy in the treatment of eating disorders comorbid with PTSD. *Medical Hypotheses, 146,* 110367, https://doi.org/10.1016/j.mehy.2020.110367.

Brooker, B. (2022, August 4). Evaluating the Pollan effect. *Overland.* https://overland.org.au/2022/08/evaluating-the-pollan-effect/

Carhart-Harris, R., Giribaldi, B., Watts, R., Baker-Jones, M., Murphy-Beiner, A., Murphy, R., Martell, J., Blemings, A., Erritzoe, D., & Nutt, D. J. (2021). Trial of psilocybin versus escitalopram for depression. *New England Journal of Medicine, 384*(15), 1402-1411.

Danforth, A.L., Grob, C.S., Struble, C., Feduccia, A. A., Walker, N., Jerome, L. Yazar-Klosinski, B., & Emerson, A. (2018). Reduction in social anxiety after MDMA-assisted psychotherapy with autistic adults: A randomized, double-blind, placebo-controlled pilot study. *Psychopharmacology, 235,* 3137–3148. https://doi.org/10.1007/s00213-018-5010-9.

Domínguez-Clavé, E., Soler, J., Elices, M., Pascual, J. C., Álvarez, E., de la Fuente Revenga, M., Friedlander, A., & Riba, J. (2016). Ayahuasca: Pharmacology, neuroscience and therapeutic potential. *Brain Research Bulletin, 126,* 89–101. https://doi.org/10.1016/j.brainresbull.2016.03.002

Fotiou, E., & Gearin, A. K. (2019). Purging and the body in the therapeutic use of ayahuasca. *Social Science & Medicine, 239.* https://doi.org/10.1016/j.socscimed.2019.112532.

Freud, S. (1912/1964). The dynamics of transference. In J. Strachey (Ed.), *The standard edition of the complete psychological works of Sigmund Freud (Vol. 12, pp. 97-108).* Macmillian.

Hillman, J. (1997). *The soul's code: In search of character and calling.* Transworld Publishers.

Krystal, J. H., Abdallah, C. G., Sanacora, G., Charney, D. S., & Duman, R. S. (2019). Ketamine: a paradigm shift for depression research and treatment. *Neuron, 101*(5), 774-778.

Labate, B. C. & Goldstein, I. (2009). Ayahuasca—from dangerous drug to national heritage: An interview with Antonio A. Arantes. *International Journal of Transpersonal Studies, 28,* 53–64.

Mabit, J. (2007). Ayahuasca in the treatment of addictions. In *Psychedelic Medicine (Vol. 2): New Evidence for Hallucinogenic Substances as Treatments,* pp. 87–103. Praeger Ed.

MacKenzie, I. (Host). (2020, November). The law is in the land (#27) [Audio podcast episode]. In *The mythic masculine with Ian MacKenzie.* https://www.themythicmasculine.com/episodes/tyson-yunkaporta.

Macy, J. (2009, June 29). *The great turning.* Center for Ecoliteracy. https://www.ecoliteracy.org/article/great-turning.

Meade, M. (n.d.). *The soul of genius.* Mosaic Voices. https://courses.mosaicvoices.org/courses/the-soul-of-genius

Mitchell, J.M., Bogenschutz, M., Lilienstein, A., Harrison, C., Kleiman, S., Parker-Guilbert, K., Ot'alora G., M., Garas, W., Paleos, C., Gorman, I., Nicholas, C., Mithoefer, M., Carlin, S., Poulter, B., Mithoefer, A., Quevedo, S., Wells, G., Klaire, S. S., van der Kolk, B., ... & Doblin, R. (2021). MDMA-assisted therapy for severe PTSD: A randomized, double-blind, placebo-controlled phase 3 study. *Nature Medicine, 27,* 1025–1033. https://doi.org/10.1038/s41591-021-01336-3.

Noorani, T. (2021). Containment matters: Set and setting in contemporary psychedelic psychiatry. *Philosophy, Psychiatry, and Psychology, 28*(3), 201-216. https://doi.org/10.1353/ppp.2021.0032.

Posey, D. A. (2002). Commodification of the sacred through intellectual property rights. *Journal of Ethnopharmacology, 83*(1-2), 3-12. https://doi.org/10.1016/S0378-8741(02)00189-7.

Thomas, G., Lucas, P., Capler, N. R., Tupper, K. W., & Martin, G. (2013). Ayahuasca-assisted therapy for addiction: Results from a preliminary observational study in Canada. *Current Drug Abuse Reviews, 6,* 30-42.

Yu, C. L., Yang, F. C., Yang, S. N., Tseng, P. T., Stubbs, B., Yeh, T. C., Hsu, C. W., Li, D. J., & Liang, C. S. (2021). Psilocybin for end-of-life anxiety symptoms: A systematic review and meta-analysis. *Psychiatry Investigation, 18*(10), 958–967. https://doi.org/10.30773/pi.2021.0209.

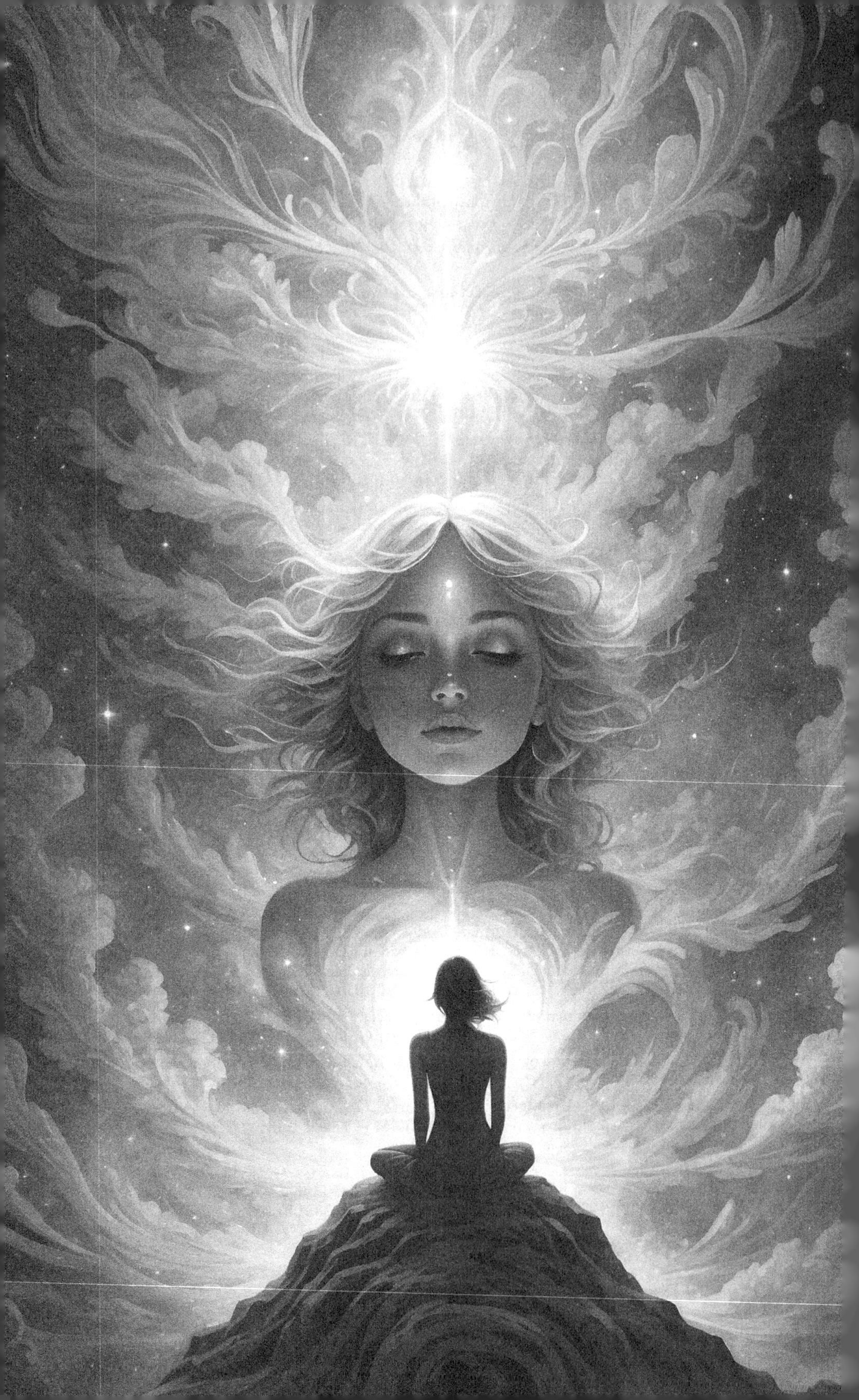

Nina Izel

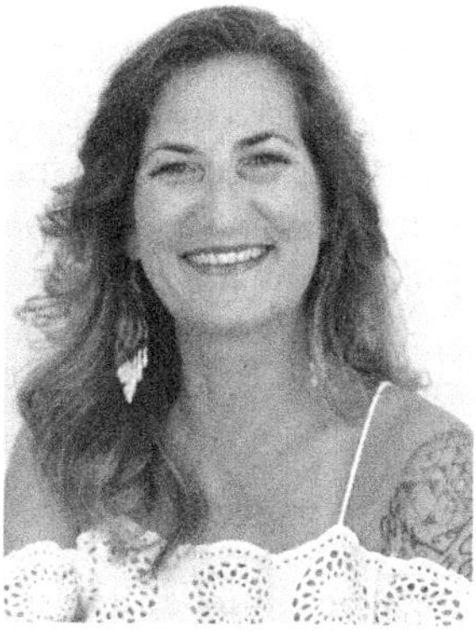

Nina Izel is a well-known pioneer in the psychedelic healing field, being a respected healer, teacher, and author worldwide. She is the founder of Avatar Healing Arts, author of the book *Heart Medicine: Ayahuasca Assisted Therapy and the Integration Process*, and host of the popular podcast *Ayahuasca Avatars*. Nina is passionate about supporting people through psychedelic-assisted therapy to heal, to reclaim their power, and to create their breakthrough results!
nina@avatarhealingarts.com

Ayahuasca Assisted Therapy: An Awakening Experience

My own suffering and my natural interest in healing and self-discovery led me to first study and practice psychology, then transpersonal psychology, holistic healing, and finally healing in non-ordinary states. This essay recounts my personal odyssey, explores the impact of psychedelics on my life and my clients, and delves into the potential and pitfalls as psychedelics gain global prominence.

Transpersonal psychology and healing in altered states

Healing in altered states was the first thing that helped me to truly heal from trauma and establish healthier behaviors. These personal experiences made it clear to me that I am more than my body, mind, and mental processes, which is the fundamental thesis of transpersonal psychology but greatly ignored by much of the mainstream.

Transcending the boundaries of conventional psychology, transpersonal psychology acknowledges the spiritual dimensions of human existence, emphasizing the interconnectedness of mind, body, and spirit. But still, these were initially just concepts I resonated with, not yet my personal experience, until my journey with ayahuasca.

When in 2012 I received my call from the Mother Ayahuasca [1] and decided to leave behind my country, my continent, and my known life, little did I know that I was embarking on a journey of death and rebirth that would shatter my ideas, beliefs, and preconceptions about myself and life in general.

Redefining healing

In the past, the focus was always on how broken and dysfunctional we all are, how much we have to work on

1 The often-used term "Mother Ayahuasca" refers to the plant medicine derived from the plant Banisteriopsis Capi or ayahuasca vine and incorporated into the spiritual practices of the Indigenous people of South America.

our shadow side. Nobody ever said a word about how amazing, divine, powerful, and connected we all are!

In school I was taught that healing was about discovering our dysfunctional parts and trying to fix those aspects. But now I understand that healing really is the integration of our different aspects back into our original state of wholeness and connectedness. This was a whole new level of understanding for me but reflects ancient wisdom rooted in shamanism.

Shamanism is an ancient spiritual and healing practice found in various Indigenous cultures around the world. Despite global attempts to wipe out Indigenous populations and their cultures, shamanism survived by being passed down in oral tradition through the generations.

According to the shamanic worldview, everything is conscious, connected, and alive. This view implies that invisible life force energy, otherwise known as consciousness, is the source of all life, referred to also as the Great Spirit. Rituals and ceremonies to access non-ordinary states of consciousness and the careful use of mind-altering plants are important and integral parts of any shamanic tradition.

Shamanic healing assumes that all problems, including physical illness, have spiritual and energetic roots. Intervention and healing happen on the spiritual, soul level, in other words in the invisible, energetic realms, which are accessed with the guidance of a master healer or shaman.

The shaman works with other invisible entities, such as plant spirits, animal allies, or ancestors, to restore balance and wholeness and to clear one's energetic being. Most shamanic traditions believe that the root cause of illness is a loss of power—in other words, a loss of life force energy—that is caused by the fragmentation of our soul due to traumatic events. Soul retrieval is a common shamanic practice to integrate these lost soul parts.

If this sounds crazy and completely unbelievable, I know exactly how you feel. If you think this is more like a fantasy or fairy tale and doesn't make much sense, I completely understand because that's what I thought too. I believed what most people around me believed: that if you talk with the plants, you are just crazy. There is no way to really understand these concepts with our Western conditioned minds, until we have a personal experience that takes us beyond our traditional thinking.

My journey into the unknown

They say, when you are called by ayahuasca, trust and follow that call. It is a call to adventure, an irresistible desire to journey into the unknown. For me, it came as an opportunity to go to Peru, deep into the Amazon jungle, and participate in a traditional ayahuasca dieta. My calling by Mother Ayahuasca was so powerful that even though I had no idea what to expect, I felt very deeply that my life wouldn't be the same after this journey. So, I decided to let go of my life in Ireland, take a year off from my therapy practice, sell all my belongings, and take a leap of faith toward a new beginning.

Although my first dieta (plant-medicine retreat) in Peru was quite intense and challenging, my time with Mother Ayahuasca created a fundamental shift in my life that unfolded in quite unexpected ways. Before my ayahuasca experience I thought of myself as a human being having a soul or a spiritual aspect, but this understanding was really stuck on an intellectual level. I believed it, but it wasn't a deeply felt experience.

Since my ayahuasca dieta I know beyond a shadow of a doubt, in all my cells, on every level, that I am a spiritual being having a human experience. How do I know that? During my ayahuasca ceremonies, I experienced many times what I imagined death would look like. I felt all my power, all my life force energy, leaving me, leaving my body until nothing was left, not even one breath. But I was still there. I was still present and conscious of myself, but from the outside, my body seemed lifeless and dead. After some time, I felt myself coming back, regaining control over my body again, and slowly grounding back into this Earth and into the present moment. This is what we call a death and rebirth experience. When you go through this experience over and over again, you start to lose your fear of death and start to really live and enjoy your life in the here and now. At least that's how I felt.

After my initial experience, even though I had some big breakthrough moments, I couldn't really translate them into my daily life, and I continued to feel miserable and even more challenged than before. Because I didn't feel better, I thought I needed more medicine and more ceremonies. This is the most common mistake for first timers by the way; the concept that more is better is a common Western mindset.

I kept drinking more medicine until I ended up in a spiritual emergence that could have easily turned into a spiritual emergency if not for a beautiful healer who came to my help. My experience was very intense, very scary, and I felt like I was going crazy and losing my mind—which I did, but it turned out to be a gift.

This healer, a Mexican medicine woman, helped me to move through my dark night of the soul, and the first thing she told me was to stop drinking ayahuasca and start focusing on my integration process. Now that was a new concept! What is the integration process?

The integration process

Integration is the process of making sense out of your psychedelic experience, receiving deeper insights, and integrating them into your everyday life to create real, lasting transformation. There is not enough space in the scope of this essay to describe my journey in detail. But I want to share some important lessons I learned through my integration process.

Most importantly, I started to understand more deeply what healing really is. It felt like Mother Ayahuasca expanded my awareness, and I saw myself from a higher perspective that allowed me to perceive and embrace myself with compassion and love. This was my first powerful experience of the healing power of love. I understood how when we heal trauma we bring our fragments together, making ourselves whole again, and this is a process of integration. This inclusion can be only accomplished with love and acceptance.

Healing our relationships

When we are in a state of trauma and blame, and we hold emotions like sadness, resentment, and anger, we can't heal. What the medicine helped me with the most was to see certain events of my past from a higher, more detached perspective and to understand the deeper reasons behind a chain of events. In other words, I could make peace with my past and let go of the blame, guilt, shame, and never-ending fear and worry that I did something wrong and am somehow faulty, not good enough to be happy, not deserving.

The healing didn't stop with me. I started to feel at peace with my parents and my family. I could see their lives with compassionate eyes. I could understand that nothing is personal, and I could feel the love between us, underneath all the pain and suffering. I connect to that love every day since and bring that into my relationship with my parents every time we interact. I feel deep acceptance of myself, of them, and of everything that happened between us in the past.

They don't trigger me anymore. Today, when I visit my family we have a good time and enjoy each other's company without any drama or conflict. For most of my life this seemed impossible. Home was always a source of stress and anxiety, but now it's a source of love, joy, and gratitude. Now that's what I call a miracle.

Healing our relationship with our ancestors, letting go of our anger, blame, shame, and judgment, is a major milestone of the integration process when working with sacred plants. For me this healing doesn't mean justifying or normalizing what happened, nor does it mean suppressing or denying the past, but rather finding a different perspective, a loving perspective that naturally leads to acceptance and deep inner peace.

Once this reconciliation happens in family relationships we can open our hearts and receive the power and wisdom of our ancestors and feel their support in everything we do.

Healing our body

I was learning and experiencing how thoughts, emotions, and memories affect the physical body. They can make our body sick but also can heal it. I discovered food as medicine and a major factor in health and well-being. I felt more energetic and woke up around sunrise without an alarm feeling rested, which for a long time was a struggle in my life.

For the first time I started to feel safe in my body. I started to feel at home, and I started to feel love and appreciation. I used to hate my body and treat it very badly: putting junk food and toxins into it, putting alcohol, pills, and drugs into it, often without limit, until I wasn't aware of my body. Then I wasn't aware of myself anymore. I used to party hard and be promiscuous. But I made sure that from the outside you didn't see this at all; all you saw was just glam, façade, and false confidence.

I know that a lot of people will relate to this. I am still learning to treat my body with even more love and respect, treat her as an ally, not the enemy she used to be. I have to say I prefer love over hate; it just feels better.

A new beginning

As I continued my deep and devoted work with Mother Ayahuasca and learned more and more about the integration process, I felt a deep pull to share my experience and to bring awareness to the importance of the integration process. At the time integration was not even a commonly used term. I wrote a blog, started a podcast, and eventually wrote a book called *Heart Medicine: Ayahuasca Assisted Therapy and the Integration Process* (Izel, 2020) to educate people about the integration process and help them navigate their own plant medicine integration, especially if they are working with Mother Ayahuasca for the first time.

I also pivoted my therapy practice into ayahuasca-assisted therapy as a result of my personal life-changing experience with this medicine. My first client was an ex-Olympic athlete, a 27-year-old woman with a Xanax addiction to manage her eating disorder, depression, and anxiety, among other things, who was in a great deal of pain and desperate for a change.

Her story is nothing short of a miracle. With less than a year of holistic therapy and personal guidance of her ayahuasca integration she was able to rewrite the story of her life, shift her behavior, and experience a full recovery! She truly had an awakening experience when she was able to see things from a different perspective, looking for the gifts and learnings that were hidden in each challenge. She realized that her experience of abandonment by her father could be seen as the greatest gift that helped her to awaken to her power and liberate herself from suffering. And when I say full recovery, I mean coming off all pharmaceuticals after over 8 years of addiction, leaving behind depression and anxiety. Her eating disorder was just gone, nothing left to control or manage. She started to take good care of herself physically, mentally, and emotionally. Her whole life changed fundamentally, and she ended up moving to Peru and learning to work with the medicine in a ceremonial setting. In her own words, "I am imperfect, and I am loved anyway. I am a divine being. I can't be more perfect. Loving myself is inevitable" (personal communication).

I was amazed by what was accomplished within such a short time even compared to alternative therapies or psychotherapy or deep psychoanalysis. Mother Ayahuasca has the power to rapidly break down internal obstacles and resistance and lead us to the root of the problems where we can uproot our suffering and change the trajectory of our lives. I never saw any other healing technology before that works in such a tailored manner, so effectively, and so fast to create transformation in the life of an individual.

Personal integration support

Personal support and a safe container can make all the difference between reaching your desired results or eventually falling back to old habits and patterns. The advantage of this work with sacred plants is to deepen and accelerate the healing process, and everybody wants that. But on the other side, this process is more intense and mentally, emotionally, spiritually, and physically taxing on every level at the same time.

We instinctively want to move away from pain and toward pleasure. To surrender to discomfort requires conscious choice, courage, deep commitment, and specific tools and resources that most people do not have. Through the personally guided integration process people learn how to work with this medicine. They learn about their own personal gifts and challenges, triggers, traumas, and shadow aspects. They learn practical tools and skills so they can navigate their own journey with confidence. That is one of the goals of the integration process.

Breakthrough results

Since my first client I have supported many people in ayahuasca-assisted therapy and pivoted my practice to support plant medicine integration. If you want to hear more breakthrough results and full recovery stories from chronic disease, anxiety, depression, addiction, and PTSD, let the people talk for themselves in the video testimonials on my website (Avatar Healing Arts, 2024).

To create breakthrough results I believe it is essential to have these four elements:

- Safe container (including preparation and integration process)
- Personal support of an experienced integration guide
- Safe and integral ayahuasca ceremony
- Deep commitment, openness, and willingness to change.

Providing support during the whole healing process, before and after the ceremony, increases the chance for people to make the most out of their experience. It's important that people understand that they cannot bypass the deep inner work required to create transformational results. It's more likely that they succeed when they are guided and supported.

As a therapist, I used to have an agenda of healing people and this way of elevating myself above them. As a healer, thanks to working with sacred plants, I humbly step aside and look at the innate intelligence unfolding in front of my eyes. I just observe, listen, and ask questions, and only when I feel guided and sure that my actions are for serving the other and not my ego mind, when I am sure that my words are coming from my heart, do I contribute to their process.

In my work I use a variety of tools, skills, and approaches I learned and experienced as part of my training and healing journey. Breathwork is one of my favorite tools, supporting emotional release and regulation of the nervous system. Somatic experiencing is also a good tool to include body intelligence in the healing process. Compassionate inquiry is a great way to uncover limiting beliefs and clear the mind.

Who is a qualified guide?

You can only take people as deep as you have gone.

—Nina Izel

The most important characteristic of a guide is extensive personal experience. You simply can't relate to a client's experience and provide accurate guidance if you have never been there. Imagine going for brain surgery, and hearing the doctor is say, "Don't worry, I have read lots of books about this; I think I am ready to operate."

The deeper I go into my own journey of healing and self-discovery, the more intensity I can hold space for, allowing people to go deeper in their own process. People can feel what you are ready for, how much you can bear to hold, and if you don't have plenty of training and personal experience, you won't have the necessary confidence to hold space for others.

Of course having a lot of experience is necessary but not enough to guide others. It's also important that guides have different skills and are trained in various traditional or non-traditional healing modalities, especially focused on trauma healing, to effectively help others in the psychedelic healing space.

Of course, you can have the best guide, but if you are not willing to move forward, if you are not fully committed to your own transformation, if you are not open to seeing different points of views, nobody can help you. No one can force people to change; that will result only in conflict and resistance. Therefore, for successful healing with psychedelics it is vital to have an open mind, willingness to change, and full commitment to showing up for yourself and your process. This is a warrior path, not for the faint heart.

Death & Rebirth

Psychedelic integration commonly refers to making sense out of your experience and integrating your insights into your everyday life. But for me it goes deeper than that. It means integrating the fragmented self back into our original state of balance and wholeness. In other words, integrating the different aspects of the psyche, especially the unconscious, but also integrating the body, mind (intellect, emotions) complex with our heart and with our eternal, spiritual self.

The longest journey you will make in your life is from your head to your heart.

—Sioux Indian saying

Mother Ayahuasca is a powerful ally who helped me in this process and reminded me of the power of the heart and the true medicine, which is love. I see this over and over again in my program, and it never ceases to amaze and inspire me how powerful we are and how we can make the impossible happen, how we can overcome the unspeakable and not just survive but thrive again. This is why I am doing this work. There is no deeper fulfillment and bigger privilege than being a spiritual midwife and assisting people to birth their new life and happiness.

I was taught in the West over and over again that the best we can do is to learn to cope with dysfunction (living with depression, a life with diabetes, etc.). Sometime we can cure things, which means eliminating the symptoms, but often during this process we create new illnesses.

What I learned from illiterate shamans who live without running water and electricity, what I learned from the Spirit of the Ayahuasca, is that we can fully heal ourselves. We can heal the Earth. We can heal the world if we can open our hearts and are willing to let go of the control of the mind. I learned that this is possible.

Plant medicine helped me to love and accept all parts of myself, the beautiful and the ugly, and as I was doing this I lost my anxiety, addictions, and compulsions. The pain from my body just vanished for good, and I truly felt I was reborn. I was a different person, not broken anymore, but most of all I started to see myself with the eyes of love: all that I have overcome, all the past pain, all the joy, all the heartbreak now didn't touch me at all; I just felt grateful, renewed, and free.

My deep work with Mother Ayahuasca, both as a student and as a guide, totally changed my view of myself, the world, what healing is, and how the mind works. It allowed me to find deeper healing, freedom, love, and joy than I ever thought possible, helped me to serve on a higher level and create a greater positive impact and find deeper meaning, passion, and purpose in my life.

Before my work with Mother Ayahuasca I used to think that there was something wrong with me: that's why my life sucked. I felt that I was a sinner and that my life was a punishment, and I wasn't even Christian.

Mother Ayahuasca helped me to understand that I am just a spiritual being having a human experience like everybody else. I am not better or worse. I am not a sinner or a saint. I am a unique expression of the divine, full of love and potential, and most of all with the gift of choice. Free will to create as you wish, individually and collectively, because everything is connected. And that's a big responsibility and honor and privilege.

Ayahuasca-assisted therapy proved to be an effective way to let go of lifelong suffering and fundamentally transform one's life. Mother Ayahuasca not only made me leave behind my country, my culture, and my known life but inspired me to dedicate my life to psychedelic-assisted therapy, something I never even thought was a thing.

Our Responsibility

Working with clients in a therapeutic container with the Mother Ayahuasca allows the healing process to be deeper and significantly shorter as she helps us to access the root of our problems by expanding our awareness and breaking down natural resistance. Definitely deserving of the term breakthrough results, and it's exciting to know that we are only at the beginning of this beautiful journey.

Sacred plants are powerful tools and amplifiers with no agenda. It is up to us whether we use them to bring harm or work with them for healing and spiritual growth. Healing in altered states creates more vulnerability for possible harm to occur so we have even more responsibility to make sure that we have the highest level of standards, integrity, humility, and transparency when we decide to work with these powerful plant allies, within or outside the ceremonial setting.

Psychedelic therapy is on the rise and it is our responsibility to steer the wheel of this movement. For inspiration and to start a much-needed conversation, I have developed a Code of Ethics and Best Practices for Ayahuasca Professionals, available on my website (Izel, 2024).

Imagine a world....

Where we remember all this and more. How would that world look like?

Where love, compassion, kindness, service to others, protection of all life, purpose, and meaning are our main values and highest priorities instead of money, power, sex, fame, status, and prestige, what kind of world would we live in?

References

Avatar Healing Arts (2024). Testimonials [videos]. Retrieved from https://avatarhealingarts.com/psychedelic-therapy-testimonials/

Izel, N. (2020). *Heart medicine: Ayahuasca assisted therapy and the integration process.* Bloomington, IN: Balboa Press.

Izel, N. (2024). *Code of ethics for ayahuasca healing professionals.* Avatar Healing Arts. Retrieved from https://avatarhealingarts.com/code-of-ethics/

Shannon Gendron

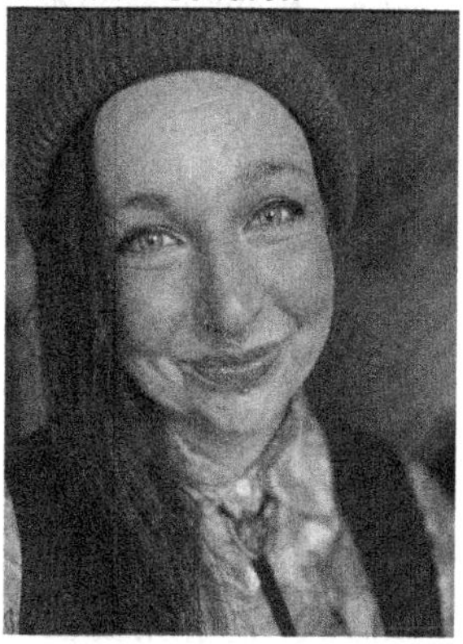

SHANNON GENDRON is ultimately an illusion. When not exploring realms of the mystic, they can be found investing in trans advocacy and community soul care initiatives. Residing on the stolen lands of Anishinaabe, Haudenosaunee, and the Huron-Wendat, currently known as Kingston, Ontario, Shannon is a Queer, non-binary, Métis Creative who is passionate about queering mental health. They are working as a psychotherapist and specialize in providing trans and gender diverse care.
shannon.hope.gendron@gmail.com

On Nesting and Love:
How Working With Plant Medicines Informed My Clinical Identity

COLLAPSED IN THE FETAL POSITION, DAMP WITH MY OWN SWEAT, TEARS, AND VOMIT—raw from my own screams—the shaman rocked me in his arms. He softly sang icaros (medicine songs) in my ear and pressed his forehead to mine. All of me was only tremble. *Me* was gone. It was hour 7 of my first ayahuasca journey. In my reality at that moment, the shaman's arms were giant, feathered wings. I was pressed against the breast of Love's own beating heart. The maloca that held the ceremony was a cosmic nest. I was only just hatching. It was the summer I finished grad school to become a psychotherapist. I was exploring plant medicines to better integrate my own trauma so that I could best hold gently the traumas of others. I spent that summer working with plant medicines at an ayahuasca retreat centre/eco-village in the Andes. There, I held space during ayahuasca and San Pedro ceremonies for folx on healing journeys from around the world. I lead integration circles and meditations. There, I was introduced to the teachings of the Ecuadorian shamans and their lineage in holding ancient plant wisdoms. I had the honor of holding hundreds of stories of medicine journeys, discoveries, horrors, and marvels. I also had the honor of cleaning toilets and making beds. Emptying purge buckets. Chopping carrots and harvesting San Pedro. All of it felt like Love alive in my being.

My first experience with ayahuasca obliterated *Me*. All my life had known up until that point was the egg. I was me. In an egg. My sense of Self and reality was an insular shell: containing and limiting, yet it felt so real. The plant medicines shattered my egg and showed me my soar. They taught me the power of nest, of rebirth, of seeing a reality that exists outside the eggs of our own projections and interpretations.

I was told that in that first ceremony I wept loudly the entire night into the morning. *I* was not there; I had no idea Body was weeping. I was only a wee bird, feathers slicked from fresh birth, being rocked in the feathery bosom of Love. Prior to this moment, I was told, I had been screaming so loudly into my purge bucket that helpers had to intervene because it was disrupting the ceremony. I had blasted into a space where I was no longer my body or mind, or even an Earth dweller. I blasted into a space where I was met with the deepest horrors of my heart. I spiraled into the darkest crevices of my being, and vision after vision unfolded. I felt only terror. I was being sliced from the forehead down to the navel. Pain radiated, and Grandmother Ayahuasca appeared as this old, stout woman who reached into my gaping chest, pulled out my Self—all I had ever known to be true—and started scrubbing Self away on a washboard in the river. I could feel my entire being rung through the washboard's slots. Every part of my identity scrubbed away. I then saw everyone I loved being obliterated. Everything I valued named meaningless. Everything I believed, built my Self around, hoped for, hid. All of it. Obliterated. Absorbed into this river.

And then suddenly, in the midst of my horror: stillness. My *I*-ness became swept into an expansive state of euphoric Unitive Love. Then bright dazzling light. Then no-thingness.

The shaman had come to rock me because Body would not stop convulsing. At that point, there were moments when I could hear those around me who had drunk the medicine purging and crying out. I felt deep love for each of them. I could hear their cries but had no desire to remove them from their suffering. I knew they, too, were hatching. I felt only love. Deep Oneness. I was experiencing everyone purely as energies in shells in the same nest. Hatching into a new layer of aliveness. Raw. Overwhelming. Marvelous. I was in a space where everything else had been stripped away, and all that remained was Love. Only Love holding. Only Love existing. Everything else, illusion.

Working with entheogens taught me the power of radical acceptance before Tara Brach and the Buddhists did. In the medicine ceremonies that followed, I learned to bow in reverence before surrender: I learned to release my agenda and comfort and trust the process of the plant teachers. I learned to not resist the horror of my own heart or the heart of the world. The moments I stopped fighting what the plants were trying to teach me, were the moments I was able to be enveloped by the Love Source. Suffering truly is the resistance to pain. Entheogens, and later meditation and other transcendental practices, showed me I don't have to spend my Earth-time suffering. I can spend it making nests for Love to rest. Nests made from twigs of compassion and attuned presence. As I see it, compassion is turning towards suffering with tenderness. I feel enormous tenderness towards suffering within my Self and others because psychedelic and transpersonal practices have taught me that all wounds are portals into this unitive state. All pains are portals home—home to this Love Source I believe we are born from and return to and are infinitely already part of.

When I returned to Canada that fall to begin my work as a psychotherapist, I was eager and inspired; I was filled with purpose. Within a week back, I crashed. I crashed hard. I didn't understand how to reconcile all I had learned. I felt desperate to be enveloped by the same Love I had felt when working with the medicines. I didn't know how to embody what I had learned and felt like a failure for understanding the teachings in a cerebral sense yet not in a lived body sense. I felt discouraged by my flawed and finite vessel. In the Andes, I had been surrounded by a rich interdependent community, was deeply connected to the land, and had been existing in a space where non-dual states were understood, held, and practiced. I had spent months feeling robustly connected to my Self energy. Now I had left the nest, I felt far from Self, far from God, far from Love. Without proper integration support back home, I plummeted into a thick depressive episode. My soul yearned to be returned to a unitive state, and I could only feel panicked separation. Everything within my internal world had shifted. Identities that were burnt to ashes rose anew into facets of Self that now felt even more robustly me than ever before. I was in the midst of a crisis of faith, as my theological orientation radically shifted, and I could no longer find peace in the faith tradition or community I had spent my adult life devoted to. I felt alien, with ideas no one around me seemed to understand or take seriously. My pansexuality and authentic gender, which had previously been exiled due to trauma, was now begging to be seen and integrated. Everything practical felt meaningless. This reality felt like an absurd cosmic joke I didn't want to participate in. I was in, as my therapist cheekily coined, an existential blitzkrieg. I cocooned for weeks, unable to leave my bed. Unable to move Body. I floated in and through dissociation trying desperately to be re-united with Love state. My first dark night of the soul led to a catatonic state.

The following spring, I was diagnosed with bipolar II.

As someone who is reluctant to pathologize spiritual emergencies and is skeptical of the egg cartons of the medical model, getting—let alone accepting—this diagnosis was harrowing and shame-inducing for me. I spent the following years trying to not dismiss my favourite parts of my Self as symptoms or a disease. Times when I wanted to unalive my Self the most were times shame took over. Where shame convinced me that all the beauty, wonder, horror, and pains I experienced so intensely and with such profound depth were simply my sickness. That the unconventional life I'd built around my sense of God was in fact delusional. Shame and my suicidal part told me I could never be a therapist because I couldn't even fix my Self. While it remains a daily effort, I refuse to not see the God in my bipolar experience. I've since grown to appreciate the beauties of this neurodivergent brain I have by seeing it as a lifelong invitation into ceremony and communion with God. I've grown to accept this piece as a valid and sacred part of who I am and how I have come to know my Self and the mystic and the world. I refuse to pathologize or apologize for the dark and light I travel on a regular basis. While it is challenging and painful, it is also wildly interesting, richly creative, and deeply meaningful for me. I now have affection towards madness. I have profound reverence for psychosis. I have deep awe for the altered states of our built-in drive for survival. I know now my illness would teach me more about how I wanted to show up as a therapist than any book or lecture hall ever could.

After my diagnosis, I was told it was no longer safe for me to journey with psychedelics. I was crestfallen and believed I'd never again be able to access the magnitude and beauty of Unitive Consciousness. In desperation to further connect with altered states of consciousness sans plant medicine, I grew passionate devotion to exploring holotropic breathwork, Wim Hof breathwork and cold exposure, various traditions of meditation, tantric philosophy, ecstatic dance, sound healing, journeying through my inner world in trance states, and experimenting with my own ways of playing in transpersonal spaces with curiosity and reverence. I spent many depressive episodes in bed binge listening to talks on Sufism and Christian mysticism and Buddhist philosophy.

I'd always felt my emotions deeply. I'd always experienced God deeply. Psychedelics and transpersonal play/travel taught me that the more I learn to find the God in my emotions, the more I get to experience Love. My soul doesn't have to suffer because I am protected by and infinitely connected to Love Source. I am contained and part of a stillness and dazzling spaciousness of the nondual. My experience navigating the depths of my depression and hypomania as if it were a medicine journey taught me to trust symptoms as teachers and guides. My darkness is a portal to Love. I learned to nest my Self through these intense times so I could integrate what I learned once I returned to humanning.

No matter how dark a wound's voice might be, I now know my way back to the stillness of Love. No matter how much I am struggling with the intensity of my Earth experience, I trust my ability to return to nest space within my Self. When I'm depressed, my wounds convince me I will never feel Love again. My wounds tell me if I am this far from compassion's gaze now, I will never feel Love again. In fact, Love never existed. Shame violently arrests me and sends me to trial. My rage deems me guilty. My suicide parts warrant death sentence. My despair says the nest never existed in the first place.

When I surrender to the pain, I see my Self as separate from the voices who try to convince me I am separate from Love. I then can become my own parent bird gathering the various states of my inner-eggs and chicks with my wings and pulling them close to my own beating heart. I hold the tension of being simultaneously a bird and egg. I know if I allow my Self time to nest, I eventually return to the cosmic spaciousness within and around my Self.

There were times in my process, however, when I felt the goal was to transcend the body so I could transcend the pain and burden of body, especially as someone who at the time struggled with complex trauma and unacknowledged dysphoria. As I've been connecting more with somatic work and embodied mysticism, I understand more and more the great power of our bodies as conduits of Love in the present moment. While my preference is to travel through dimensions free from space/time, the real work is integrating those teachings in how I show up for the present moment. How I show up with clarity and openness for what is. How I show up and live this Love as flawed, struggling human and clinician with Soul integrity.

Medicine integration work for me has looked like creating a world for my Self where I can live and embody my authenticity and laugh at the cosmic joke alongside others. Integrating Love gave my Self permission to live my queerness out loud, to take up Earth space, to embody and embrace my non-binary identity, pansexuality, and polyamorous heart without shame edits. Love also gave my Self permission to own and practice my pan-spirituality with intention and in intentional community. Love helped me make peace with and understand my former faith tradition with even more richness, beauty, and reverence. By embodying my values and learnings from the psychedelic world, I began naturally orbiting more and more like-minded folx who made me feel understood and inspired. Folx who knew the horrors and joys of hatching. I have now found my Self organically nuzzled in a deep, supportive community of mystical comrades, deep feelers, and wounded healers from varying spiritual traditions all drawn by the same passion for collective hatching. I am nourished by the nests others have already created.

I am energized by the nests I get to create for others. I began investing in community soul care initiatives, volunteering at psychedelic integration circles, running my own queer cannabis circles in the forest to teach others how to somatically connect with this medicine. I started a queer meditation group called Queer Yer Mind. And I began experiencing more and more synchronicities as I did. I began to let my Self be fully human: eager and willing to experience it all: the glory, the heartbreak, the grief, the sorrow, the electric bliss.

I now know depression is not a truth-teller. Anxieties are not prophets. Shame is not a death-sentence. Despair is not a prison cell. My own inner-nest time helps me connect boldly with the inevitable pains that consume me. I now know I am more than body, more than pain. I know pain herself is an illusion of separation from Love Source. My suffering tells me I am egg. Love reminds me, I'm already born. I'm already head nuzzled in the chest of Love. This is my home state: Love. I do the human things now with awareness that no emotion and no person, no politic or policy, no social construct or life circumstance can ever separate me from my nest or tear me from the bosom of Love. My invitation is to reflect this belief in how I attune with and experience others as a therapist and member of an aching humanity.

I am now a psychotherapist at a university and work exclusively with queer and gender diverse/trans students. My clients have deep spiritual and psychic wounds. Many are in touch with what life outside an egg feels like yet have been told by so much of the world that because of their queerness, they are not worthy of nest or God of Love to snuggle into. My creative intentionality within the therapeutic relationship is how I make nests for others to encounter the Love that already exists inside them.

One of the first questions I ask new clients, before we address their therapeutic intentions or identity constellation is "Tell me about one thing that makes your eyes light up." Then I ask them to describe what color the sensations they notice in their bodies are when answering. Often, I notice a visceral shift in energy in our space. Their inner posture softens, even if only for a moment, to curiosity and connection—something more infinite than their pain. I get to meet them closer to their Self energy than their wounds because when they describe and embody what they Love—whether it's the stars, or a favorite animal, a song, a pretty rock they found once—I get a deeper invitation into their inner-worlds, their values, their meaning-system, their spark. They get a deeper invitation into felt sense, body, and inner medicine that already exists. How I weave whatever they answer into our unique nest is how I deepen my connection with them. Their passions inform my interventions. I incorporate their color into breathing exercises and customized grounding rituals. I try to underpin my metaphor work in imagery most relevant to their Loves. I base guided meditations and visualizations on themes that emerge from this first encounter. I also adapt my session integration invitations based on their eye-sparkle. I offer unique journal/poetry prompts to further integrate our nest time.

I heard it said that trauma separates us from Love. At this moment in time, my sense is that if God is Love, it is through bringing God to our traumas and self-hatreds, fears and self-limiting beliefs, that we heal. To me, all nervous system regulation strategies are prayers calling out for God—rituals of returning to body and to a state where Self can better access compassion, connection, and Love.

I'm reminded through my practice that we're all in this nest together. We are all going to inevitably shatter. All of our eggs are going to split in some way, to some degree over time. Some of us might stay in the egg because of its familiarity and comfort. Some might see Love's pure light through the cracks from within the egg and yearn to break through. Some might feel stuck and deny the egg even exists. The more time I spend with God through transpersonal practices, the more fluent I become in Love's first language: compassion. Compassion accepts others exactly where they are in their egg process. Compassion can turn towards the horrors of suffering with a calm presence because inevitably compassion knows we are all one. We all will hatch. Someday. Love knows everything other than Love is an illusion. Ultimately, the eggshells don't really exist. We are all trying our best to return to Love. All emotions and attempts to cope with emotions are trying to protect us from feeling far from Love or rejected from Love. Trauma work, in my opinion, is helping people's bodies and internal parts return to Love, so their souls don't have to cry out.

Because of this my clinical work weaves a nest of internal family systems with polyvagal underpinnings with gentle breathwork, somatic metaphor play, and guided collaborative visualization. I believe my work is helping clients connect with an embodied sense of Love in how they integrate their parts by unburdening the illusion of being unlovable. When parts become unburdened, they hatch. They hatch into the truth that they were always held in a whole. We cannot unburden our wounded parts until we let ourselves break through the darkness of our shells and illusion of separateness to experience Love. Experience connection. Experience Self-energy. I try to lead inner journeys that help my clients compassionately encounter and transmute their pains. I cultivate creative spaces for them to experience their emotions as guides and their wounds as portals, so that they, too, can someday learn to create their own nests.

Every time I share nest with someone who is suffering, I swell with the depth of Love I felt that first time I had experienced ayahuasca. My Soul knew in that first nest experience that when it returned to Body, it would devote Earth time to creating nests. Nests in community care. Nests in therapeutic relationships. Nests in holding space for those on transpersonal journeys. Nests for my Self. Nests for lovers and beloveds. I trust Love is the benevolent mother bird holding us tender in our hatchings. My calling is making mindful nests as a therapist, so there's space for love to welcome us in our breaking downs and breaking throughs. Psychedelic medicines and integration have taught me life is a series of hatchings and often re-hatchings. My responsibility is to prepare loving space for these ongoing hatchings so that bit by bit we can return to love. Before every session, my Soul whispers to God, "Here. Please see these twigs of attuned presence and compassion as a place to land. Please gather me in your breast feathers, so that I may invite others into the nest to rest." It's only through learning to hold Love to my suffering and my hatchings that I was able to then hold the sufferings of others with that same Love. Afterall, plant medicines taught me we can only know and befriend Love to the depth at which we have learned to know and befriend our own wounds. ▼

Float On: A Journey with Ketamine

Danielle Sukenik

I was quickly swept away by the effects of the medicine,
rushed down a fast-moving river with high walls like a canyon.
I attempted to cling to the red sand-colored walls and exit, but there was no exit.
How will I keep myself alive if I let go?
The only option was to float on, flow, move with the water.
I felt the soft waves underneath me.
Struck by the beauty in the peace I was experiencing.
Is this what dying feels like?
Transcendental.
Rocking with the music filling my ears.
Floating.
This journey was brief.
I soon returned to my thinking brain, wanting to resist the peaceful stillness.
Ah, this is what I do.
I find discomfort here and then create distress, attachments.
I cling to the internal chaos.
Otherwise, there is boredom, dullness.
How much time is left? Am I witnessing the isness? Being? Or letting go enough?
Do not cling to the walls of the canyon or the banks of the river.
Go with the water.
Float on.

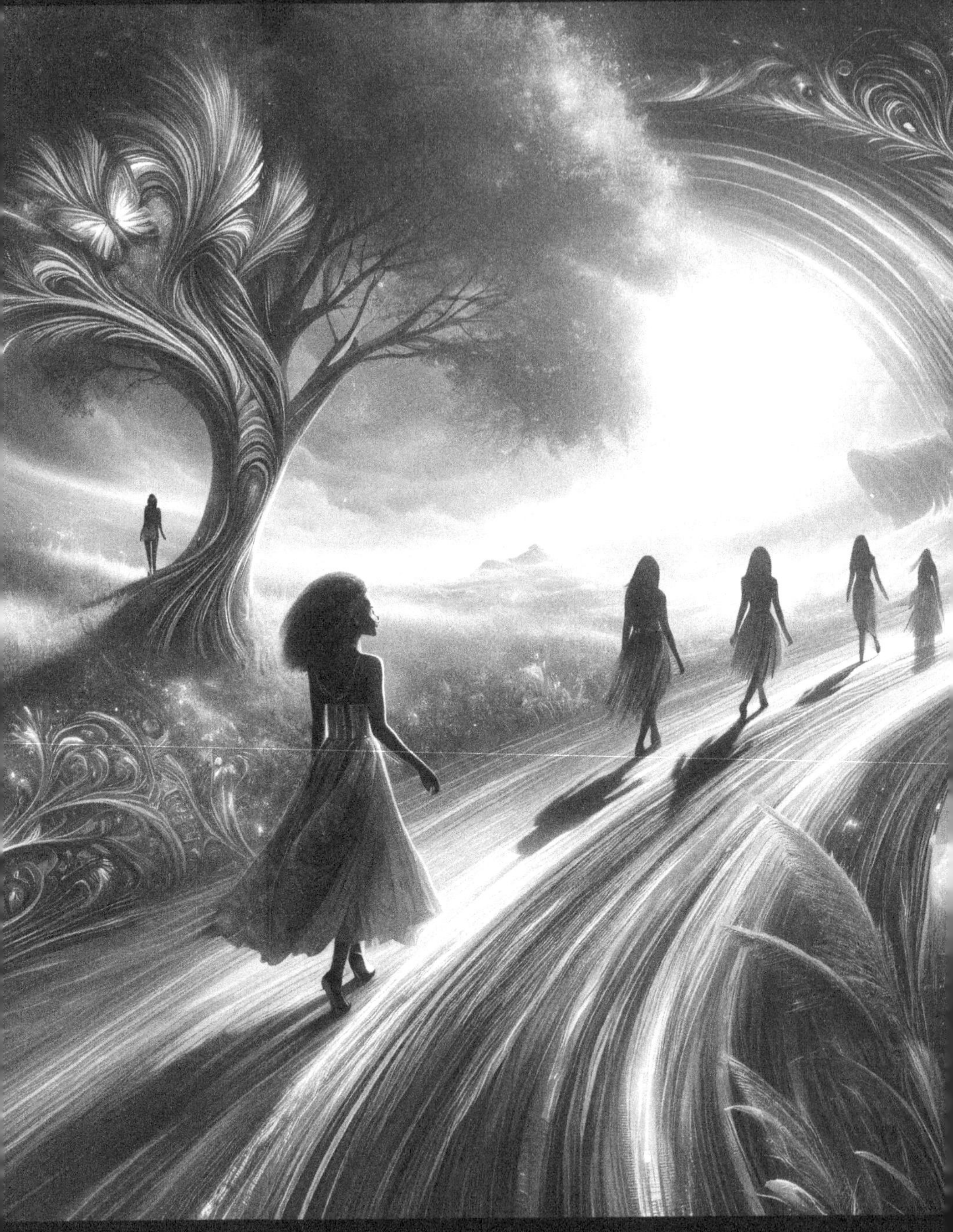

Laura Hutchins

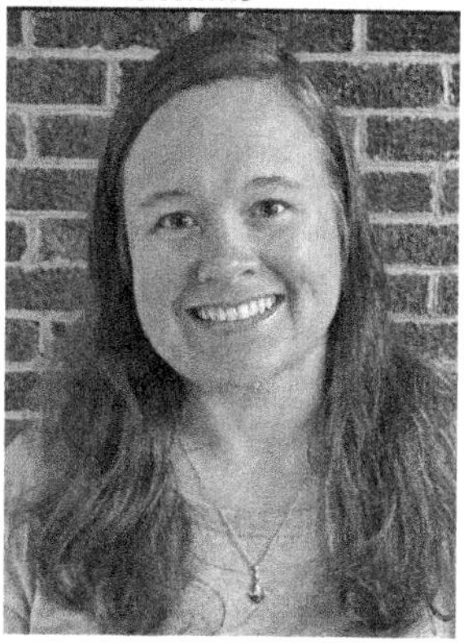

Laura Hutchins MA, LCMHC, LCAS, is a therapist, educator, advocate, and explorer who is deeply passionate about helping those with treatment-resistant symptoms find hope and relief through creative and evidence-based approaches. Laura received her graduate and undergraduate degrees from Lenoir-Rhyne University in Hickory, North Carolina, and is dually licensed in mental health counseling and addictions. She currently works in private practice, where she serves as the ketamine-assisted psychotherapy (KAP) program director and lead therapist.
laura@salemcounselingandconsulting.com

A Psychedelic Therapist's Journey Home

I fell so naturally into the world and work of psychedelic therapy that I am often amused by the long and winding road it took to get here. Nevertheless, I am a firm believer that even the most unexpected or uncomfortable journeys can offer opportunities for growth, insight, and reflection if we choose to accept the challenge.

The Long and Winding Road

My current work as a psychedelic therapist is the product of years of searching for meaning, both personally and professionally. After graduating with my master's degree in clinical mental health counseling, I accepted a job working as a substance abuse counselor. Substance abuse counselor was close to, if not at, the bottom of my Jobs I Would Be Interested in Exploring After Graduate School list. In hindsight, I can clearly identify my then-hesitance as directly related to experiencing firsthand the effects of loving someone with a severe substance use disorder; at the time, I only knew it would be a very temporary job until I figured out what type of work I really wanted to do.

Perhaps naive about the complexity of the process of "figuring out what I want to do with my life," I spent the next several years working as a substance abuse counselor, eventually obtaining a second professional license (licensed clinical addictions specialist) and becoming lead counselor at the clinic where I worked. Despite my initial reluctance, helping people who are struggling with substances and working on recovery turned out to be work I truly enjoyed.

Still, I knew this was not where I was meant to remain for the duration of my career. After resigning from my job as a substance abuse counselor, I shifted into working with a private group practice. The first few years of private practice went really well. I found myself working with individuals with various mental health diagnoses and providing sex offender evaluations and DWI assessments. My job was never mundane and usually fulfilling. During this time, I also pursued advanced training in various areas such as DBT and EMDR. I found these to be great interventions, and I still value and teach DBT skills to clients regularly.

But something was still missing. I began to wonder if I simply had unrealistic expectations about being able to do work I am deeply passionate about, or if I was perhaps just restless and needed to settle into the role I had. As it turned out, anything less than pursuing work I love felt complacent. Eventually, I made the decision to stay at the job I was in, while exploring my options, staying open to opportunities, and trying to be patient.

A couple of years ago, after a season of practicing much patience and mindful gratitude, an opportunity presented itself. I received a phone call from a dear colleague that sounded something like, "A ketamine provider I know and trust contacted me to see if there are any therapists in my group practice who might be interested in working with her patients; I know you don't work in my practice, but being a therapist who is open to exploring new opportunities and who has experienced ketamine firsthand, you're the first person that came to mind. Do you have any interest in discussing this further?"

In my early years as a clinician, I had experienced difficult mental health symptoms that did not respond to traditional methods of treatment. I learned about the use of ketamine to treat various mental health symptoms, pursued treatment, and experienced significant relief. Even then, I knew there was something special about this medicine, though I had no idea at the time it would later play such an intricate role in my daily life.

Coming Home

As you may have guessed by now, the answer to my colleague's question was a resounding, "Yes, let's talk!" And so, we did. We discussed and planned and within a short time span, wheels were in motion for me to start working with clients who are receiving ketamine treatment for mental health symptoms.

Prior to this new opportunity, I had completed a few continuing education courses on the subject of psychedelics and therapy, but not enough to consider myself competent in this area. From the time I decided to take this job, I knew that I had a responsibility to be properly trained. Immediately, I began taking all the low or no cost trainings I could find while researching more advanced training programs. To date, I have completed somewhere north of 200 hours of training and education on the use of psychedelics for mental health treatment, including completing postgraduate certification in ketamine-assisted psychotherapy (KAP) and psychedelic therapy and integration (PTI) through Fluence (n.d.) and MDMA therapy education through the Multidisciplinary Association for Psychedelic Studies (MAPS) (n.d.). I dove head first into my new role with a fire and excitement I'd never experienced in my professional life, and I remain excited about continuing to learn and grow into this role.

Since this was a brand-new role for all parties involved, I was able to create a KAP program from scratch, using information from my training program, researching, consulting, and learning everything I could about how to create a successful KAP program. Fast forward a couple of years, I work in partnership with some amazing medical providers, where I provide preparation and integration sessions to infusion patients and ketamine-assisted psychotherapy to those using oral routes of ketamine administration. I also provide psychedelic harm reduction and integration (PHRI) services to those using psychedelic medicines in other contexts and consultation services to other professionals who want to learn more about this area of mental health treatment or to better support their client who is engaged in such treatment.

Additionally, I have recently expanded the KAP program to include a support group, as I have learned that many clients are hesitant to tell loved ones about their treatment—usually due to things like fear of judgment from others or uncertainty whether the medicine will even help them—and going through this intense treatment can feel very lonely at times. Group is a place where people can experience a sense of community, connection, and support from others who are also addressing mental health concerns, while being able to practice providing that same sense of support to others in a safe environment.

When I did my own ketamine treatment, there was no option to sandwich an infusion with psychotherapy. Starting this work was all still relatively new to me, and yet, somehow, it felt so right. I no longer felt restless or uncomfortable in my job; I didn't find myself longing to do something more—something deeper. It felt like coming home, and for the first time in my professional life, I knew I was exactly where I was supposed to be.

The Responsibility of Doing Meaningful Work

Working with people who use psychedelics, whether natural or synthetic, to improve their well-being is an incredibly special space. It can be a space that provides safety and connection; it can facilitate healing—often rapidly—and a hopefulness that things can get better.

In my practice, KAP and PHRI are short-term treatment models. I typically have a very limited number of sessions prior to a client starting treatment; oftentimes, I hear from people who are seeking help after a difficult experience with using psychedelics on their own. Being able to quickly build rapport and establish trust is of utmost priority.

I have a deep level of empathy for others, as I assume (or hope) many people in the helping profession might. One of my strengths, regardless of setting, is the ability to earn the trust of others and build deep connections quickly. This is a gift that gets to shine in this work, and one I do not take lightly; I am continually humbled by this work.

Meeting people where they are has also always been at the center of my professional work, regardless of setting—to accept others fully and wholly, exactly as they are. I also value being authentic and transparent with clients, to whatever extent is appropriate and beneficial in a given situation.

Some of the best advice I received was shortly after completing graduate school. A wiser, more experienced clinician told me that I should always be mindful of why I'm speaking in a client's session—is what I'm about to say going to help me or the client? And, of course, if it's the former, don't say it. I've heard several different ways of saying this over the years, but the meaning at the core of this advice has guided my work over the years.

Prior to my work as a psychedelic therapist, I rarely self-disclosed in session. More specifically, I never even fathomed disclosing anything as personal as my own mental health treatment. To be fair, I still don't self-disclose often, and I still use much discernment in this area, but now when I do self-disclose, it is a powerful tool.

When working with ketamine clients, they occasionally ask me, "Have you ever experienced ketamine?" I was told before starting this job that it was likely for clients to ask if I'd ever been through ketamine treatment, so I spent time reflecting and consulting with more experienced providers about how I'd answer when the question arises.

If I answer "no," or reflect the question back to the client (i.e., "Why is my treatment experience important for you to know?"), I am not responding in a manner that supports increased trust or strengthened rapport. Answering "no" means not being authentic, and clients can usually tell if their therapist is not being real with them. "No" can support a client remaining guarded and create a greater feeling of isolation on their healing journey. Reflecting the question back is simply rhetorical—I know clients ask out of uncertainty and fear.

What if I can help calm that fear by just being honest? I have found that, in this particular setting, the use of careful self-disclosure is typically more beneficial to the client than saying no or reflecting the question back to them. What does this look like in an actual session? When I answer, "Yes," there is a look or a felt sense of realization that "Oh, this therapist really does understand the range of mixed emotions I'm experiencing around starting this treatment." And that is usually the extent of questions from clients about my own experience with ketamine. I don't volunteer this information without the client asking, and interestingly, I don't get asked this question as often as I anticipated; however, when I do, I see the use of brief and thoughtful self-disclosure as a tool to support increased trust, decreased fear, and stronger rapport. This use of self-disclosure can also help instill a deeper sense of hope that this treatment could help them, too, as they see their therapist who has been through the same treatment is healthy, happy, working full time—areas in which clients often hope to experience improvement.

This is what works well in my practice and is a decision that was made after much contemplation and consultation; when used in this way, self-disclosure can be a powerful tool in my toolbox. Still, this can be a tricky area in which we always need to be mindful of our intentions when sharing.

The Challenges of Psychedelic Work

I find my work as a psychedelic therapist to be exciting, rewarding, and deeply meaningful. Many clients experience rapid symptom relief, and witnessing such a transformation is nothing short of mind-blowing. However, this rapid relief often presents with its own set of challenges.

Many of the clients I work with are pursuing ketamine or other psychedelic medicines as a last resort; often, they have tried countless psychotropic medications, various therapy modalities, transcranial magnetic stimulation (TMS), electroconvulsive therapy (ECT)—all without sufficient symptom relief. When a client experiences rapid improvement with the use of psychedelic medicines, it is sometimes a feeling they've never experienced, and this unfamiliar feeling can be quite overwhelming and even exacerbate anxiety symptoms. Learning this firsthand from clients, I have been able to discuss this potential and be better prepared to help clients manage the situation if it arises.

Another challenge of this work is when the medicine does not prove to be an effective (or effective enough) treatment. If a client views this treatment modality as a last resort and they do not experience relief, it is easy to understand their feelings of defeat and increased hopelessness and helplessness they might experience. As the therapist, this can certainly create challenges, but it can also create opportunities for me to stretch myself and grow, as it often takes much creativity to find ways to best support the client who feels defeated. Helping clients find motivation to keep moving forward and not give up when they've lost all hope is not for the faint of heart; it requires patience, determination, and creativity. This particular challenge is an excellent example of how therapeutic work can be both an art and a science, and the balance between the two is where change and growth can transpire.

Although I work with a short-term treatment model, to terminate a client because they did not respond to the medicine would be irresponsible and unethical; I will continue working collaboratively with the client until there is a plan in place for the next steps of their care. Therefore, challenges such as these can be an opportunity for the client's growth as well, as it allows the person to see that they are not alone in the process, that someone else is on their team, and that they are not going to be abandoned in moments of such despair.

Looking to the Future

After years of working with diverse client populations, working in various settings, taking countless trainings—diligently searching for an area of mental health treatment that I am passionate about—the work of psychedelic therapy found me. Only after I made the conscious effort to focus more on being than doing, did everything start to fall in place for me professionally. I no longer feel restless or complacent; I am exactly where I'm supposed to be.

I am hopeful for the future of psychedelic therapies and the potential benefits they hold. At the same time, I have concerns about the accessibility of such therapies, as well as accessibility of adequate training for providers. Increased access to and inclusion in psychedelic therapy and training is an area I feel strongly about, and I continually seek ways to become more involved with people and movements that are working to increase access and inclusion.

It is important to note that knowing where I'm supposed to be does not equal complacency. Rather, it indicates a dire need for continued dedication and hard work. For me, this includes staying up to date with current research; ensuring adherence to the highest standards of ethical client care; having solid self-care practices and keeping myself healthy; setting boundaries, both professionally and personally; continued training and education; and ongoing consultation, community, and connection with other psychedelic providers.

The ways in which my previous professional experiences support my current work leave me with no doubt that, despite past hesitations or feelings of restlessness or yearning for something more, I was exactly where I was supposed to be every step of the way, from my very first job working in a harm reduction substance use setting to better prepare me for later doing psychedelic harm reduction work to dual licensure that allowed me a wide variety of work opportunities. Without these experiences, I would not be the clinician that I am today; every single experience has been valuable and supported my future work in some capacity.

In the very early days of my work as a psychedelic therapist, I found a way of talking about psychedelic medicine in a pretty relatable way; I explain that the medicine itself does not give the answers; rather, it can help provide access to the information and more insight and clarity around what is needed for healing. In the movie, *The Wizard of Oz*, Dorothy sets out on a long journey in the effort to find her way back home, only to eventually discover that she held everything she needed to get home all along (Fleming, 1939). Everything that is needed for us to find healing or relief, or to discover how to live authentically, or whatever "going home" looks like for an individual, is already within each of us. We may just need help accessing the information, which can often be provided by psychedelic medicines and the therapeutic process.

Even in the most challenging of times, I find much joy in my work as a psychedelic therapist and I am grateful for the opportunity to share about my experience. In closing, I urge readers to remember and reflect on, perhaps from a brand-new perspective: "You've always had the power, my dear, you just had to learn it for yourself" (Fleming, 1939).

References

Fleming, V. (Director). (1939). *The Wizard of Oz* [Film]. Metro-Goldwyn-Mayer.

Fluence. (n.d.). *Professional education in psychedelic therapy* [training and certification]. https://www.fluencetraining.com/

MAPS. (n.d.). *MAPS' international therapist education program.* Multidisciplinary Association for Psychedelic Studies. https://maps.org/

It is never too late to be who you might have been.

—George Eliot

Dr. Adekemi Oguntala

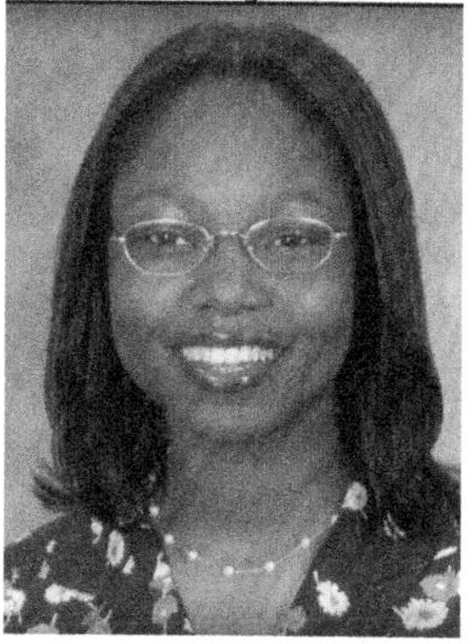

Dr. Adekemi Oguntala, or Dr. O, is a teen physician who received an undergraduate education at the University of California, Berkeley, a medical degree from what is now Drexel University, and her pediatric residency at St. Christopher's Hospital for Children, both located in Philadelphia, Pennsylvania. She also did an adolescent medicine fellowship at Stanford University. She is available for teaching and speaking opportunities.
theteendoc@gmail.com

Psychedelics and the Role of Shame in Medicine and Psychotherapy

I trained in allopathic medicine and therefore know the importance of pharmaceutical medicine. I had family members who needed medicine to get better. And then as a physician training in the ICU, I saw patients who were there only because their parents did not believe in medicine, a belief that often cost them their child's health, if not life. My training shunned the use of drugs not prescribed by a clinician. This changed when opiate use increased in middle America and changed again when psychedelics proved a way to advance the emotional work desperately needed by so many to survive what we know now is the shame of relational trauma. As a trauma-informed medical clinician, I now know opiate use was never just about over prescribing any more than the diseases I treat were just about having asthma. Failure to recognize the role of shame in human behaviors that eventually lead to medical disease limited the impact I could have through medical intervention.

I trained in adolescent medicine and was always in the position of seeing the fork in the road for teens, where a series of changes could make their lives go either way: inner peace or anxiety and depression. Stanford trained me to look for eating disorders but never discussed shame. So each appointment with a teen and their parents was me speaking to a co-conspirator I never realized was in the room: debilitating shame. That is, until I started reading books by neuroscience doctors like Dan Siegel (2012). This changed how I practiced: I started asking questions about how events and interactions affected patients and soon realized that the impact of diseases, pregnancy, and grades were not dependent on my ability to order a lab or ensure a birth control method, even though this was what I was tested on. Addressing these symptoms was dependent on whether I could get my patients to see that they mattered: that they were worthy of love and belonging despite how they believed their parents or anyone else felt about or treated them. This was no small task. You can't just tell a person they are worthy and have them believe it, and you can't ask a parent to change a parenting practice that has been passed down like an heirloom. It turns out the debilitating shame that is part of not believing oneself worthy is the cause of what adolescent medicine typically dismissed as noncompliance and teen rebellion. So now the question was how to get a teen to care about themselves when they think they don't matter.

To answer questions of healing or treatment, medicine will always ask about cause. What causes this disease process? Shame was never considered a medical illness so it was never evaluated as the cause of so much disease. It's still not clear that clinicians consistently make a connection between childhood shame and disease process, despite saying they are trauma informed. Shame occurs in our relationships with others. The feelings of worthlessness, not feeling good enough, fear, and as one patient described it, feeling like trash come from being in a relationship where we are not seen or heard for who we are. Instead, our value is placed on our utility, productivity. This leads to self-criticism and perfectionism in the struggle to attain an unrealistic ideal. When we fall short, we have an inner critical voice that internalizes the emotional and psychological violence of our relationships. Shame is created in our relationship with others, and the first relationships we have are with our caretakers and families. Emptiness, unlovability, and loneliness are healed the way they are created: through relationships that are healthy or secure attachments, as explained by researchers John Bowlby and Mary Ainsworth (Bowlby, 1969; Ainsworth & Bell, 1970). The concept of shame became a key element that I sought to integrate into my medical practice.

I read *The Body Keeps the Score* by Dr. Bessel van der Kolk (2014), and the pages on internal family systems (IFS) caught my attention (p. 283). After reading and finding any course possible, I began using IFS to elicit the part of the teen that carried the worthlessness that allowed protectors or coping mechanisms like substance use, sexual promiscuity, and school failure to be the most visible signs of the teen's shame. When I could get teens to understand their story from a place of compassion, there was less interest in high-risk coping skills, and behaviors changed. They no longer used weed to numb, and these teens had a greater sense of what they wanted to do with their lives, no longer doubting their worthiness and gaining confidence that comes from knowing they matter to themselves. This was great for another set of patients who found the changes in how they felt about themselves decreasing their need for ADHD medication.

When I was able to discuss key parenting issues that were really legacy burdens with parents, I saw even more things change for not just the teen but the parents and family as a whole. Still, there were students whose pain was so intense that the fear of looking at it was too overwhelming. They sat mute in sessions. They were unable to utter any part of their story in order to process it. They could nod or look at me if I was able to guess what was in their head, but they could not speak. This is how severe their shame was. That's when I signed up for a psychedelic conference and decided to listen to what they had to say about psychedelics and mental health. I knew I could extrapolate the information to medicine.

Accounts of the patients who had experienced psychedelic journeys using MDMA and ketamine were incredibly impactful. They were mentioning the exact type of patient I was having trouble with: those who had a story of chronic or toxic shame, who could not see themselves as worthy and had no hope of relieving that burden. I thought about the patients I couldn't work with anymore because they didn't make enough progress to convince themselves that the emotional work was worth it. Talk therapy was not enough, and somatic therapy was hard because they were so numb that the progress was achingly slow. They would shame themselves for not being able to do the emotional work. I made the decision to see what ketamine was about.

I found someone trained in ketamine-assisted psychotherapy (KAP) to help me with a long-time patient of mine who struggled to get past dorsal vagal collapse no matter what we tried to discuss. There were three sessions done, and initially it didn't feel like anything had happened, but then I noticed that they (my client's preferred pronoun) could endure more difficult questions and we could talk without their collapsing into a dorsal vagal slumber. Something had indeed changed. They didn't remember a lot from their ketamine journey, save the concern that their parent would think it was a waste of money if they didn't "do it right." This was one of the few things the ketamine practitioner jotted down, but not much else could be recalled. As far as I could tell, no opportunity was taken to ask about any concerns around the parent-child dynamic, gender, or other beliefs that were most likely preventing my client from completing tasks. This was why I wanted an IFS practitioner for them. Instead, during my session with them, I brought up those issues, and to my surprise, they were able to talk about some of this stuff, finally! They were able to start feeling something as they talked about their shame in this and other situations. This meant they could begin to recognize the warning signs of hypoarousal in their body and pause to check in with themselves before complete collapse. Over time, they could offer themselves more kindness as we worked toward compassion or recognize how they used anger to block the compassion toward what was really sadness. The moments of collapse became few, and when they appeared, it was more obvious that something difficult was happening for them. This was critical because they were about to leave for university away from home, and the potential to feel shame and not good enough was risky in an engineering program. But, these baby steps were starting to lighten their shame burden.

What I recognized with the person who helped me do the ketamine session with this teen client was that the practitioner did not use the internal family systems (IFS) model as well as I had hoped. This was the modality with somatic elements that had really impressed me at the conference. The impact of IFS, which already has a structured framework for connecting with Self-energy, is intensified with psychedelics on board. The combination boosted compassionate feelings through elevated oxytocin, in the case of MDMA, and dissociation or observation, in the case of ketamine, which made space for the client's compassion to be guided toward their traumatic event. The ability to unblend from the emotional burden of shameful past experiences allows us to revisit them with new perspectives and knowledge and save ourselves. When shame, in the form of fear, threatens to revisit that moment of trauma with the same overwhelming feeling that incapacitated our younger selves, we are paralyzed and immediately become stuck. Using IFS during the latter part of a ketamine journey is a great opportunity to put the patient in the seat of the observer of the suffering, as Michael Singer (2007) describes, instead of being overwhelmed by it. This perspective comes with the gifts of Self-energy as described by Dick Shwartz (2020) as the 8 Cs: calm, clarity, confidence, compassion, courage, connection, curiosity, and creativity, plus kindness (p. 45). This perspective reflects those of many Indigenous and other spiritual traditions, further resonating with the history of psychedelics.

I use this concept of the observer in conjunction with ketamine to allow the client to take topics they could not talk about and use the latter half of the ketamine session to process difficult things. Our worth is not dependent on a grade, romantic partner, or accomplishment when we can offer ourselves radical amounts of compassion and validation when we are hurting. These steps seem intuitive with psychedelics. This is different from the pseudo-positive self-talk of entitlement. Psychedelics potentially allow access to the space of our mind-body connection, where compassion overrides criticism. It allows some space between our thoughts and who we think we are. People heal as they are able to create a relationship with themselves where they believe they are worthy of love and belonging.

I wasn't there to pursue these directions with my initial ketamine client during their first session, though I knew the client better than the person who conducted that session did. Shame is created in a relationship, and it is healed in securely attached relationships, first with an external person; further healing then occurs when the client begins a securely attached relationship to what IFS would call their parts or themselves. So I took more classes and did the subsequent KAP sessions myself.

Since that time, I have seen psychedelics like ketamine and MDMA allow people to truly heal toxic levels of shame that have inhibited emotional and psychological growth, especially in a way that gives them a sense of Self-energy. When patients are able to experience what worthiness feels like, the emotional work makes more sense. And it makes more sense that we have to heal the past through decreasing shame, which is done through compassion. This is how my clients get to see the impact the past has on the present moment. It is how the past gives clarity to current abusive or traumatic situations that are feeling implicitly familiar. The ability to name the feeling and recognize the etiology empowers my clients to recognize the uncertainty or manipulation of the past. These concepts were also appreciated sociopolitically in various isms of exclusion that they could see were now based in shame and childhood trauma and not personal: like a boss humiliating them the way a teacher might have in grade school. This information was priceless when discussed in the latter part of ketamine journeys. These were buried memories my client had not had explicit access to. They logically understood the events might have happened in the past, but to tie it together let them see they were not overreacting. This is critical when validating anyone, but especially BIPOC and otherized groups. And for White men in particular who refused to see they had been harmed by fathers they worshiped or mothers who were complicit, it created understanding of extreme protectors, IFS language for ego states (Schwartz, 2020), to never be controlled by anyone, including the perceived emotional needs of their children as controlling.

I kept fine-tuning the psychedelic experience for my clients who gave me feedback in small ways about the taste of the medicine, the issues associated with it like indigestion, and the music, because sometimes a song would really bother them and they would have to say it in the middle of sessions. As I did this, each experience for the client got better!

I learned new ways to decolonize psychedelic sessions that added to my clients' well-being irrespective of gender, ethnicity, or religion. One place this showed up was in the choice of music. I initially had a typical music offering, but clients sometimes gave feedback that the sounds were very Eastern, or words I thought were inspirational were jarring depending on the part of the journey. The music became distracting or pulled them out of the initial onset of the medication. I did what was suggested or used playlists given to me. With each journey, I saw how critical this part was for the experience.

Entering and exiting the journey would have lyrical songs at very low volume. For example, "I AM" by Stan Walker (Indigenous New Zealand, Māori), "Shinunoga E-Wa" by Fugii Kazi (Japan), "Unbound" by Robbie Robertson (Indigenous American), and "Without You" by Teeks (Indigenous New Zealand, Māori). Here, I needed the words to be a source of validation, invoke curiosity about themselves, or be calming if clients were anxious. I often asked clients for a song that I placed first to ensure that they could anchor in familiarity if it was very important to them or they were nervous. One client, knowing how important the session was to connecting with her inner kids, asked for "Te Guardo" by Silvana Estrada (Xalapa, Veracruz, Mexico) knowing the artist discusses this theme in the song. The actual journey was marked by songs also at minimal volume like "Kothbiro" by Ayub Ogada (Kenya), "Why Not?" Jónsi (Iceland), "A New Day" by Ludwig Göranson (Swedish), "Agape" by Nicholas Britell (American), "We Bring Tribute" by Terence Blanchard (American), and "The Belt of Faith" by Jung Jae-il (South Korea). These songs in a certain order allowed me to represent the global diversity in sounds so there was an audible representation of connection or oneness with the global community. We know this feeling of connection is part of Self-energy and makes us see the role we have in caring for more than ourselves and seeing how we fit into the world, the universe. This was a core concept of Indigenous communities who did not understand not sharing or the ability to sell property. This trait of Self-energy changes the attachment to the world: instead of disconnection, there is connection. Self-energy transitions many clients from I, me, mine to what Siegel (2022) calls Mwe, an integration of self, identity, and belonging. This made for a natural transition to discuss clients' parts around racism, prejudice, and otherization.

The music became important because clients could later listen and recall the feelings of spirit, ātman, and Self obtained in the ketamine-induced state without ketamine, just using music, the body scan, and the awareness of being in the seat of the observer as practiced in session. They could use the IFS tools to find the part of them that was suffering, hear their story, validate the feelings brought up from past events, offer compassion, and learn to be there for the parts of them that were hurting. Knowing so much of their story made perceived shameful stories opportunities to connect with what they experienced rather than just how it made them feel. Gentle reminders I could provide underscored that when these events initially happened, the client was powerless and alone, but such tools as ketamine, IFS, and music let them feel empowered to help the part of them suffering rather than distract from their suffering. This is a gamechanger for those who experience toxic shame.

The ketamine session soundtrack became one more emotional regulation tool, and this meant my clients could use the playlist to be in that low shame and high compassion state while connecting with themselves beyond the KAP session. They were developing secure attachments with parts of themselves. This is the difference between giving someone a fish and teaching someone to fish. The client could continue emotional processing after the session, without ketamine on board. They would remember the way I promoted curiosity about an incident, connect with those parts more deeply, and be able to process another feeling the same way. When they got stuck or couldn't figure it out, the sessions pushed them along; because I knew their story, I could offer them moments from their lives they may have minimized or forgotten. These became easier because all the tools implemented together create what IFS calls a critical mass of Self-energy to show themselves more kindness rather than shame causing avoidance and isolation. Repeatedly, clients would remark in and after sessions that having a guide they could trust was so important. Again, I could see that secure relationships heal shame and improve outcomes.

Of course, it's not all rainbows and unicorns. Some clients who described using psychedelics did not do IFS or did not talk at all or did not have someone there when they took medication that was prescribed by a provider but self-administered. So often those with a heavy shame burden opt to do the prescription instead of integrating sessions, and this is not as impactful. My clients who got psychedelics online or did a group experience noticed that a guided session changed what they got out of the experience. This didn't mean other clients who chose a different method got nothing out of it, but clients noticed that what I described in our consent sessions was different from previous information that came from someone who had done KAP in a non-guided way. Others would dismiss ketamine as something that got people addicted because that was what the news had been reporting. They didn't see the potential, and this helped me see that there was something else those clients had in common that I worked with: a foundation of trauma therapy.

Clients' previous non-KAP sessions with me gave them an idea of where they were stuck, so they had a very clear intention for the KAP journey. When trauma therapy continued after ketamine, I could point out the effects of ketamine in session by noticing how they had been open to processing information they would have been too afraid of before the KAP session. To me, it defeats the point of a lived experience when we have not processed the events that ultimately shape who we are. Yes, someone could say this is the power of integration sessions, but integration is potentially even more powerful when the relationship of someone who knows you can help you make connections that might otherwise be missed.

There is true possibility in the tsunami of psychedelics to come, but we can't forget that the foundation of so many conditions is the shame of relational trauma. IFS training asks if the practitioner is Self-led, or in a state of awareness. IFS draws on Indigenous concepts that understand that the role of the shaman or healer is someone who is fully present and can regulate emotions. Coregulation is what gives clinicians the intuition to know if a client is in distress or needs to work something out on their own. Mindfulness and connection with the universe permit a low state of shame and higher state of compassion, and this is what is essential for shame in another person to heal. People recognize this state with comments like "It felt bigger than myself." The relationship is where the injury happened, and the relationship between the practitioner and the client models a secure attachment that can open a person up to accessing their own healing qualities. Psychedelics together with the secure relationship enhance that process, creating an emotional environment where the person feels safe enough to listen to the parts of them that have needed to be validated, heard, and seen.

Psychedelic therapies have true potential to heal people so they are connected to their emotional body and can feel what Porges (2017) calls "neuroception," neurological safety (p. 19). This is part of trauma therapy that has shown that when we help clients understand their family history and the sociopolitical context of that history, they can be more compassionate towards themselves. They can heal layers of shame that are not theirs, while taking responsibility for what they can and should be doing for themselves emotionally.

References

Ainsworth, M.D., & Bell, S.M. (1970). Attachment, exploration, and separation: Illustrated by the behavior of one-year-olds in a strange situation. *Child Development, 41*(1), 141-61.

Bowlby, J. (1969). *Attachment and loss.* Basic Books.

Porges, S. W. (2017). *The pocket guide to the polyvagal theory: The transformative power of feeling safe.* W. W. Norton & Co.

Shwartz, R. C. (2020). *Internal family systems therapy.* The Guilford Press.

Siegel, D. (2012). *The developing mind: How relationships and the brain interact to shape who we are (2nd edition).* Guilford Press.

Siegel, D. (2022, October 3). Dr. Dan Siegel talks IntraConnected—MWe (Me + We). *The Science of Psychotherapy* [Video]. YouTube. https://youtu.be/TrgjF9xLaGg?si=oA8h5nJTUcAAJMi.

Singer, M. (2007). *The untethered soul: The journey beyond yourself.* New Harbinger Publications.

Van der Kolk, B. A. (2014). *The body keeps the score: Brain, mind, and body in the healing of trauma.* Viking.

Once we believe in ourselves, we can risk curiosity, wonder, spontaneous delight, or any experiences that reveals the human spirit.

—e.e. cummings

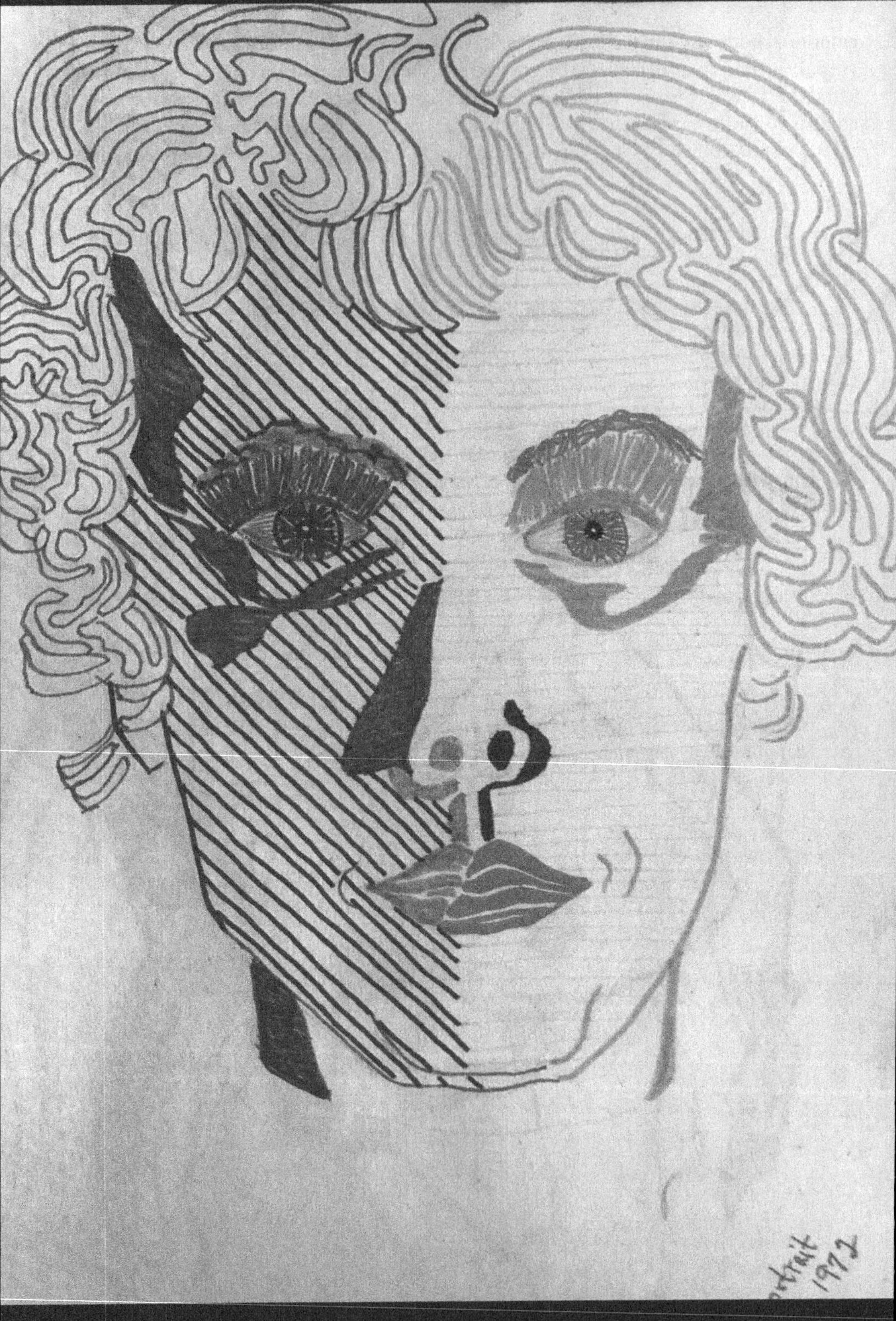

trait
1972

Heidi J. Dalzell

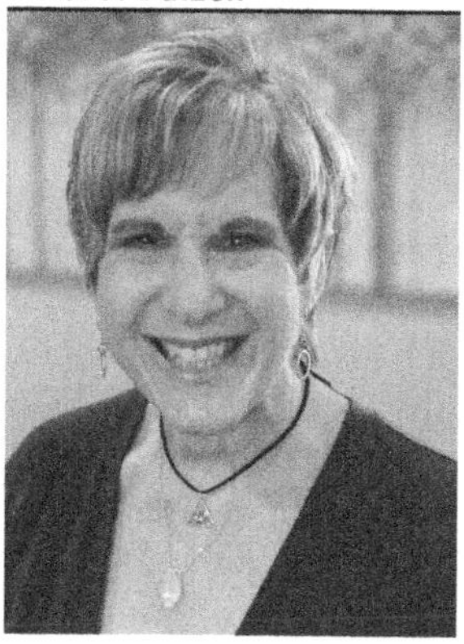

Heidi J. Dalzell, PsyD, is a licensed clinical psychologist with over 30 years of experience, specializing in trauma and eating disorders. Particular interests include non-ordinary states, psychedelic medicines, and mid-life eating disorders. Dr. Dalzell is certified in ketamine-assisted psychotherapy through the Polaris Insight Center. She is also a trained psychedelic sitter/guide, through The Guiding Presence, and is completing training through the Integrative Psychiatric Center for additional certifications in ketamine-assisted psychotherapy, working with psilocybin, and as a MAPS-trained MDMA facilitator.
hmdalzell@verizon.net

An Embodied Path

Begin to see yourself as a soul with a body, rather than a body with a soul.

—Wayne Dyer

While I have few memories of childhood, one that stands out is the painting hanging above my childhood bed. The painting is of a young girl holding a stray cat. Tears leak from her large brown eyes. The artist, Margaret Keane, understood secrets as well as I: She, not her husband, painted the popular big-eyed waifs. Each night, I would stare at the painting, keeping my feelings and grief carefully concealed. They remained buried deep beneath the delicious food I'd consume, offered in lieu of comfort by my well-meaning grandparents.

Fast forward more than half a century; I'm now an adult participating in a Peruvian plant medicine ceremony. The *Despacho*, a traditional Indigenous gratitude ceremony, has ended, and our guide—part shaman, part therapist—encourages us to quickly drink the sweet earthy liquid. The cacao doesn't fully mask the psilocybin's mushroom (Steel Magnolias) earthiness, vaguely bringing to mind Campbell's soup.

The pungent flavor lingers. Our facilitator also consumes the sacred cacao, allowing her access to the realms we will visit. We set intentions: mine to heal my grief connected to the death of my father a little over a year ago. Since setting that intention, I'd started to feel angrier about the deathbed promise he had extracted—care for a family member with whom I have a difficult relationship. This role and the need to attend to her emotions rather than my own hasn't allowed me to grieve. I was also grieving the decision to leave the therapy practice I'd built with a colleague.

As I finished the cacao, I reminded myself to hold the intention loosely with an openness to whatever might arise. Every journey is so different.

I counsel a fairly stoic therapy clientele. Many are Boomers or Gen Xers, who have been schooled in the art of repression, conflating stoicism with strength. Family secrets could easily topple the image of the perfect family. I often hear stories of secrets such as job loss, deaths, alcoholism, and mental illness. Some echo the secrets in my own family-of-origin that the big-eyed girl in my childhood painting held in our shared silence.

I specialize in eating disorders, where such emotional restriction accompanies food restriction or binging. Most people with eating disorders live in their heads, as logical as *Star Trek's* Spock, instead of in their bodies where they feel. Embodiment is the sense of feeling safe to connect to one's body and practicing body mindfulness: noticing physical and emotional sensations connected to the body in a present nonjudgmental way.

But how many of us are truly embodied? During my psychedelic journey I recognized that I struggled with disembodiment much like my clients.

The effects of the mushrooms came on quickly. My senses were staggeringly acute, so much so that it was virtually impossible to ignore my body. The medicine did not leave the barest possibility that I could. I was nauseous from almost the first sip of cacao; I alternated between focusing internally on my body, and externally on my surroundings. The music appeared to be blaring; those around me emoted a cacophony of laughter, tears, and occasional exclamations of ecstasy. I was both fascinated and repelled by the depth of emotion.

I felt angry at them. How were they allowed to show such emotions?

Embodiment opened the gateway to memories. That night I dreamed about my mother's fatal car accident. I saw myself as a child on the porch of our house, playing out the accident with toy dolls and trucks. The porch door opened and my father and stepmother rendered a stern lecture, forbidding me to play that way.

Upon waking, I reflected on how my father's deathbed promise again curtailed my grieving. Watching other group members fully express their own emotions was profoundly healing. As I opened my journal to reflect on how profound this dream was, my emotions opened up as well. Tears streamed down my face as I described—and experienced—the sadness, confusion, and anger that little girl felt. I was also aware of the physical sensations: rumbling stomach slowly settling, and the peace I felt as a clearing of these emotions and an opening in my chest.

My clients relate similar experiences. Starving, binging, and purging numb their emotions well, but their bodies bear the ravages, becoming an unwelcome place. Ketamine, the only legal compound that can act as a psychedelic, allows emotion to arise safely and uncensored.

Consider my client Anna (all names changed). A diminutive woman in her 40s, Anna had struggled with anorexia most of her life. Anna was raised in a wealthy home. As a child she was often compared to her paternal grandmother. Her grandmother had been frequently moody and depressed; she'd struggled with a severe eating disorder and ultimately took her own life. This comparison was not wholly unwelcome; Anna's father loved his mother immensely and still seemed to be grieving. "His mother's death seemed like the one thing he did care about," Anna said. "Besides that, all that mattered to him was his work." Anna craved his approval to little avail.

Anna made the unconscious decision to become more like her grandmother. By the time Anna graduated from high school, her family was burned out by her frequent eating disorder hospitalizations and precarious health. Her father issued an ultimatum: get well or move out. Desperate, Anna turned to a teacher at her school. He offered Anna a place to stay, with the condition of secrecy about their relationship. The significant age difference and need for secrecy further distanced Anna from friends and extended family.

Desperate to escape from the eating disorder and this relationship, Anna contemplated suicide. Then she read Michael Pollan's (2018) book, *How to Change Your Mind,* which kindled a spark of hope. Ketamine-assisted psychotherapy (KAP) seemed like a great fit.

Anna's mood was brighter after only a few KAP sessions. She described this as a shift in her body; she felt more relaxed than she had in years. "I never even noticed how tight my muscles were, how I clenched my jaw and face." While experiencing the medicine journey, Anna described this as "a softness in my body. I've never welcomed softness before." I suggested that she spend time each day returning to this feeling. As she did so, the constant thoughts of suicide diminished.

The physical feeling of ketamine is difficult to describe. It feels gentler than many psychedelic medicines I've tried. While not everyone finds this a pleasant feeling, my experience of the medicine—a dissociative—was of floating on a cloud. There was a sense of freedom and expansiveness, a simultaneous connection both to the universe and to the me that was not body. Body was no longer important, soul was.

Even clients who are not particularly spiritual often experience similar insights. My client Megan's impetus to seek therapy was her father's sudden death from complications of COVID-19. Their relationship was complicated. He'd been a demanding parent, seeking perfection in the form of high grades and low body weight. Megan was not a naturally thin child, but constant low-calorie diets ensured that she met his weight expectations during their weekly weigh-ins.

Since her father's passing, free of his restrictions, Megan's abandon around food has become a constant hunger she freely satisfies. What at first felt like a reclaiming has now morphed into a helpless sense of rebellion and feeling out of control.

Megan opted to do a series of KAP sessions, progressing to a higher dose in which she began to actively confront her traumas. During one impactful session, she experienced her father, seemingly contrite, apologizing for how harsh he'd been with her. "I didn't know how to do things any better," he said; "I just wanted you to be happy." Megan recognized that the image she first thought was her father was actually her body, and it was irate about Megan's binge eating. As Megan continued in the ketamine journey, tears fell freely. She described the experience thusly: "I noticed a light, and I was floating, and it got brighter, and the voice got softer." The hatred "seemed to float from my body," replaced by "softness." In our debrief, I asked how this might apply to her intention of body kindness. Megan struggled to find the words, finally settling on "It's finally time to change."

During her integration sessions, Megan focused on mindful self-compassion and body attunement. Some of the more concrete changes Megan made included daily gentle movement, yoga, and lovingkindness meditation. Change was slow and steady.

I also often recommend family constellation work, a method created by psychologist Bert Hellinger (2011) and based on family systems therapy and Indigenous South African beliefs. Family constellation techniques incorporating psychodrama, family sculpting, and energy psychology are helpful in processing and integrating insights from the psychedelic experience. I've found these helpful in integrating my own psychedelic journeys. Family constellations tend to have no explanation as to how they promote healing. They are energetic in nature. Anna, while a skeptic, is remarkably open to trying even more woo-woo approaches. Anna continues to see change as a result of her hard work. She interacts more freely with family members. She's maintained her weight at the lower end of normal. She's slowly gaining confidence that she can move on from her eating disorder and a relationship she now sees as unhealthy.

Psychedelic medicines, while not a cure-all, are helpful, and while their mechanisms are not fully known, the process of embodiment may be part of the reason for their efficacy. I'm an advocate of their possibilities.

References

Hellinger, B. (2011). *Laws of healing.* Washington, DC: Hellinger Publications.

Pollan, M. (2018). *How to change your mind.* New York: Penguin Books.

Psychedelics are a way of shaking up the snow globe.

—Robin Carhart-Harris

Tali Silver

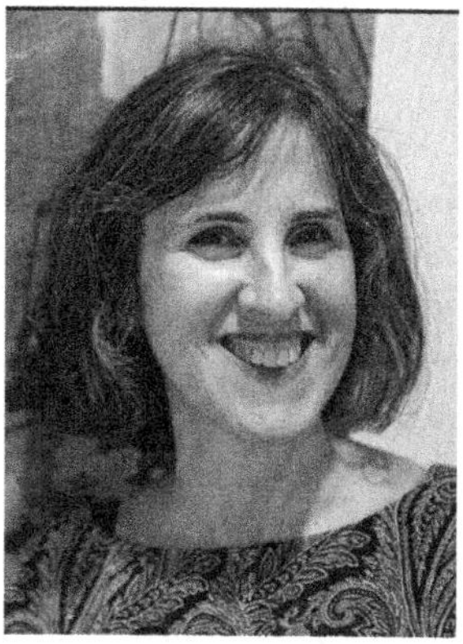

Tali Silver, MA, IAAP, is a Jungian analyst in private practice in Stoneham, Massachusetts. She immigrated from Israel to the United States to complete her master's in expressive therapy and raised her family near Boston. She was an adjunct at Endicott College and currently teaches and serves as a training analyst at the C.G. Jung Institute of New England. She enjoys writing, painting, nature, and the miracle of walking.
silvertali21@gmail.com

Just Going Not Knowing

With permission and deep gratitude, I present a case-based inquiry into psychedelic-assisted therapy in the treatment of a severely traumatized woman. In the following account and analysis of a single psilocybin retreat, her words are quoted in italics. Pertinent images are symbolically mined in the integration process.

Deidre's narrative and mine co-create a screen upon which her complex, dissociative inner world is projected and illuminated. Jung (2016) spoke of the essential task of bringing to consciousness imagery that holds the opposites, toward a new synthesis. I elaborate on images from Deidre's hallucinations that contain vivid oppositions and show how their processing increased awareness. I point out tensions between her hope to heal through psilocybin and co-occurring blows to her health and functioning. This case begs the question of the experience of patients with severe dissociation, who disregard recommendations and pursue psilocybin.

Background Information and the First 3 Years of Analytical Psychotherapy

Deidre began analysis with me in her mid-50s. She had an earlier 10-year Freudian-Lacanian analysis. She is a worldly, educated immigrant and a competent professional in a committed relationship. An only child of Jewish survivors of World War II, she suffered an insulating childhood, bullying, torture, and multiple rapes. She presented with lacerating despair, dissociation, self-harm, and self-medication. Hospitalization was avoided due to it triggering the medical environment in which she had been tortured. In-session flashbacks externalized what she had endured. To increase containment, a one-a-day exchange was established: a photo by her and a brief text response by me. It became part of the frame, a non-verbal channel of communication and an outlet for her unacknowledged creative gifts. She said, *When your response hits the mark, I feel seen.*

Deidre was caught in a cycle of exploding and collapsing. She called herself a stray bullet. It was miraculous that she maintained the external trappings of a functional life. She felt trapped in a tyrannical regime with a looming death sentence. She pitched the idea of psilocybin as a last resort. Considering her history of poly-substance abuse, it seemed risky. Contraindications were spelled out; that she had survived so much was no guarantee against a breakdown. Even though it is classified as a hallucinogen and not a dissociative drug (National Institute on Drugs, 2014), psilocybin might worsen her dissociation. On the other hand, in a safe setting, with proper preparation and integration, it might help her get unstuck.

Deidre felt compelled to go for it. Rejecting the legal route of clinical trials, she found a guide and mustered the trust to sign up. She sobered for a few weeks and read extensively about psilocybin. She knew that the trip could only bring up what was already inside of her and that her reaction would be critical. She formulated intentions: *To free myself from the grip of pain and helplessness. To stop running and find a way to just be. To see myself from a different perspective.*

The journey took place during our 4th year of treatment. Deidre said it was rough and disappointing but not traumatizing. She had no flashbacks to it, nor delusions or psychotic reactions from it. Her response fits with adverse reaction to a difficult journey (Aixalà & Carlos, 2022). *It was a bad trip that was actually good. Good because it felt spiritual, life became a tad less grating, sleep improved, cravings ceased. Bad because it was brutal and oppressive just like the rest of life,* and because the symptomatic relief lasted only 1 month. She regressed to previous levels of despair under a surge of painful memories.

Six weeks after the retreat, Deidre had a stroke. Speech and movement of her right limbs were compromised; hospitalization was traumatizing. Doctors refused to rule out a connection between psilocybin and her stroke. She did her own research and didn't find science associating psilocybin with strokes. However, because it could act as a vasoconstrictor, a possible connection couldn't be denied.

During her months of recovery, Deidre made plans to take more psilocybin, despite the debatable risks and my objections. Since she had barely processed the first retreat, I wanted to salvage from it as much as possible before the next one. I asked her to record it in detail. In addition to its therapeutic mental health value, this exercise would aid in speech and motor recovery. The idea grew into hope that by sounding-out her voice, she would listen to it and maybe even pick up warnings from within. Deidre was not eager to cooperate. In childhood it hadn't been safe to write, and she didn't want to leave a word-trail. Only after I said that I would compose this essay, did she get on board.

A Condensed Version of Deidre's Writeup of her First Journey

The setting was a rustic accommodation in a remote, rural environment filled with natural beauty. Four strangers got together with two facilitators in a cozy, welcoming cabin. Dining, rituals, setting intentions, journeying, and integration were communally shared. The trip was 5 hours long. I ingested three doses of dried psilocybin mushrooms: an initial dose of 1.5 g, followed by separate boosts of 1 and ½ g. I lay on a mat with eyes covered throughout. Music was integral to the journey. By listening to the soundtrack later, I was able to reconstruct it.

I experience and see myself experiencing at the same time. I am calm, awaiting in mystery. I start to walk, not sure where to. The territory feels sad and dark. The first time the tempo of the music builds up, thorny fractals appear and dread sets in.

I am split into four: One part slowly starts to walk through the fractals. Another passes through dark, cold, obscure passages, still sensing wonder and exploration. A third part feels intense sadness and oppression. A fourth part sees all; it is omniscient and empathic. It tells the others not to resist, as it will only make things worse.

I am stuck, waiting with no movement. The tempo increases, the visuals become more unpleasant, anxiety intensifies. The calm me tries to soothe the tense me and reminds her that she needs to remain open with curiosity. She is unable to let go of fear; it is unbearable. A powerful female voice lifts me up momentarily. It turns aggressive and nasty, I reject it and run through the fractals, looking for something — not sure what. It is a maze of cavernous, brown, black, and gray horrors. I am lost in desolation with no port or anchor, no direction, and no end.

The fractals stop. A little boy appears. We walk together on dirt roads through a green countryside. He wants something, a toy. We're going somewhere, to a store. I go back and forth between being the boy and the adult holding his hand. Alone again, I pass a road sign with an image of the kid. I know that he was murdered. Sandy Hook comes to mind. I question myself: why does it come up? It must be the constant media ads about the litigation. I stop looking for reasons; it's wasting time. I get back to desperately searching through the fractals, not knowing what for.

Something is blocking my vision. I can see only half of the field; the other half is black. It is so bothersome that I tilt my head and try to lift the side of the eye-cover. I immediately realize that this will not help, as I'm hallucinating, not looking with my eyes. It adds to my frustration. My rational mind insists that something must be pressing on my eye, because seeing only half makes no sense. The block is intermittent; it alternates directions up-down and side-to-side. It changes into a theater curtain that comes down and leaves just a slit. I tiptoe to the opening, peek through, and wait in suspense. I see the entire field again.

I look around and move slowly. I can't find the expansiveness that I need. I feel defeat, resignation, and impotence. I beg for clemency: Why? Please let me feel different; I don't want to be lost, no more pain! Engulfed by annihilation, I want to scream my rawness. I explode. I see myself lying prostrate on the floor, broken and exhausted. It's like watching a character in a play surrender to defeat at the end of the final scene.

Needing some care for cuts, bruises, and the pained body, I stop. Mantra music invokes unconditional compassion. The tempo increases, I cycle — running through the maze, searching, splitting into parts that talk to each other, and flashes of the murdered boy on signposts. I am condemned to just keep going, not knowing, in eternal damnation. It is a post-apocalyptic journey through the ruins of my life.

For a second, there is no more music, and I'm dropped. Cuckoos break the silence. Their playfulness is a relief, then they mock me. The other me joins the birds in the laugh of myself, laughing and crying at the same time: "You're crazy, you're looking in the wrong place; stop silly, find yourself first. You're killing yourself without even knowing what you're looking for, ha, ha, ha!"

All stops. I yearn for people, lost friends, my lost life. If I could only go back and be some-

one else. Soft music helps me ride the feelings. It ends with a deep lament, a scream and a return to anxiety and searching. With a crescendo, I am oppressed, subjugated, shoved, slapped, and punched. Lyrics come through: "Be like water, my friend; you shall find a way around or through it" ("The Waves We Give"). I fluctuate between defeat, going in for a last chance, and being done. I am scared of ending without an answer. I finally accept that it's over. A Russian Jewish cradle song resonates with my need to be held. As I lift the eye cover, a communal experience unfolds: interactions with other group members, smiles, looks of reassurance and welcoming, a bonding togetherness. There is some lightness. We listen to soft music and feel connected to each other. It's ok. I feel tranquil, nostalgic, and sad. That's it, I will not find a way out. "Somewhere Over the Rainbow" is playing.

Images, Insights, Integration

Integrating a psychedelic trip is tedious work. Like weaving tapestry or burnishing a mirror, it requires much repetition for images to crystalize. We worked with several images and themes that stood out in Deidre's experience.

The image of thorny fractals: Deidre stated that what stayed with her most was *just going, not knowing, through thorny fractals, with intervals of running, waiting, and flickers of memories of trauma.* The cycles of freezing, speeding, and collapsing have a flavor of the fight-flight response. It brings to my mind type D attachment style, disorganized and disoriented. This attachment style has been proposed as a predictor of adult dissociation (Chefetz, 2015, p. 20).

Deidre's *interminable journey through post-apocalyptic ruins* reminds me of Samuel Bak's paintings. A child survivor of the Holocaust, his life's mission became to paint his shattered world in endless variations. Deidre associated the fractals with the unending sorrow of the concentration camps. She created an image of herself as a child in the fractals. I see it as a portrait of intergenerational trauma, a disaster long ended but never ending. The inability to arrive at completion and the accompanying sense of failure were reenacted in her repeated re-entries into the fractals. A similar pattern occurred in our sessions, with difficulties parting and feelings of abandonment triggered at the door.

In the group integration, Deidre was labeled as a victim. She objected vehemently but couldn't shake off the sense of victimhood left over from her trip. Addressing this was a thorny affair. Reflecting on her continuous accrual of trauma in late decades of her life brought up feelings of blame and shame. Reckoning with the archetype of victim/persecutor opened the door to looking at herself as being on the path toward becoming a survivor.

Running without a purpose, captures Deidre's reactivity; even the stroke couldn't slow her down. Life in the fractals mirrors a lack of conscious choice, a fight-flight response gone amok. We looked at this as an inner trap that hijacks and robs her of choices. She recognized her inability to pause and ask, "Do I need to run into this situation; is it safe?"

A sadomasochistic feel is echoed in *shoved, slapped, and punched.* In my mind, it links with Deidre's abuser's periodic reemergence via social media. His communications kept her raw and sent her spiraling down. She thought she allowed them in order to confront him once and for all, *to just stand up to him.* This was a tall order, similar to

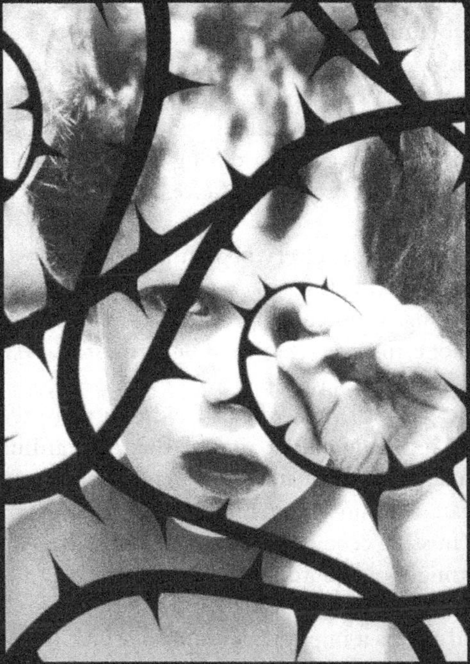

the unrealistic intention *to let go of fear.* We discussed her nervous-system's restrictive impact on how she responded to him. Eventually, she finally blocked him.

The cuckoos could have been a nice interlude in the fractals, but they weren't. Like the female singer, they tantalized and mocked. The cruel female voice hints at a malignant maternal realm. A part of Deidre joins in with self-negation. It brings to mind her confusing parents: loving, but unable to keep her safe and happy.

The retreat was Deidre's first attempt beyond analysis to reach out for healing. In the fractals, she had a novel experience, a brief pause for self-care. This seems like a gift, a message that it is possible to slow down in self-kindness. She still bristles at the suggestion of self-care, but having experienced it during the trip offers hope. It might usher a revision of her belief system that excludes self-love.

The theme of splitting: At the very beginning of her trip Deidre split into four parts. The description of splitting reads like a progression through fight-flight. Her first part is neutral, just walking. The second part is cold. The third is gripped by terror. The fourth, the omniscient one, instructs the others *not to resist and make it worse.* Warnings go unheeded; survival instincts take over.

The group setting was a positive factor for Deidre. It consisted of four individuals. The number four is often called upon in rituals. The four cardinal directions stabilize and center the individual. Four, the quaternio, is an important Jungian symbol of wholeness (Jung, 1959). It can show up as a premonition of a future coming together or as a compensation for the missing center, as in the case of Deidre. When splitting extends long past an assault, it might obliterate the center.

The fourth part urges Deidre *to let go and just be open.* It sounds like a well-intended witness, or a misguided ego, as it imposes an impossible task. We learn to let go by sensing gravity and consciously re-directing muscles to release its pull and relax. But Deidre is dissociated from her body and has limited ability to direct it. Driven by torment, she begs for clemency. This brings to mind the first step of Alcoholics Anonymous: We admit that we are powerless. In dissociation, consciousness is rendered powerless. Witnessing herself split in the fractals mirrored to Deidre her prolonged exile from her body. Increased body awareness would help her re-inhabit the interrelationship between psychic and physical phenomena. "The patient experiences a shift where their perception of matter is complexly interlaced with their psychological and philosophical psyche" (Swank, 2020, p 28). The empowering process of embodiment was seeded in the retreat.

The split-screen divides the field in half, partly visible and partly black. It becomes a theater curtain, an artifice separating perception from reality. Deidre falls, like an actor on a stage. She feels her adult life is *fake and empty,* real life concealed. The halved screen conjures the cup half-empty/half-full and the tension of opposites: concrete/symbolical, light/dark, yin/yang, conscious/unconscious, in-sight/outer-vision. I associate this duality with our bi-hemispheric brain and its specialized functions. It is possible, however, that the split-screen was caused by an actual obstruction inside Deidre's brain. What if the right/left, top/bottom alterations of the split-screen hallucination were induced by fluctuating vaso spasms? Was it a physiological response to pressure from pooling blood in her skull? Could it be both an image of her mind and a symptom of an incipient stroke, and a warning of what would come 6 weeks later?

Deidre's interpretation of the split-screen is pertinent. In a typical dismissal of ambiguity, she said, *the split isn't true; it's a hallucination.* Similarly, she rejected her spontaneous association of the murdered boy to Sandy Hook. Discarding her associations reveals a conscious ego bent on splitting off intuitive, nonlinear leaps. This supports an understanding of the split-screen as an image of psychic division. Dissociation breaks up affect, knowledge, and sensations, preventing one from grasping the whole field.

As an adult, Deidre joined her parents in the field of science. To my best understanding, linear thought, dissociated from feelings and behaviors, dominated her default mode network (DMN). Psilocybin is known to disrupt the DMN (Carhart-Harris & Friston, 2019). It exposed her over-reliance on left hemispheric logic over right hemispheric intuition and imagistic grasping. This split is captured in the sensate-visual experience of the split-screen. In lieu of clinical language, it offers a useful reference in our conversations. When she expresses dissociation, I call out the split-screen. Perhaps as a long-term consequence of the stroke, or the psilocybin, or both, Deidre left science. This may have been a positive act of separation from an unconscious matrix, individuation in Jungian parlance. Sadly, it unraveled with chaotic wounding.

The image of the murdered boy: The boy walks with an adult on a road with signposts. The signposts hint at an atrocity. Deidre felt herself as both the adult and the child. This is significant, as both parts are missing in her life. The parental protector can prevent trauma from recurring and help her become her own guardian. The child can play, imagine, and renew her ability to know and express what she needs. The boy wants a toy and asks for it. Perhaps he represents her young animus, the opposite within, an energizer of purpose, agency, and regeneration. Since she experienced both, there is hope that she will reclaim these parts in the future.

Deidre was spared from an explicit apparition of the boy's murderer. Was the culprit the psychopath who tortured and killed her innocent spirit? Or was it the inner defense system that protected her through dissociation since early childhood? Internal guardians show up as monsters in nightmares of trauma victims (Kalsched,1996). Since her life-saving dissociation extended through many years, the original guardians attacked her from within. They blinded her to her self-worth and invited self-destruction. Built-in protection mechanisms can be as virulent as external persecutors. In her trip, both remained sequestered from sight and were merely hinted at in signposts. Her abuser's shadow and her own merged in her dark unconscious.

Deidre's narrative yields positive elements, but overall, it captures a dark numinosity. Her confrontation with intolerable psychic content was devastating. The mirror held up was perhaps too stark, certainly harsher than psychodynamic sensibilities. She sensed more intensely what she already suffered, and as a result, she was pushed deeper into the nigredo of dissociation. During months of reckoning, her intention *to see myself from a different perspective certainly materialized. I was shredded, but it left a crack through which to see myself differently.* The cost, however, was insufferable abreaction.

It is meaningful that Deidre valued her journey despite the pain it inflicted. She said it delivered *an existential truth and something spiritual that nothing else offered.* After the retreat described above, her first, she sought two more against my objections. Her resulting profound perturbation brings to mind Jung's admonition that psychedelics can overwhelm with unconscious material (Lammers & Cunningham, 2007).

Reflections

To use Deidre's image, we were caught in a split screen, each of us holding a different half. Her half wanted a psycho-spiritual transformation through mushrooms at all cost. My half felt an ethical responsibility to protect, slow her down, and deepen the insight. I was concerned with how and when dissociative barriers were broken. In empathy for her suffering, I called for self-care. I doubted that running into the darkness was a good approach to healing. Her triple tripping, originally an expression of agency, felt like unconscious chasing. I am relieved that she didn't break down. I suspect that acting in opposition to me had value. The uncharted process is humbling. I am left with some insight and many questions:

- These days, when patients with severe dissociation elect to trip, professionals may have little influence over the decision. Safety and pacing considerations will be left in the hands of the patient, who might be unable to evaluate them.

- Multiple journeys may facilitate significant brain plasticity. Sometimes, a quick succession is recommended. I suspect optimal pacing for the profile of my patient ought to have been much slower.

- Context is important (group, rituals, food, shared environment), but integration is indispensable. The journey is only the beginning of the process. Commitment to integration necessitates much added time and effort.

- Hallucinatory drugs externalize the unconscious matrix in ways that can be either traumatic or transformational (Grof, 2001). It seems to me that it is not one or the other, rather both. Psilocybin is a powerful medicine, but it is not kind nor gentle. Ought there be some protections for patients like Deidre?

- Will Deidre's unmoored state lead to the benefit she seeks? The mythological suggestion that there is no creation without destruction might be apropos.

Jung said that the purpose of the transcendent function is to incorporate conscious and unconscious material towards a new attitude (Jung, 1916). This process cannot be hurried. Deidre's haste has yet to yield a new attitude: *just going not knowing* prevails. Meanwhile, I am honored to assist her. She inches her way with tenacity and creativity, running through darkness. Her narrative of the hallucinations is our GPS, a sacrament, and a transcendent function. Perhaps like a herald dream, it illuminates what might still unfold. It is a bridge that keeps us connected, steadfast as we hold the tension of much unknown. Very slowly, Deidre musters the courage to read and heed the signposts. It is a long road. It is her ride. The trip described in this paper is real. It is all hers, and she embraces it. I am left pondering: Is this real, vital quality the magic of the mushrooms, and is it worth the risks for her?

References

Aixalà, M. B., & Carlos, B. S. J. (2022). *Psychedelic integration: Psychotherapy for non-ordinary states of consciousness.* Santa Fe, NM: Synergetic Press.

Carhart-Harris, R. L., & Friston, K. J. (2019). *Rebus and the anarchic brain: Toward a unified model of the brain action of psychedelics. Pharmacological Reviews, 71*(3), 316–344. https://doi.org/10.1124/pr.118.017160

Chefetz, R. A. (2015). *Intensive psychotherapy for persistent dissociative processes: The fear of feeling real.* New York: W.W. Norton & Company.

Grof, S. (1975). *Realms of the Human Unconscious: Observations from LSD research.* New York, USA: The Viking Press.

Grof, S. (2001). The potential of entheogens as catalysts of spiritual development. In Roberts, T. B. (Ed). *Psychoactive sacramentals: Essays on entheogens and religion* (pp. 27-45). San Francisco: Council on Spiritual Practices.

Jung, C.G. (1916/1969). *The transcendent function* (R.F.C. Hull, Trans.). In H. Read et al. (Eds.), The collected works of C. G. Jung: Vol. 8. Structure and dynamics of the psyche (2nd ed., pp. 67-91). Bollingen Series XX. Princeton University Press.

Jung, C.G. (1959). Aion. (R.F.C. Hull, Trans.). In *The collected works of C. G. Jung: Vol. 9. Part II. Bollingen Series XX.* Princeton University Press.

Kalsched, D. (1996). *The inner world of trauma.* NY: Routledge.

Lammers C., & Cunningham, A., Eds. (2007). *The Jung-White letters.* New York: Routledge, Philemon Series.

National Institute on Drug Abuse. (2014). *Hallucinogens and dissociative drugs* (NIH Publication Number 14-4209). United States, Department of Health and Human Services, National Institutes of Health. https://nida.nih.gov/sites/default/files/rrhalluc.pdf

Swank, M. (2020). *Mercurius ubiquitous. International Journal of Jungian Studies, 13*(1), 13–40. https://doi.org/10.1163/19409060-bja10006

Music:

Cradle Song (Russian Jewish). Kitka Women's Vocal Ensemble. (2009).

Somewhere Over the Rainbow / What a Wonderful World. Israel Kamakawiwo'ole. *Ka 'Ano'i* [Album]. (1990).

The Waves We Give. Beautiful Chorus. Rhythmic Meditation. (2012).

Pierre Bouchard

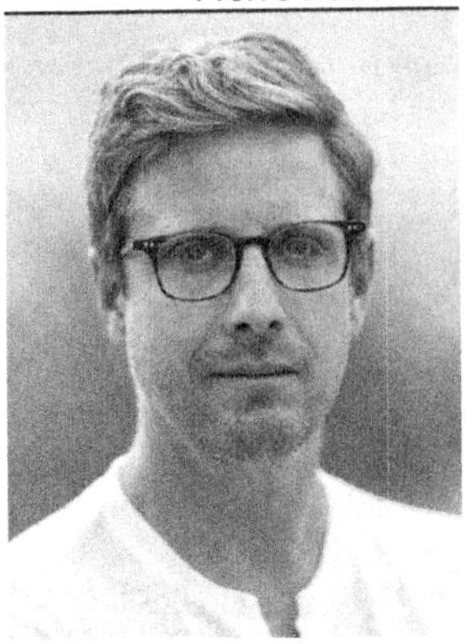

PIERRE BOUCHARD is a licensed professional counselor and minister with a group practice in Boulder and Lyons, Colorado. He integrates interpersonal neurobiology and trauma therapy with in-depth studies in Buddhist psychology, transpersonal depth work, ritual, and consciousness exploration through psychedelic psychotherapy and ministry. He is a lead trainer for the Congregation for Sacred Practices, and has operated as faculty or guest lecturer in psychedelic-assisted facilitator programs for organizations such as Naropa University and SoundMind.
PierreRBouchard@gmail.com

Ketamine-Assisted Psycholytic and Somatic Psychotherapy for Treatment-Resistant Depression: A Case Report

I (Pierre) found myself viscerally feeling like I was underground, buried in my own unlit earthen chamber of dissociation. My awareness felt dull. I felt hopeless, caked in fatigue. In the present moment, I was safe, receiving facilitated guidance by a colleague during a period of clinical practice trades. But within my psyche and body, I was reliving the protracted state of overwhelm following the sudden death of my father when I was a teen. As I stayed with these sensations, waves of aliveness returned to my body; my limbs suddenly started to feel less like concrete and a lot more like flesh. Continuing to stay with my somatic experience, anger slowly started to arise, beginning to light up this cavernous portion of my psyche. I wanted out. I could feel myself coming back to life as the tension in my muscles returned. Contractions accompanied the anger as it crested into rage. I surrendered to the process, allowing the somatic charge to follow its natural rhythm. The more my body shook, the more alive I felt, fully being with the feelings and sensations stored in my body.

This vignette illustrates a typical arc for many of my early experiences with exploring psychedelics and somatic trauma work. I had the good fortune of finding myself in community with other practitioners who saw value in the same healing paths and were willing to refine our clinical practices through experiential learning with one another. While holding space and experiencing this work in our own bodies, we learned so much more about healing trauma and the nervous system first hand. Through numerous psychedelic-assisted sessions, I learned from the inside the map of my nervous system and my pathways to healing. This map became an indispensable tool in understanding myself and my clients. Over the years, I encountered depths inside myself I had never been able

Alyssa Gursky

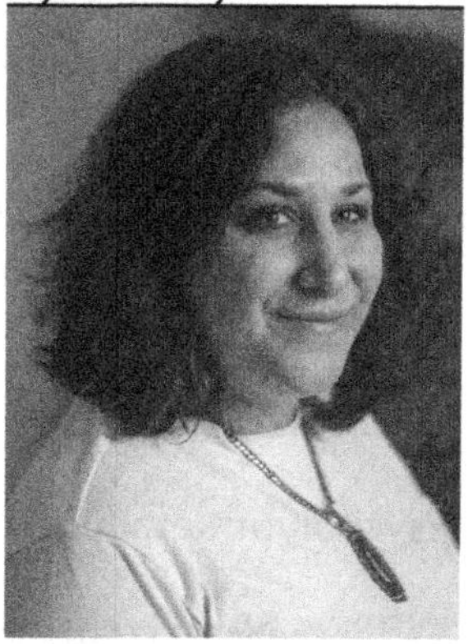

ALYSSA GURSKY, LPC, is a queer art therapist, researcher, educator, and mentor based in Portland, Oregon. They are the owner of Psychedelic Art Therapy, a psychotherapy practice and education hub legitimizing the intersection of the creative process and psychedelic healing. Currently, Alyssa mentors at Naropa University's psychedelic certificate program and is a research associate at the Portland VA's SNaP Lab, focusing on group MDMA therapy and psilocybin for depression.
Alyssa@PsychedelicArtTherapy.com

to access by other therapeutic means. I had been holding the grief of my father's early departure for so long, and nothing had helped me contact the depth of these age-old feelings trapped within my body and their impact on my view of the world. While undergoing countless psychedelic-assisted sessions I encountered dissociative realms within my psyche, fragmented and lost, as well as sympathetic states with their mythic battles against long-gone foes both known and unknown. I wasn't just expanding my capacity to feel suffering. I also expanded my capacity to feel joy. As time went on, I became less anxious, more settled in myself as both a man and a growing therapist. I witnessed similar pattern shifts within my colleagues and clients. While it was not always clear what was integrating and shifting in my psyche at the time, its unfolding had my full attention.

By the time I began to work with James, the subject of the following case study, I had accompanied both colleagues and other clients through similar processes with ketamine. With the combination of somatic work, an understanding of developmental trauma, and a potent change agent in the form of low-dose ketamine, we were able to treat what had been a lifelong depression.

Ketamine

Ketamine is a novel dissociative anesthetic drug proven to have psychedelic properties (Wolfson & Hartelius, 2016; Dore et al., 2019). The off-label usage of ketamine has recently gained increasing popularity in the fields of psychiatry (Berman et al., 2000; Price et al., 2009; Archer et al., 2018) and psychotherapy (Kolp et al., 2007; Hasler, 2019; Dore et al., 2019). However, there have been significant inconsistencies in treatment from practitioner to practitioner without a general governing board, from route of administration to the surrounding practices and methodologies. There has also been a wave of psychotherapists integrating ketamine into their practices offering a sublingual route of administration (Kolp et al., 2007; Dore et al., 2019; Hasler, 2019). Utilizing various routes of administration, research has shown ketamine to be effective in alleviating various diagnoses including treatment-resistant depression (Archer et al., 2018; Berman et al., 2000; Vasavada et al., 2016; Price et al., 2009), suicidality (Price et al., 2009; Wilkinson et al., 2018), and bipolar disorder (Sanacora et al., 2017; Wilkowska et al., 2020). Across the literature, there is little emphasis on the relationship between the individual and the therapeutic environment. Additionally, little research exists that focuses on the relationship between the therapist and the client's experience in their own body.

Psycholytic Ketamine Treatment

The model of ketamine-assisted psychotherapy (KAP) presented in this paper highlights a case study in which low, sublingual doses of ketamine were utilized to treat treatment-resistant depression. Literature discussing utilizing psychedelic drugs at lower doses in conjunction with psychotherapy refers to this as a psycholytic model of treatment (Grigsby et al., 2021). Administering low doses of mind-altering substances allows for meaningful perceptual shifts without dissolution of ego functioning; the patient's sense of self and habitual cognitive functioning remain intact (Grigsby et al.; Wolfson et al., 2016). Psycholytic therapy has also been identified to "overcome rigid defense mechanisms in treatment-resistant patients" and "increase the efficacy of the therapeutic process… [sometimes to half of the typical time]" (Wolfson et al., 2016, p. 121; Arendsen, 1963; Leuner, 1971, 1977). Ketamine was chosen due to its legal status and previous research on its efficacy with treatment-resistant depression.

Somatic Therapy and Polyvagal Theory

The following case study utilizes a somatic approach, highlighting Stephen Porges' (2017) polyvagal theory as the therapeutic modality to pair with psycholytic psychotherapy. Somatic therapy focuses on the relationship between mind and body to access trauma and healing (Weiss et al., 2015).

Porges' (2017) seminal polyvagal theory creates a functional map to understand the somatic data in terms of trauma and healing. The theory outlines an evolutionary hierarchy of brain and nervous system function, linking emotional regulation and wellbeing. Deb Dana (2018), who has adapted polyvagal theory for therapeutic use, uses the metaphor of a ladder to describe the systemic organization of dorsal, sympathetic, and ventral vagal states. The dorsal vagal system is responsible for the capacity to dissociate when a perceived threat is present; it is the oldest evolutionary response to threat. When an individual is in a dorsal vagal state, emotional connection with another is significantly impaired. Depression and loneliness are often experienced in this state (Dana, 2018). Sympathetic is a step upward on the hierarchical ladder and is responsible for mobilizing an individual into stress responses when there is a perceived threat. This state is typified by the experience of stress and tension; emotional experiences in the sympathetic system can include anxiety, panic attacks, or anger (Dana, 2018). The ventral vagal branch of the vagus nerve is considered the youngest section of the nervous system from an evolutionary perspective. It is known as the *social engagement system*; when this is active, we feel safe and socially connected, able to connect to the bigger picture of life and feel happy, fun, and peaceful (Dana, 2018). In clinical practice, the polyvagal theory provides both therapist and client with a functional map to locate one's self in the present moment, in addition to learning one's habitual responses to environmental and relational stressors.

As Dana (2018) teaches, thoughts follow nervous system states. This is to say, a client's thoughts and expressed sentiments can offer a mirror to their inner world. Depression feels very visceral and real to those who experience it. With this idea of expressed thoughts being informed by nervous system states, the clinician can hold curiosity about painful sentiments, using them as diagnostic information about the client's current nervous system holding patterns and potential cues to developmental trauma.

Developmental Trauma

Developmental trauma can be understood as the unique impact that relational ruptures can have during a crucial window of human growth, namely childhood and adolescence; it can occur not only through the impact of difficult experiences but also from the absence of closeness, attunement, and emotional presence (Cruz et al., 2022). Individuals who experience developmental trauma are especially susceptible to attachment insecurity, a compromised capacity for emotion regulation and cognitive functioning, and developing post-traumatic stress disorder when exposed to traumatic situations later in life (Spinazzola et al., 2021). As this wounding happens during a period of identity development, it can be easy for a grown adult to feel a conflation between their sense of self and the byproduct of the developmental trauma (Spinazzola et al., 2021).

Somatic Therapy and Non-ordinary States of Consciousness

When working to remediate symptoms of trauma that have a less obvious origin, such as individual clients who report chronic experiences of depression or anxiety linking back to early childhood, somatic modalities can provide the client with access to learn their nervous system, instead of being held captive by its habitual responses. When paired with non-ordinary states of consciousness, somatic awareness becomes more acute, as the novelty of being outside of one's habitual state creates less opportunity to get lost in cognitive thought. The particularly sedative and distancing quality of ketamine has been reported to support clients in holding curiosity about their nervous system state without experiencing overwhelm. When utilizing the polyvagal theory in conjunction with non-ordinary states of consciousness, a client can develop the ability to experientially learn more distinct reference points for the different stages of their unique nervous system and ultimately train the system to become more acquainted with the consciousness associated with the ventral vagal system.

Case Presentation

James is a Caucasian professional in his mid-30s who reported suffering from depression since grade school. He sought treatment specifically for ketamine-assisted psychotherapy following the ending of a long-term romantic relationship. In the initial consultation, James wore stylishly slim jeans, a fitted t-shirt, and short, neat hair. He spoke sparsely and articulately. He was, at times, struggling to go to work because of his depression. He was regularly withdrawn from his friends, not returning phone calls for long periods, canceling plans last minute. James reported intermittent alcohol and cannabis consumption throughout his life. He had experimented with LSD several times as well as MDMA and psilocybin-containing mushrooms, in recreational settings. At the time of his initial interview, he was not on any prescription medications for his depression.

To his knowledge, his parents were never diagnosed with a mental health condition. James reported that his father could have explosive anger, and his mother could be emotionally distant. However, he reported no known history of traumatic experiences. On the Adverse Childhood Experience (ACE) scale, he had a score of 0. He reported often feeling like he was left alone as a child. However, given his reports, this was far more of an emotional experience than one that would qualify as neglect. He reported often feeling "that there is something wrong, but we can't talk about it." He reported experiencing that his parents would disengage when he would have difficult emotions as a child, thus leaving him to deal with the experience on his own. James reported that he had felt depressed quite consistently since he was in grade school, with fluctuating degrees of severity. James reported having several meetings with a child psychologist between the ages of 7 and 10. However, he reported not being interested in talking to her, and treatment was concluded. As a teenager, he was placed on several different SSRIs, none of which were beneficial. In his late 20s James had several periods of being in therapy, with periods of weekly therapy lasting 6 to 12 months. While he could not remember what each specialized in, he recalled engaging in evidence-based practices, like cognitive behavioral therapy. However, he reported that none of it improved his depression.

Discussion

James partook in 26 3-hour-long ketamine sessions over 15 months. Seven months consisted of weekly ketamine-assisted sessions. The remaining 8 months were weekly therapy sessions integrating and practicing the new skills he had learned, with intermittent ketamine usage. His dose started at 100 mg, sublingually self-administered troche lozenges. Roughly halfway through treatment, dosage increased to 150 mg per session. When sessions first began, his depression was highly acute, causing him to withdraw from every aspect of his life, minus his career. The initial course of treatment began with James cognitively identifying and somatically learning that most of his life operated from within a dorsal vagal state. Examples include withdrawing from his social community and reported feelings of hopelessness and helplessness. This psychoeducation aided in building safety through familiarizing him with the map for this unfamiliar, dissociated portion of his psyche. Throughout our time together, this intellectual safety acted as a building block for the risk taking inherent in James being open to experiencing embodied relational safety.

Approximately four ketamine-assisted sessions into James's treatment, he was able to use the psycholytic state to focus on the somatic experience of depression, or this familiarized dorsal vagal state. He came to understand that his implicit patterning was how he saw the world, versus how the world is. He said, "There was a whole other world for me to enter if I would have chosen it," and continued, "[I'm] always trying to fit in. So why am I trying to make myself fit in? Fitting in feels very compressed. What if I just don't try? Feels vulnerable, not fully formed, raw."

Through careful attunement and awareness of his developmental patterning, I was able to offer James an invitation to experience connection with me in his difficult state. I said to him, "You can be not fully formed and raw, and I won't leave." He responded, "[There's] lots of possibility here. I feel like I could be okay alone, or I could go meet someone and not be too concerned with how others thought of me. [There's] spaciousness in [my] chest. It can still be painful and okay at the same time."

As he gained this awareness over time, he drew parallels from his relationship perils to his wounding by his mother. He once stated, "I'll stay in bad things just so I don't feel left." His inner working model of love that he learned in childhood taught his nervous system that it is normal and necessary to be in a dorsal vagal state in a romantic connection. From a polyvagal perspective, this is a critical insight. Neurobiologically speaking, James was living in the branch of his nervous system that protects itself with immobility. Within this habitual dorsal vagal state, the nourishment of interpersonal connection is actually physically unavailable. Even if he received the nourishment he wanted while in that state, he physically could not feel its impact in his body. Without access to his ventral vagal system, James was missing most of what he was looking for.

Moving up the polyvagal ladder through periods of sympathetic arousal was critical in a ventral vagal state becoming available to him beyond our session time. We explored his capacity to be with sympathetic arousal. While in a non-ordinary state, this included various forms of pre-negotiated, consensual physical contact with me and various props for pushing and punching. His ability to take this risk in embodiment, though highly uncomfortable for him, was a massive jump up the evolutionary ladder into the sympathetic portion of the nervous system. It was no longer an unknown territory for James. Once here, James had closer access to his ventral vagal system.

With time and repeated sessions, clinicians can learn where their clients' developmental woundings are and take calculated risks to expose a client to a new way to not only see outside of the familiar state but also see its implications and a potential new way of relating. What followed in our year of intensive sessions were similar instances of repeated exposures to this missing developmental experience. Over time, his internal map of connection changed as these new experiences became integrated inside him. They went from being a novel possibility of change to a grounded way of being in the world.

As treatment progressed and the end of the year-long intensive approached, James began to gain more autonomy and awareness of his depression. James had self-reported that he no longer thought of himself as a depressed person but rather experienced the symptoms in a transient, infrequent, and manageable manner. He shared that he felt access to these new ways of being and relating that he could apply in other areas of his life. When feeling stressed, he now had other options besides diving into dorsal vagal activation. When in distress, he could now tend to himself with a sense of kindness, offering himself the kind of nurturance and support he desperately wanted as a child and did not get enough of. He also grew in his capacity to reach out to the right people in a way that was more likely to result in satisfying support and human connection. As outlined by Deb Dana (2018), "thoughts follow state," and the way he was showing up in his life was indicative of his access to his ventral vagal state. As his capacity to tend to himself grew, so did his perspective on the world. The world now no longer seemed so barren and inhospitable. Many relationships were safe, and he could now partake in them.

Conclusion

This case report outlines the potential advantages that psycholytic therapy has to offer. These psycholytic experiences allow the client to experience their mind and body outside of its baseline state and test new ways of being. Repeated access to these states of consciousness can allow for more in-depth levels of somatic knowing and, ultimately, alleviate some degree of suffering. From this state, there is a significant possibility of re-wiring early childhood wounds and providing missing experiences in development. By doing this work, the client is pointed toward new, healthier ways of relating to himself and others.

There is a tendency in psychedelic literature to highlight instances where a single experience changes everything. While there is both qualitative and quantitative evidence to substantiate this claim, other healing methods differing in dose and length of sessions with non-ordinary states of consciousness should be explored in psychological discourse. In James' case, the early sessions often contained insights regarding aloneness. The treatment arc consisted of repeatedly deepening into that insight. It started as a conceptual insight and became over time a deeply embodied knowing. I got to model for him the relational nourishment that he did not receive, subsequently teaching him that he could offer it to himself and receive it from the world around him. Through the lens of polyvagal theory, James' treatment arc was one of moving from living in the depressive depths of the dorsal vagal, to accessing the mobilizing qualities of his sympathetic nervous system, to then finally learning how to be in connection with himself and others in the ventral vagal branch. This emergent modality can be best understood as a non-linear style of working. It becomes a practice of stabilizing states as new more durable personality traits once the initial wound has been contacted and healed.

It cannot be overemphasized how important the experiential practices I underwent myself were for my ability to do this work with James. Allowing my body to express old repressed emotions and illuminating my own inner caverns gave me the capacity to offer light to James in healing his own inner darkness. It is crucial to highlight that though ketamine was a remarkable vehicle in this treatment, it is not the main mechanism of what created success in this case. Instead, the ketamine acted as an amplifier for the vividness of the relational and somatic work happening in therapy, fundamentally transforming the early developmental wounds causing his depression.

From the lens of many clinical intakes, there would appear to be virtually nothing wrong with James. He had no major documented trauma and experienced no relief in his depression throughout numerous therapies and drug treatments. Most typically, case presentations such as his are currently treated under the notion of faulty brain chemistry. Unfortunately, this is not a unique experience for people within the medical and mental health care systems. This case report hopes to provide an alternative view to this currently accepted paradigm. Careful assessment with clients, following specialized training, should be done before working with developmental trauma, psychedelics, somatic healing, or any fusion of the modalities. Children do not develop secure attachment from a single attuned experience. It happens from thousands of experiences across an entire childhood. So too does deep healing with our clients happen across time. Various factors, including a therapist's warmth, presence, understanding of the nervous system, and capacity to trust that one's baseline is capable of change create room for this transformation to occur. This is the backbone upon which we can build psychedelic therapeutic work that goes far beyond the psychedelic itself.

References

Archer, S., Chrenek, C., & Swainson, J. (2018). Maintenance ketamine therapy for treatment resistant depression. *Journal of Clinical Psychopharmacology, 38*(4), 380–384. https://doi.org/10.1097/JCP.0000000000000894

Berman, R. M., Cappiello, A., Anand, A., Oren, D. A., Heninger, G. R., Charney, D. S., & Krystal, J. H. (2000). Antidepressant effects of ketamine in depressed patients. *Biological Psychiatry, 47*(4), 351–354. https://doi.org/10.1016/s0006-3223(99)00230-9

Cruz, D., Lichten, M., Berg, K., & George, P. (2022). Developmental trauma: Conceptual framework, associated risks and comorbidities, and evaluation and treatment. *Frontiers in Psychiatry, 13*. https://doi.org/10.3389/fpsyt.2022.800687

Dana, D., & Porges, S. W. (2018). *The polyvagal theory in therapy: Engaging the rhythm of regulation.* W.W. Norton & Company.

Dore, J., Turnipseed, B., Dwyer, S., Turnipseed, A., Andries, J., Ascani, G., Monnette, C., Huidekoper, A., Strauss, N., & Wolfson, P. (2019). Ketamine assisted psychotherapy (KAP): Patient demographics, clinical data and outcomes in three large practices administering ketamine with psychotherapy. *Journal of Psychoactive Drugs, 51*(2), 189–198. doi.org/10.1080/02791072.2019.1587556

Grigsby, J. (2021). Memory reconsolidation in psycholytic psychotherapy. In C. S. Grob & J. Grigsby (Eds.), *Handbook of medical hallucinogens* (pp. 134-159). The Guilford Press.

Hasler, G. (2019). Toward specific ways to combine ketamine and psychotherapy in treating depression. *CNS Spectrums, 25*(3), 445–447. https://doi.org/10.1017/s1092852919001007

Kolp, E., Young, M. S., Friedman, H., Krupitsky, E., Jansen, K., & O'Connor, L.-A. (2007). Ketamine-enhanced psychotherapy: Preliminary clinical observations on its effects in treating death anxiety. *International Journal of Transpersonal Studies, 26*(1), 1–17. https://doi.org/10.24972/ijts.2007.26.1.1

Krupitsky, E. M., & Grinenko, A. Y. (1997). Ketamine psychedelic therapy (KPT): A review of the results of ten years of research. *Journal of Psychoactive Drugs, 29*(2), 165–183. https://doi.org/10.1080/02791072.1997.10400185

Liebrenz, M., Borgeat, A., Leisinger, R., & Stohler, R. (n.d.). Intravenous ketamine therapy in a patient with a treatment-resistant major depression. *SWISS MED WKLY, 4.Snapshot.* (n.d.). Retrieved December 11, 2020, from https://www.tandfonline.com/doi/full/10.1080/02791072.2019.1587556

Passie, T. (1997). *Psycholytic and psychedelic therapy research 1931-1995: A complete international bibliography.* Laurentius Publishing.

Porges, S. W. (2017). *The polyvagal theory: Neurophysiological foundations of emotions, attachment, communication, and self-regulation.* W. W. Norton & Co Inc.

Price, R. B., Nock, M. K., Charney, D. S., & Mathew, S. J. (2009). Effects of intravenous ketamine on explicit and implicit measures of suicidality in treatment-resistant depression. *Biological Psychiatry, 66*(5), 522–526. https://doi.org/10.1016/j.biopsych.2009.04.029

Sanacora, G., Frye, M. A., McDonald, W., Mathew, S. J., Turner, M. S., Schatzberg, A. F., ... Nemeroff, C. B. (2017). A consensus statement on the use of ketamine in the treatment of mood disorders. *JAMA Psychiatry, 74*(4), 399. https://doi.org/10.1001/jamapsychiatry.2017.0080

Spinazzola, J., van der Kolk, B., & Ford, J. D. (2021). Developmental trauma disorder: A legacy of attachment trauma in victimized children. *Journal of Traumatic Stress, 34*(4), 711–720. https://doi.org/10.1002/jts.22697

Vasavada, M. M., Leaver, A. M., Espinoza, R. T., Joshi, S. H., Njau, S. N., Woods, R. P., & Narr, K. L. (2016). Structural connectivity and response to ketamine therapy in major depression: A preliminary study. *Journal of Affective Disorders, 190*, 836–841. https://doi.org/10.1016/j.jad.2015.11.018

Weiss, H., Johanson, G., & Monda, L. (2015). *Hakomi mindfulness-centered somatic psychotherapy: A comprehensive guide to theory and practice.* W.W. Norton & Company.

Wilkinson, S. T., Ballard, E. D., Bloch, M. H., Mathew, S. J., Murrough, J. W., Feder, A., ... Sanacora, G. (2018). The effect of a single dose of intravenous ketamine on suicidal ideation: A systematic review and individual participant data meta-analysis. *American Journal of Psychiatry, 175*(2), 150–158.

https://doi.org/10.1176/appi.ajp.2017.17040472

Wilkowska A, Szałach Ł, & Cubala W. J. (2020). Ketamine in bipolar disorder: A review. *Neuropsychiatry Review,16*, 2707-2717. doi:10.2147/NDT.S282208

Wolfson, P., & Hartelius, G. (2016). *The ketamine papers: Science, therapy, and transformation.* Santa Cruz, CA: Multidisciplinary Association for Psychedelic Studies.

Wolfson, P., Hartelius, G., Kolp, E., Friedman, H. L., Krupitsky, E., Jansen, K., ... Kolp, A. (2016). Ketamine psychedelic psychotherapy: Focus on its pharmacology, phenomenology, and clinical applications. In *The ketamine papers: Science, therapy, and transformation* (pp. 97–197). Multidisciplinary Association for Psychedelic Studies.

It's a very salutary thing to realize that the rather dull universe in which most of us spend most of our time is not the only universe there is. I think it's healthy that people should have this experience.

—Aldous Huxley

Jason Konner

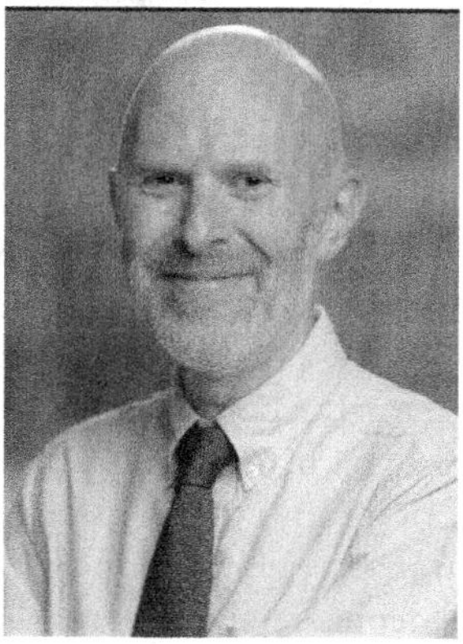

Jason Konner, MD, has worked as a medical oncologist at Memorial Sloan Kettering Cancer Center since completing fellowship in 2004. He is a member of the Gynecological Medical Oncology and Early Drug Development Services. He earned his BS from Yale and MD from Stanford. His prior research interests involved clinical drug development. He is now working to help advocate for the use of psychedelics for cancer patients, which he believes is best achieved if we start with cancer care providers.
konnerj@mskcc.org

How A Shaman Dog Relieved Me of My Burnout:
An Oncologist's Psychedelic Tale of Personal Healing

The growing prevalence of physician burnout—a syndrome involving emotional exhaustion, depersonalization, and a sense of reduced accomplishment related to work—has reached troubling magnitude and is coming to increased attention, yet effective and feasible solutions remain elusive. Doctors ensnarled under the administrative yoke, grappling with inefficient and burdensome clerical duties, can sense a loss of agency, prompting demoralization and a sense of worthlessness. Burnout can lead to depression, substance abuse, and suicidal ideation. This crisis has ripple effects on patients, families, colleagues, and the very nature of our identity. Despite its negative effects on mental health and quality of life, burnout is not recognized as a distinct mental disorder in the DSM-5. Many of the factors contributing to burnout entail the prosaic bureaucratic and logistical burdens of practicing modern medicine—long hours, stressful and difficult work, lack of appreciation—and are largely outside of doctors' control. Oncologists face the added challenges of managing very sick patients going through extremely challenging and often fatal events. The pandemic added jet fuel to this fire, stoking exhaustion, fear, conflict, illness, isolation, loss, family strife, and financial distress for many.

And so it was that I found myself, in the fall of 2022, feeling hopeless and depressed, cast into the burnout abyss. As the pandemic waned and its destructive wake became more evident, institutionally and personally, its effects continued to linger in a hobbled clinical world, even while the rest of society appeared to have moved on and returned to normal. I saw that my research interests had yielded to immense clinical demands and my academic prospects were fading. Endless, inefficient, soul-crushing documentation weighed down like an albatross. I was looking into pharma jobs, more as an escape route than out of any real interest. I felt dejected and could not see a path towards improvement; I seemed to be done advancing and could only foresee a few decades of drudgery, withering towards inevitable decrepitude and death. This was conflated with turning 50, enduring a romantic break-up, finding a new left inguinal hernia, and experiencing a series of stinging patient losses. Needless to say, I was in a dark place and unable to perceive how negative a lens I was projecting onto reality.

As the light of autumn days continued to wane, my planned hernia surgery loomed ever more menacing. I blocked off 2 weeks from work, as advised, and I was told I could not do any exercise using the core for 6 weeks after the procedure. I sensed that spending 6 weeks of long nights without yoga—the salve for my soul at the time—would cement a depression I saw brewing. As my busy practice continued unabated, I was more burned out than I was able or willing to recognize. As the surgery approached, it dawned on me that I had not taken a full 2 weeks off in over a decade and had scarcely taken vacation during the pandemic. What I needed, more than inguinal mesh, was to take some time for myself. But to do what? I was too anhedonic to conceive a trip. And so, a week before the break, still without a plan, back to yoga I went. After class, I randomly overheard another yogi say the words "ayahuasca retreat," and in that moment I knew what I would do.

Several years prior, I had read Michael Pollan's (2018) acclaimed book, *How to Change Your Mind*, which discussed how psychedelics can seemingly help heal emotional wounds and heighten one's capacity to love the universe. I concluded that a substance with high LD50 (low lethality), low addictive potential, and a rapid and durable effect, that can yield spirituality and openness, might just be worth trying at some point in life. But when, where, and how to experience one of these elusive and largely illegal substances remained unknown. The moment I heard the call of the sacred vine in yoga class, the when was clear. A quick Google search and a brief phone call easily solved the where and how, as I suddenly glimpsed the world of international psychedelic retreats. There's even an app for it—who knew! I decided that, as a novice, rather than brave the uncertainties of the otherwise alluring Amazonian jungle ceremonies, I would instead go the safer and more comfortable route, at a well-appointed resort with a robust team of shamans, facilitators, and medical staff. [1] Expensive, but if "aya" could truly provide the equivalent of a decade of psychotherapy, as many have claimed, then it seemed a worthwhile investment. I canceled the surgery, and off I went, not yet able to perceive quite how vast a plunge I was about to take.

Psychedelic Substances

Ayahuasca, a Quechua term meaning vine of death, is a decoction of Amazonian plants, consisting principally of leaves from the chacruna plant (Psychotria viridis) with the ayahuasca vine (Banisteriopsis caapi). In the chacrunna leaves is found the psycho-

1 Among practicing Amazonian tribes, there are some that endorse sharing the medicine with travelers, while others do not. It is important that an explorer of ayahuasca and other indigenous sacraments ensure a mutually non-exploitive and sustainable relationship with Indigenous groups and their plants. Indeed, approaching them with humility, reverence, and reciprocity will likely enhance the benefits.

active substance DMT. If ingested alone, DMT is abruptly metabolized in the liver and gut by monoamine oxidase (MAO); however, when mixed with the sacred vine, the MAO inhibitor activity of harmine, a beta-carbolide found in the vine, allows the DMT to make its way to the central nervous system. This is chemically and spiritually analogous to ancient Middle Eastern religious blends that combined acacia coals, a source of DMT, and Syrian rue, which has MAO inhibitors. How these cultures may have determined the entheogenic consequences of these specific admixtures remains shrouded in mystery. The term *entheogen* describes a substance which can elicit a sense or experience of the divine, while *psychedelic*, coined in the 1960s by Humphrey Osmond, refers to substances that can help reveal the soul. In preparing the aya, a shaman carefully selects the appropriate plants from their area, as there are regional varieties (eg yagé, caapi, hoasca) with protean effects and spirits. They will pulverize and then boil the mixed components over many hours until a thick brew is formed (McKenna, 1992). This is a sacred and complex ritual imbued with deep cultural and spiritual meaning and ancient expertise; it is suited neither for fume hood nor dorm room.

DMT is considered a classical psychedelic, a tryptamine agonist to 5-HT2A and other receptors. Other serotonergic psychedelics include LSD, a derivative of an ergot alkaloid developed by Albert Hoffman; psilocybin, found in psilocybe mushrooms; and the intense and short-acting 5-MeO-DMT, aka Bufo, secreted by the Sonoran desert toad. Ibogaine, another tryptamine, is found in Central Africa and may have utility in treating addiction. Mescaline is a phenethylamine found in spikey, succulent peyote or San Pedro cacti, and has been used for centuries by Indigenous groups in the Americas. While opinions on this grouping vary, non-classical psychedelics might include MDMA, ketamine, and cannabis, which have significant overlap but important differences. MDMA, an amphetamine historically derived from safrole found in sassafras root, is considered an empathogen and a stimulant, eliciting a deep sense of compassion and loving awareness, while ketamine, a derivative of PCP, is a dissociative anesthetic and can produce the sense of disconnection from one's body and surroundings (Johnson et al., 2018). While these substances differ widely in route of administration, duration of effect, and risks, they have in common a tendency to expand consciousness—what my uncle lovingly terms "high-church drugs." The low-church drugs on the other hand, include heroin, cocaine, and methamphetamine, which may provide a quick thrill or transient numbing of pain but ultimately do little to encourage personal or spiritual development. Conversely, high-church drugs can also have potential for misuse by individuals or reckless facilitators; it is highly contextual. Sacred tobacco (mapacho), cacao, and toasted coca leaves (mambé) each have distinct roles in accessing spirit through ritual but are often misused and abused outside of sacred settings. I dare not attempt to categorize caffeine.

The Psychedelic Experience

Psychedelic experiences can be divided into preparation, the journey itself, and, perhaps most important, integration. Preparation can vary from spiritual or meditative practice, journaling, purification practice, or consulting with a guide. Some may study and plan for years, while others, like me (for better or for worse), might just jump into the deep end and hope for the best. A few particulars about aya preparation include a special, purifying, and restrictive *dieta*, which can engender ritual, commitment, community, and mindset, as well as avoidance of most psychotropic medicines (especially SSRIs), other psychedelics, and tyramine or serotonin-augmenting foods or drugs, due to the MAO inhibitor activity in harmine. Exercise, sleep, and hydration are encouraged, while fasting before ceremony is advised. In addition, a meeting with the shaman may be in order to review intention. In my meeting with the shaman, I was assured that "Mother Aya would present me with exactly what is needed," a prod to choose to yield to the process.

During psychedelic journeys, the mindset and intent of the participant are essential features, as is being in a safe setting. An intention can be specific and goal-oriented but should be distinguished from expectation, as it is important to trust, let go, and be open to whatever arises. A setting may vary from a clinical or personal space to outdoors in nature, or a ceremonial space, such as the maloca for aya ritual. Ceremonial tools and symbols may also help fill the container. Journeying alone is not advised, especially for the novice. A guide, be they shaman or shrink, priest or rabbi, can be critical in grounding and containing the experience, especially through rough or confusing territory. Group journeys can engender profound connection and may provide comfort and facilitate openness. Eyes may be closed, for a deeper spiritual connection, or open, especially when connecting with nature; visual imagery may manifest either way. Music can be a particularly powerful companion and guide and should be carefully considered.

Integration is where one processes what was learned from the medicine and applies it to their inner and outer worlds for sustained embodiment and actualization. It demands the most work and yields the greatest rewards. As with preparation, useful tools for a robust integration may include therapy, self-reflection, meditation, journaling, and spiritual and physical practices, to help nurture and propagate positive change. As I came to appreciate these components, it become clear that working with a psychedelic is far more complex than simply filling a prescription and taking a pill.

My journey was to begin with breathwork, a practice of intense guided rapid mouth ventilation culminating in breath holding, that helps dip one's toe into the vast waters of expanded consciousness. There are myriad breathing practice traditions, such as pranayama, with ancient roots in diverse spiritual cultures. Many modern breathing rituals have been influenced by Stanislov Grof and Wim Hof. It is thought that some of these techniques may stimulate release of endogenous DMT, which may be present in the pineal gland and as a precursor in the lungs, and can play a role in protecting cells from the effects of hypoxia (Szabo et al., 2016). Endogenous DMT has also been thought to associate with dreaming, intuition, and the dying process. What a marvelous internal pharmacopoeia we possess! Breathwork provided a glimpse under the curtain which aya would soon strip away. As I labored through the process, I felt the expected extremity tingles which can crescendo into tetanic muscle seizures and discomfort, and continued to power through (it's not an easy task). After blowing off ample CO2 came a surprisingly long breath-hold, where I found myself thinking lovingly about relatives and friends, and I also resolved, without any need for deliberation, to learn frame drumming. What just happened? A new world was about to emerge.

Each aya journey is unique and largely unpredictable. A user may experience so-called body (physical sensations), pinta (visuals), consulta (heard messages), or nada (imperceptible); or combinations of these. Aya can induce vomiting, which I had presumed was a predictable drug toxicity. Off-putting as it understandably appears, I later came to appreciate that the purge is an important physical, spiritual, psychological, and metaphorical element of the aya journey, and can also take other physical forms, such as crying, sweating, shaking, laughing, etc. Journeyers are provided buckets and instructed on proper vomiting ergonomics. These are not experiences for pure enjoyment; there is a good reason ayahuasca is not a club drug.

My aya journeys would be at times exhilarating, exasperating, glorious, and terrifying. Neither a pleasure cruise nor a horror show, they shared elements of each. Accessing the subconscious is an extraordinary opportunity, which is inherently attended by risks of encountering challenging elements of one's shadow side. Depending on set and setting, the dark night of the soul could constitute a bad trip or can present powerful opportunities for self-knowledge, healing, and growth, perhaps through the confronting and befriending of our well-meaning but over-protective parts. In encountering repressed memories, one can address and resolve the traumatic effects of difficult experiences in a safe space, temporally detached from the event itself, which may have been too much to bear or process at the time and was protectively sealed off in the subconscious, like a festering abscess needing a psychic lance. Acknowledge, engage, seek to understand, and embrace the darkness, then move forward and start to heal. As Hopkins psychologist Bill Richards (2016) put it when speaking at a conference in summary of his book, "In the diamond of self, one may need to enter a facet of despair to reach the inner light." The stages of the spiritual journey are understood to include awakening, followed by purgation, then gradual illumination. Without this middle step, one risks a spiritual bypass, which may be the path of the many religious leaders we have seen taking downfalls.

As I reflect on the retreat, I perceive three key events that related to healing my burnout, namely an awakening, a death, and a purge. The first night of aya changed my life profoundly and sustainedly. Along with dozens of others, I took my place on a mattress in the maloca, dressed in white linens, with a cup (for drinking) and a bucket (for puking). The live music was joyful and inviting as I queued up to fill my cup with the Peruvian shaman's brew, a mix of excitement and apprehension in my heart and gut. After drinking the thick, earthy brown decoction, I lay down to wait and meditate, while the music played and the shaman team read and adjusted the energies in the maloca. After 40 minutes, the vomiting came. It felt as awful as it might seem. I assumed the recommended position, and as I furiously wretched, I couldn't help but think, "This must be what cisplatin (chemo drug) feels like." After a few bouts, I somehow looked at my own body from above and declared, "You don't need to do that." In an instant, all nausea ceased. I was stunned at that moment by how powerful the connection between mind and gut could be. Soon it was time for the second cup. After some time, things started to get pixelated, a preview to the sacred geometry which would later manifest. I was portaling into the subconscious. In quick succession, during what seemed like just 10 minutes, I gained new and resonant insights into family and personal relations, and engaged in ancestral healing to salve intergenerational trauma. None of this was intended or expected but it felt meaningful and relevant and continues to inform my life to this day. From there, I ventured into what I chose to call the spirit world. It was a mystical and transcendent experience that is difficult to adequately describe with words. I experienced a sense of calm, bliss, and clarity as I viewed the nature of reality from a radically different perspective. It seemed truer than the consensus reality to which we are accustomed. I felt profound amusement at the folly of life and the majesty of existence. Moments like this can produce what is called ontological shock, but was for me—a secular Jewish atheist and STEM adherent—a beautiful revelation, a moment of metanoia. It may be that atheists are more prone to accept such experiences, as we tend to be more open and curious, and less constrained by dogma. Whether I remain an atheist is a question of semantics. As for science, my appreciation of it has only grown stronger, though I now better recognize its blind spots.

How does this relate to my burnout? It would be some time before this became more clear. Several days after my first journey, I was talking with a rolfer from California who was my mattress neighbor in the maloca. He told me, to my surprise, that in the depths of my journey, my outer body was talking incessantly. What was I saying? The rolfer, sensitive to the fact that I was undergoing a spiritual transformation at the time, hesitantly informed me that I kept repeating, "I need a day off." A doctor friend later pointed out to me that "experiencing unity with the universe while your outward body is asking for a day off was the most profound illustration of burnout [she] had ever heard."

On my third night of aya, I was introduced to yagé, an aya blend from Colómbia known for its potency and power. The music on this night was noticeably less inviting than before. The shaman's ways can be subtle yet potent. Less than an hour after my first cup, I became progressively tremulous and nauseated. A pressure developed in my head, accompanied by tinnitus and dread. I felt a dark foreboding as disturbing visuals began to present themselves. As the physical and visual phenomena crescendoed, I found myself hurtling helplessly towards a wicker bassinet buried in soil. Then nothingness. I collapsed. I lay there in shock—empty, spent—for probably an hour until I was able to pull myself up and consult with a member of the shaman's team. "That is your ego dying," I was told. Though at the time it felt to me (a concept that was starting to blur) like abject suffering without meaning. The aya ethos is to keep drinking more medicine as long as you are able. After what came from the first cup, I was terrified of taking a second. I mustered the courage for a refill. I told the shaman about my death experience, and he mercifully filed my cup just halfway—an adaptive dosing strategy that I recognized and appreciated.

The days after ceremony consist of recovery and preparation from and for journeys, but also the digesting and unfolding of what was and will be learned. Having one's channels open and being surrounded by others who are just as open and present, and having a shared experience, is immensely helpful for the process. On day 4, one of my many new friends looked deeply in my eyes and asked me how I was. Unaccustomed to being on the receiving end of such a query, my eyes welled up, and I started beathing heavily. He suggested we meet later that afternoon to sit and talk. I had no idea what we would discuss, but I knew it needed to happen. Later that day, sitting on the ground in the yard, under the open sky, surrounded by trees, birds, stones, and paths, a monumental outpouring of grief ensued. This was to be my purge. Through a steady cascade of tears, I told tales of loss and pain and hurt, memories of patients and their loved ones, and their suffering and demise. A cathartic discharge of accumulated grief from a career's worth of unspoken trauma spewed unabated. It's hard to say how long I sat there with my empathetic new friend, but near the end, I saw a small, dark figure approaching. A four-legged one. I had heard of and briefly glimpsed the shaman dog, but there had been no reason for us to meet until now. He said very little as he approached with an air of seriousness in his demeanor. He proceeded to circle me three times, before heading off into the distance. I'll never know to where he sent my pain - to wind, to water, to fire, or (most likely) buried into the earth - but I know that with him it had finally departed.

Psychedelic Healing

The medicine, as it is sometimes called, has helped me reconsider and adjust my core beliefs. The challenges of work are inevitable and unavoidable. but the suffering we experience as a result can be mitigated by recognizing, reducing, and replacing fear, judgment, shame, regret, resentment, and other maladaptive reactions which can impair our resilience. The medicine has connected me with the idea and practice of connecting with my inner healer, capable of auto-repair of the psyche, when allowed. It has helped me cultivate agency and live with intention, to advocate for self and for patients (which go hand in hand), to acknowledge limitations, and to learn to accept whatever remains.

I have adjusted my view of reality and am more able to not take most things, including myself, too seriously. The medicine has taught me to believe in the inherent good in all people, call it Buddha nature, Atman, or what psychologist Richard Schwartz terms The Self, it appears that we are all blessed with an indestructible and inexhaustible core of love and benevolence. The challenge is to get past the external and internal barriers to connecting with these best parts of ourselves; plant and fungal medicines can be great allies for this. Further, the medicine has allowed me, previously a lifelong thanatophobe, to heal my relationship with death, and along with that, to enhance my enjoyment of life and to show up for my patients in a more present and connected way. My relationships with loved ones have deepened and improved. I have been more mindful of how I treat my body and am in the best shape of my life. Plant medicines can also inspire biophilia; I now find myself at various times embracing trees, talking to plants, and apologizing to insects. On the downside, I still have a hernia.

Through my experience, I have come to believe that we all share a boundless capacity for compassion, which can be nourishing to embrace. It can feel fatigued, not because the well runs dry, but due to the barriers to accessing it that can be formidable and exhausting. Faced with the burdens of clerical work, long hours, repeating exposure to pain and loss, and governed by (often soul-disconnected) administrators, the clarity and calm needed to connect with compassion can be badly obscured. It is therefore imperative that we work on ourselves to nurture and cultivate the best features of being a healer, that imbued in us the love for medicine that brought us here to begin with. In a field increasingly dominated by 3rd parties, we must be the guardians of compassion, for our patients and for ourselves. Our jobs can be our spiritual work if they align with our sense of purpose. For some, the plant medicines may reveal a misalignment and illustrate the need for a new path. For me, I now appreciate my job with renewed passion. My patient interactions are deeper and more gratifying than ever, and I am imbued with a renewed sense of fulfillment. I hope the day comes when more of my colleagues can avail themselves to these marvelous and healing gifts of nature.

References

Johnson, M., Hendricks, P., Barrett, F., & Griffiths, R. (2019). Classic psychedelics: An integrative review of epidemiology, therapeutics, mystical experience, and brain network function. *Pharmacology & Therapeutics, 197,* 83-102.

McKenna, T. (1992). *Food of the gods.* Bantam Books.

Pollan, M. (2018). *How to change your mind.* London: Penguin Press.

Richards, W. (2016). *Sacred knowledge.* Columbia University Press.

Szabo, A., Kovacs, A., Riba, J., Djurovic, S., Rajnavolgyi, E., & Frecska, E. (2016). The endogenous hallucinogen and trace amine N,N-dimethyltryptamine (DMT) displays potent protective effects against hypoxia via sigma-1 receptor activation in human primary iPSC-derived cortical neurons and microglia-like immune cells. *Frontiers in Neuroscience, 10,* 423.

In DSM V, the diagnostic and statistical manual of politically sanctioned terms used by mental health providers to label patients for insurance reimbursement, the diagnosis 'fear of joy' is noticeably absent.

—Bill Richards

Rob Cole

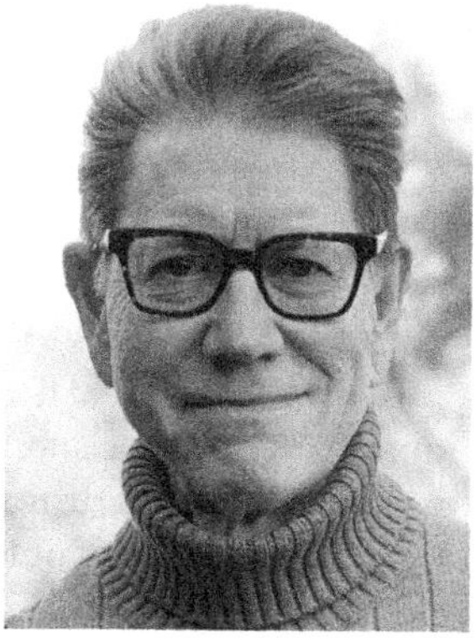

ROB COLE, MD, is an associate medical director of Hospice East Bay. Dr. Cole practiced obstetrics and gynecology in Walnut Creek, California, for over 20 years. Currently he maintains a private practice counseling patients with life threatening illness. As a stage four cancer survivor, he remains cancer free and lives in Orinda with his wife, Dale.
robbcolemd@gmail.com

Mortality Rising

MY EXPERIENCES WITH PSYCHEDELICS occurred primarily over a 3-year period in my early 20s. They formed a framework of reassurance and clarity about my relationship to self, the universe, and death. More recent psychedelic experiences continue to support many of the conclusions I came to as a young man. The insights are still fresh in my mind and heart 50 years later.

I suppose all lives are unexpected. Certainly, mine was bumpier than I anticipated.

I first heard about the disease, melanoma, from my father in the fourth grade when we built the model kit of the Visible Man. While we were painting the organs, he started explaining to me what each one of the organs did. He was not a doctor—he was an engineer—but he had an intense interest in medicine. Dad loved a great teaching moment. While we painted the lungs, Dad started talking about lung cancer. He talked about cigarette smoking and how it was a carcinogen, and then he talked about sunlight being a carcinogen and something I hadn't heard of before: melanoma. He explained to me that it was one of the worst kinds of cancers, very malignant; it was black, and if it was not removed very early when it was really small, it would always kill you. It would metastasize, another new word for me, which he explained meant that cells from the tumor could spread to any part of the body. Despite his good intentions, he told me a real-life horror story. I was 9, and it terrified me.

My relationship with melanoma continued in medical school, where it was one of the diseases I found most unsettling. The large disfiguring surgical excisions for such small tumors upset me during my surgical rotations, striking me as gothic and primitive. Fortunately, I rarely saw melanoma in my OB/GYN practice. It was not on my mind when my hairdresser moved out of town and my friend referred me to a new stylist. After the shampoo she began to comb out my hair.

"Rob? Do you know there's a spot on the top of your head?

"No."

"It's black, like ink; you should have it looked at."

There was a sensation of falling, followed by diaphoresis; I could feel my moist palms. What I had heard was "You have cancer."

In my first round of diagnosis and treatment I had a wide excision of my scalp, removing my stage two melanoma, and a negative sentinel lymph node biopsy. Nothing left to do; just to see if it returned.

Living from that moment on felt like waiting. I was 49.

Having a serious disease as a physician complicates anxiety. There is no sanctuary of ignorance. We all just know too much about what we have. One thing I knew was that if my melanoma returned it would most likely arise in one of the lymph nodes in my neck. I began to check the nodes in my neck a couple of times a day. It became an unconscious tick for me, but it kept me calm.

During a surgical procedure I was performing about a year after my diagnosis, my anesthesiologist shared a most disturbing tale with me. A man in his 20s had been diagnosed with stage one melanoma. It was excised without complication and did not return. In his 40s, he died in a motorcycle accident. His organs were donated: a heart, a liver, and two kidneys. All the recipients received cyclosporine, a drug that suppresses the immune response. All the recipient patients died of melanoma within the year.

The significance of this story is difficult to over emphasize. The implications are that the man with melanoma had been completely infested with the disease. Cells had metastasized to all his major organs, and they were sitting there dormant waiting for the opportunity to grow and multiply. When I got home that evening, I looked up the case and did in fact find it to be true. I found the case horrifying. Had my body already been completely corrupted?

All these experiences primed my anxiety. I felt like my sympathetic nervous system had been permanently activated. I was always in a fight / flight state because the threat was there, inside me; there was no escaping it. As I worked to find calm, I returned to a high dose LSD experience I had in my early 20s. During those experiences I became aware that my consciousness is both unique (singular, mine only) and ubiquitous (universal, nondual, beyond self). These two viewpoints are contradictory, yet both true. The viewpoint rooted in self is required for survival, and biological success limits perception. The physical world demands singular focused attention. But a deeper truth is that I am a part of a massive biologic whole, as we all are. Finding consciousness, within and part of that whole, was the discovery in that psychedelic experience. This collective view is complex and embodies consciousness, memory, and love. My experience of it was fleeting but intensely powerful. The truth of that experience was undeniable to me and, at its core, reassuring.

Thinking more deeply about the experience in my 20s, as well as in more recent experiences, it felt like a shifting of the location of consciousness to a place outside of self. It is difficult to describe, but in the moving of the center of my awareness my sense of self became smaller, while my consciousness became larger. There is bliss in selflessness. Returning to that memory is deeply calming for a number of reasons. The sense that I am something more than my physical body consoles me. In that thought I am more than a body corrupted by cancer. A glimpse of consciousness beyond the corporeal opens a door to metaphysical possibilities that provide hopefulness of a reality beyond death.

The question was—would that truth hold for me as I was tested?

Three and a half years had passed since my surgery. My anxiety about the return of the melanoma was in a manageable place. We had planned a trip to Cape Cod. We were staying at a bed and breakfast, and my wife, Dale, was taking a nap. I was reading, and I checked my neck—and there it was, just a firm little sphere of tissue deep to my sternocleidomastoid muscle, about a centimeter in diameter. It is always odd to experience a moment in time that you have spent so much time thinking about before it actually happens. I sat there drinking my gin and tonic, deciding what to do next. We had dinner plans at a nice restaurant, and there would be no point in telling Dale and ruining the evening. And even as I was defining the outlines of the mass with my fingers, I was wondering if it was really there.

Three weeks later, after the pet scan and biopsy were complete, the results showed a 1 cm melanoma in a lymph node deep in my neck. I would now need a radical neck dissection to remove any remaining cancer and other lymph nodes.

Changes started happening within 2 days of the biopsy. The node that I could barely feel exploded; it was now at least 2 to 3 centimeters in diameter, and I could see changes in the mirror. There were more nodes palpable as well. There is a phrase I had heard many times in the past: "Making the cancer angry." It certainly seemed like something like that was happening.

We met with my oncologist a few days later to talk about the biopsy results, the upcoming surgery, and the whole situation. I had worked with him for years. I had absolute trust in him. Before he examined me, his words were profoundly reassuring. Unfortunately, after he examined my neck, his eyes betrayed him. I could see his fear.

The darkness and overriding sense of doom that swirled around me over the next weeks were difficult. I scheduled an appointment with a psychiatrist. I started on an antidepressant, Paxil (paroxetine). I started feeling much better in just a few days. Work was tolerable, and we were getting closer to the surgery. After about a week had passed, I started feeling terrible. I was dizzy and nauseous, and it reached a crescendo on the weekend. I spoke with the oncologist on call, and we decided I needed to get a brain MRI to rule out brain mets. Fortunately, the scan was clear, and I was fine, but I had reached a new place in my struggle with this disease; it was now capable of killing me.

When I woke up the morning after Christmas, my jaw was hurting, and my tongue felt slightly swollen. It was a subtle sensation in the morning, but it became more intense throughout the day. The calmness that I had felt at Christmas was melting away. I started trying to get my brain around losing part of my tongue, but I was overwhelmed. So much for not being afraid. This cancer was assaulting my head, my neck, and now my mouth. I was starting to feel like soon there would be no place to retreat to. How much would be left of me after this operation was complete?

I returned to my mortality and my connection to the wider biologic whole. It still calmed me. Death did not frighten me, rather it was the path between now and then that terrified me: the deconstruction of my face and neck, the inevitable return of my cancer, the relentless disfigurement and consumption of me.

My operation was 2 days later. When I woke up from surgery, there was a heavy smell of chemical anesthesia on my breath. I had drains coming out of my neck, and I was nauseous. The surgery had taken a long time, and Dr S came by the next morning and explained that all my nodes were matted down and that he had to do a comprehensive neck dissection. I had lost my external and internal jugular vein, my sternocleidomastoid, and spinal accessory nerve, which would affect my shoulder and my right arm. I realized practicing obstetrics was probably over, which at the time was not the issue because I probably had little time left anyway.

When I got home, I realized I had not looked at myself in the mirror. It took 2 more days to do so. My tongue and my jaw were intact but my neck? The gaping defect in my neck was covered by tightly drawn skin pulled into position and held in place by a line of heavy nylon sutures. The tissues were angry and inflamed. The loss of mass and symmetry was unsettling.

When I was healed enough to travel, my oncologist and surgeon encouraged Dale and I to travel to melanoma centers around the country to investigate the next best treatment option for me. We visited several university hospitals. After hearing all the options offered to me, I realized every approach was different. I tried not to think about the insight that emerged: If no one can agree on what works, most likely nothing works.

I continued to struggle with sleeping and staying calm. I had unrelenting thoughts of disease progression, resulting in episodes of anger, depression, and anxiety. I began reading *Man's Search for Meaning* by Viktor Frankl (1959). The story of Frankl's experience surviving in the concentration camp in Buchenwald was stunning to me. We cannot control the events of our lives, but we can control their meaning. We can find our grace and dignity despite terrible situations. It gave me hope.

I found cannabis calmed me. It is a medication with profound psychedelic effects, and it reset and reframed the difficult days for me by pulling me out of the future. The future is a dangerous place to dwell for a stage four cancer patient. Cannabis is effective in bringing awareness to the present moment. For myself, and for so many cancer patients, looping negative thoughts about an imagined event at some point in the future can consume large swaths of time. It can become a default mode of its own. Once a pattern is established, it is difficult to disrupt. For me, as a pet scan approached, worry loops congealed in my head. A simple framework example: worry = vigilance, vigilance = protection, protection = safety, safety = worry. This structure tightens in on itself, consuming hours and hours of my life, exhausting me. I found cannabis could pull me out of these thought patterns and place me in the now.

Two years passed.

The appointment was well planned on Valentine's Day. Dale and I would go into San Francisco to see my oncologist at 2:00 p.m. We always wait, so we should be finished by 4:00 p.m., then head down to North Beach for dinner. We had come to enjoy these appointments because the visits were always encouraging and every good checkup meant I was closer to being out of the woods. Having a nice dinner together was our way of appreciating the moment of doing well and being together.

I took my shirt off and got on to the exam table. Both Dale and the nurse practitioner were looking at me from several feet away Evelyn pointed to my right shoulder, walked over, and touched it, asking, "What is that?" How could I have missed it? There it was, the enemy, a diffuse black spot less than a quarter of an inch in diameter, centrally quite dark, fading to a light gray at the perimeter. I looked at it; we all knew immediately what it was. Dale knew the second she saw it, before I sat down. How did I miss it? It must have come up so fast. Dale stood there working hard to say something reassuring. I could feel myself sweating and sticking to the paper on the exam table.

While we were driving home, I was trying to understand how I was feeling. I was sad, but that was not all of it. It felt like I had failed. I would never see 60. I would never see my children get married. I would never hold a grandchild. My wife would mourn me appropriately, then she would find new companionship. Everyone would be sad, but they would move on, as they should. I would become a memory. My grandchildren would only know me as a photograph and a few stories. I was going to have to let all of that go. I was not sure how I would do that.

After a PET scan and fine needle biopsies, the hidden infestation was completely revealed—a total of six new tumors were confirmed in my chest, leg, upper back, lower back, shoulder, and clavicle.

I had heard of experimental immunotherapy at the National Cancer Institute. It was the most promising light in a dark therapeutic landscape. We got an appointment, and within a week, Dale and I were flying back to Washington, DC. I was accepted to their program and began a year and a half of flights every few weeks. There were many hospital stays and infusions to stimulate my immune response to my invading cancer. Ultimately, one of the tumors growing in my body was harvested, and the immune cells growing in that tumor were grown in a lab and given back to me to attack my cancer and, hopefully, cure me.

The therapy was given to me after more than a year of preliminary therapy, and my tumors were shrinking as we headed back to DC for our third follow-up appointment. A new fellow walked into the room. She did not know me. Her presentation centered on a lymph node in the back of my knee that had increased in size. The change was measured in millimeters and provided the prognostication that would terminate my relationship with the institute. There were sounds emanating from her, but they were not being reconstructed into words in my brain as she spoke. Three complete sentences had been uttered before I reinstituted my ability to interpret language. She was telling me the therapy was no longer working and they had nothing else to offer us. I had reached the end of the line. It was very quiet in the room.

Surprising how things had ended so abruptly. They had nothing else for me. This was the last time they would see me. The speed of the change in my status was dizzying. They recommended a new drug, Anti CTLA 4, and that I should find a trial somewhere. It would be up to me to find a study protocol.

I was stunned at my own naiveté. I thought these people would be taking care of me forever. I suddenly had no idea what I had been thinking. I was there participating in a study protocol. It had not worked, and I was done. I had so wanted to be a good patient, and now what that meant was that I should collect my things and go. Walking to the elevator at the clinic was an out-of-body experience. I could not talk. Dale held my arm, and we just walked away.

When we got back to the hotel I lay down on the bed, and Dale got to work. She called the office of my oncologist about a CTLA 4 protocol. There was a group they worked with that was participating in the protocol. I was given the last remaining space before the study was closed. To be honest, we were not overly optimistic, but we were so grateful to have a study close to home.

The summer was coming to a close, and I was spending many days with a dear friend wandering around San Francisco, going to museums, walking in the park, and enjoying cannabis. It continued to help center me in the moment. But at the center, I was still searching for my own peace about completing my life and facing my death. I was staring out at the horizon of the Pacific Ocean at the top of Sutro Park, and it was clear to me that there was a part of me undefined and amorphous that would continue beyond my physical end. That would be enough for me. There had been so many disappointments in this journey. I was disengaging from the outcome. My attention was moving to the day I was living. I began focusing my gratitude on a good day.

Over the next year, I slowly responded to my treatment. I stopped waiting. I stopped worrying. I assumed my disease would return and consume me. In an attempt to find my own grace and normalize death for myself, I began my clinical work as a hospice physician. My own cancer journey helped me connect to my patients. Some conversations were remarkable; however, I was surprised to find many patients committed to a path of denial, unable to conceive or contemplate their own passing in ways that they could find comfort in. Traditional theistic structures were ill suited and secular or scientific narratives lacked the emotional support to carry them to their journey's conclusion.

One of my first patients was a man in his 50s. When I met him in his home he was deeply jaundiced, cachectic, in a robe and slippers, and unsteady in his gait. He was an intelligent man, an engineer. I was there with our chaplain to talk about what lay before him and how we might help.

Early on, he said, "If this cancer kills me..."

The conversation continued, but I was stuck on that phrase.

"If this cancer kills me..."

Really? An intelligent man with months to absorb the medical reality of his diagnosis of advanced metastatic colon cancer and he could not comprehend he was going to die?

It was a strange and uncomfortable conversation. Three days later, I was in that same living room where he lay in a hospital bed, in a coma, actively dying.

I remember walking to the car with our chaplain, Elizabeth, when we first met him saying, "He has no idea where he is, does he?"

This death deeply affected me. He had two children, and he never said goodbye. I felt that his fear kept him from fully completing his life. It was simply a leap that he could not make. He had found his situation so stark that his commitment to denial was total. Over my 11 years in hospice work, I saw this many times. In palliative care it is our job to help people to become situationally aware around the time of their death. My experience with these patients and my own journey convince me that the present cultural, religious, and spiritual structures in play are inadequate to fully support many of us as we complete our lives. With many, increasing doses of benzodiazepines being the central instrument of reassurance.

I have come to believe there is an important role psychedelics can play to help us confront our mortality more directly. The religious dogma that was so central to the culture for the management of terror of death has become anachronistic, rigid, irrelevant, and most importantly, unbelievable. As our lives are enlightened by science and technology, we yearn for new narratives: a modern mythology and spirituality, if you will, to serve us as we bridge the gap between our present naturalistic view and the next uncharted realms of enlightenment. Psychedelics have long been a tool for reframing consciousness. We need to begin to integrate them into our care and culture to provide existential and emotional support as we face life threatening illness.

I am deeply grateful for the cumulative impact all of my experiences have had on me. In many ways I credit them for providing me a foundation that allowed me to fully embrace my mortality as I engaged with a cancer that had fully corrupted my body. Throughout that engagement I was able to find calm, humor, meaning, and hope despite deep darkness and being convinced much of the time that my death was inevitable. So much of life is a manifestation of perspective, and I am thankful for the frame of reference these remarkable substances have provided me. They continue to inform and support me as I endeavor to embrace life fully, gracefully, and gratefully. The best preparation for death is a life well lived. These tools may help free us from fear, anxiety, and depression as we live and as we die.

References

Frankl, V. (1959). *Man's search for meaning.* London: Hodder & Stoughton.

> Throughout human history, as our species has faced the frightening, terrorizing fact that we do not know who we are, or where we are going in this ocean of chaos, it has been the authorities, the political, the religious, the educational authorities who attempted to comfort us by giving us order, rules, regulations, informing, forming in our minds their view of reality. To think for yourself you must question authority and learn how to put yourself in a state of vulnerable, open-mindedness; chaotic, confused, vulnerability to inform yourself.
>
> —Timothy Leary

Anonymous

Touching Within

When my husband and soulmate died several years ago, my whole life changed completely. I was grieving. Soon after, friends from out of town came to pay condolences. They had an underground retreat center in Hawaii where they worked with plant medicine. They thought the medicine that they were trained to deliver would be helpful in my grief process.

It was the catalyst that led 3 years later to my completing a 1-year program in psychedelic therapy and research at California Institute of Integral Studies (CIIS) in San Francisco. I then sought out direct experiences in an underground training in methylenedioxymethamphetamine (MDMA) and psilocybin (psychedelic mushroom) with a psychologist who had been working in the field for over 10 years. Since then, I have been able to facilitate underground medicine work and have found it to be life changing.

So, let me tell you a story about facilitating one woman's journey.

Jill's Journey

I received a call from a naturopathic doctor who told me that her 35-year-old daughter, Jill, had been diagnosed a year before with stage four melanoma cancer. She hoped that a plant medicine journey would help Jill deal with both hospital trauma and end of life issues. I agreed to work with her.

Jill is a senior neuroscientist. She had never taken any psychedelics. At the time of her first interview, she felt that her body had failed her—and she was mad at it! She also felt guilty because she felt she could have prevented her cancer if she had worn sunscreen more frequently. She did not want to die and was anxious and afraid of death. She wanted to feel peace and acceptance of her current health challenge.

Two preparation sessions were held after the initial intake to establish Jill's intentions for her journey and to provide education about what she could expect during the journey. Preparation emphasizes trusting the medicine and the client's inner healing intelligence, as well as discussing the specific arc of the journey and the structure of the day.

At the end of the first preparation session Jill came up

with three intentions for her focus during the journey: trusting herself, accepting the diagnosis with peace, and living in the present. These intentions were simplified to three words she could hold on to and repeat to herself during her journey: trust, acceptance, and presence.

What was unusual about this MDMA session was that Jill decided to invite her husband and her mother to support her during the journey. I talked with each of them to prepare them for what to expect.

Set and setting are important in a psychedelic journey to feel safe and comfortable. I set up an altar with the four elements of nature: earth, water, fire, and air. On the altar there is incense and flowers, and on the floor there is a mattress with blankets and pillows. With the journeyer wearing a headset and eye shades, the music is specifically crafted to flow with the arc of the journey. A role that I have as a facilitator is to support the journeyer in my being present and making sure that they are feeling safe.

I gave Jill a first dose of MDMA and then a boost an hour and a half later. MDMA works on serotonin, dopamine, and oxytocin. It is an empathogen, which increases the feelings of empathy and benevolence towards others, and an entheogen, which produces a non-ordinary state of consciousness.

Here are some of Jill's direct quotes during the journey (italics taken from personal communications in sessions or follow-up calls):

"My body is saying healing — peace, presence, trust, and healing," said Jill.

"Mom, did you ever have a fear that something would happen to us?"

Mike, Jill's husband: "Did you ever have fears that something bad would happen?"

Jill: "Did you think I was going to die last summer?"

Mom: "I was open, but I didn't think it was really going to happen."

Jill: "Mike?"

Mike: "Yes."

Jill: "Mike, are you mad at me that I didn't go to the doctor earlier?"

Mike: "No."

Jill: "Trust is so healing. I haven't trusted myself; my body betrayed me, and so I wouldn't trust my body. Trust and healing are connected."

"Mom, I hope you're with me to the end whenever that might be..."

Mom: "And I you."

Jill: "Mom, what do you think happens when you die? Do you believe in an afterlife?"

Jill: "My body feels good. I feel peaceful, warm, and comforted. I'm drawing energy from Mom and Mike. Mike, are you mad at me?"

Mike: "No."

Jill: "I want you to be close to me...is there anything holding you back?"

"I'm afraid I won't be alive for a long time...I can overcome that fear! I feel warm and at peace...since the cancer I've been on edge...with thoughts about what's coming."

Jill went on to talk about how she wants better connections with other people but expressed how "everything I have to say is so heavy—so I keep it to myself. I hope people don't feel I'm not connected to them." She told me that she could hear in every song being played in the journey the words, "peace, presence, healing, and trust."

Later in Jill's journey, she said, "I feel guilty I have cancer... Now the medicine wants me to let guilt go and breathe it out..."

Jill: "Mike, would you be OK if I died?"

Mike: "I will survive."

Mom: "The family will take care of Mike."

Jill: "I hope I'm not fighting it—if I'm close to death."

Last thought before the end of journey: the things Jill would like people to remember about her... that she was smart, that she cared about other people. She was not sure if people knew this.

When I called her the next morning to see how she was doing, Jill reported that she heard:

Trust your body and it will give you what you need. That surprised me. My body knows what to do...my body doubted it...but it knows what to do. Peace, presence, trust, and healing...my body knows what to do. I felt energy and warmth.

Typically, clients have three follow-up integration sessions with their facilitator. Integration helps people digest the information and insights that transpired during the journey so that they become enduring qualities.

Here are some of Jill's words during the first integration session:

Trust and healing are at the forefront of my mind.... My life is being cut short—my body knows exactly how to live...my body won't let me suffer.... I trust myself. My body knows how long I'm going to live...it will be perfectly long enough...I trust my body...it already knows.... Trust is going to be everywhere... more trusting others...I trust you. I trust my mind...I heard to love others and trust.

Then she told me of her behavioral changes since the journey:

I started mindfulness practices in my daily life...taking a minute...what do I hear? I was breathing in the journey...Mike was lying next to me and breathing.... I'm trusting myself...I do have fears, but it's OK. My body is in control, and it knows what it's doing. I was very connected during the journey...I know I wasn't ready to die. During the journey my forehead was cold—then energy radiated out of my heart... and feeling warmer—so comforting.

In the second integration session, she said that in the journey the instructions were to be open to whatever came up, so now she finds that she isn't second guessing herself: "There is a strong confidence in trust... a strong sense of it."

She related that she used to cry when talking to others about her diagnosis. She recognizes that "most people don't have to contemplate their mortality like I do."

"I felt so connected to Mom and Mike during the journey, and it has extended to the desire for connection to others," concluded Jill.

A Second Journey

Eight months later, Jill wanted another session. This time it was going to be a combination of MDMA and psilocybin. She had changed physically. She was weaker. She had not been able to eat well because she was feeling nauseated, had lost 10 lbs, and had not been able to lie on her back because of her nausea.

As a therapist I was concerned with two things: the impact of the cancer on her body and whether she could tolerate the medicine, because ingesting psilocybin can bring nausea.

We met for the prep session on Zoom, and she was lying prone. The immune therapy, not the cancer, had attacked other parts of her digestive tract. She felt fatigued, slow, and not able to do much walking. She was on prednisone.

Her intentions for this next journey were formulating. She wanted to lighten the power of grief by acknowledging what she could still do with compassion for herself and compassion for others.

She feared that if she shared her true self with others she would be rejected. Because she had been such a high achiever, accomplished so much, and felt so good about it in the past, now she felt limited and like a failure.

She felt that she had two lives: before and after the cancer:

> *I'm a whole new person, and who do I want that person to be? It took 35 years to be comfortable with the person I was and only 2 years to be a new person. A new person that knows that I will die. As this new person I want to be a true authentic self that doesn't hold back because of a fear of rejection.*

We ended the conversation saying she was going to try more medication to help with her nausea.

In the second prep session we established three intentions: *"practicing compassion for self and others, processing and understanding how grief is shaping the new me, and connecting to my true and authentic self."* The three words she would hold on to during the journey: compassion, understanding, and connecting.

Jill's mother planned to be at the next medicine journey again. Her husband was traveling. The medicine that was given was MDMA and psilocybin.

Highlights of the second journey:

She was lying on her back. "I haven't been able to do that. It's been very difficult. Felt good," said Jill.

"If I make it 11 years or maybe even 7 years, I want to have a Harry Potter party," she said to her mom.

"Mom, have you ever contemplated the meaning of life? I think it's the connection with other people. I feel like I'm living two lives. The one before and the one after the cancer, knowing I'm going to die. I've only been diagnosed for 2 years with cancer, and it might take time to be comfortable with this."

"It's great lying on my back, and it's a good feeling lying down."

"Cancer patients should say thank you for all the support instead of I'm sorry I'm such a burden."

"So happy I can lie on my back."

I had a conversation with her about grief and trauma. She said, "Trauma happened to me, and grief resulted." I then asked her if the grief stepped aside what was left? She was quiet, thinking about it, then responded, "I feel happy and at peace...I hear breath in the music...I'm not as connected to compassion. I'm connected to the new me."

At the end of the session, Jill said:

> *I have a sense that the earth is holding me, and I feel like I am connected to nature with the mushrooms. This is the best day in a long time. I don't feel the grief—it's nice to have a break from grief though. When grief steps back, love comes forward.*

She never felt any nausea during the journey, and for the first time after months of nausea she was able to eat a simple snack I prepared.

I made a quick check-in call the day after the journey. She said she slept well and that in reflection the music experience had been different:

> *I could hear each instrument and it was breathing with me. I was able to lie on my back last night—still feeling good—that grief had stepped aside.... When I thought about the questions of what's next, if grief stepped aside, what came forward was excitement. I'm excited about what's going to happen. Let's wait and see. Maybe I'll work with cancer patients. I would be happy to connect with them.*
> *I had a great experience and felt more connected with my intentions this time.*

In the first integration session, 1 week later, Jill said, "I am still feeling much better. Nausea has lifted a lot. The medicine knew what it was doing and knew what I needed and how to direct the medicine in my body for healing."

During the session, her face was at times flushed so I would give her a cool cloth. I asked her about what that meant to her. She said it was like a forest fire cleaning out burned-out old life. "It was there for the new life to grow."

She said her grief had shifted—now she realized it was anticipatory grief and so it felt lighter. Not quite so crushing. The whole experience was overwhelmingly positive. More than she expected. More than her intentions...

In the last integration session, 1 month later, Jill said she was doing much better since the last session. She was back to work and she had not had any nausea since the journey. I asked her where she was with her goal of having peace about dying, and she said she's not at peace with where she is right now because it's hard to accept that she will die, but she doesn't feel fearful about death anymore.

As far as her issues around grief, she said that once she understood what she was experiencing was anticipatory grief and could give it a name, it no longer felt overwhelming. She's accepting where she is right now. She's gone back to physical and occupational therapy to be able to be able to work with her limitations.

Post-Medicine Journeys

Jill is employed by a pharmaceutical company that manufactures sunblock. As an act of compassion towards others, she wanted to place dispensers of sunblock in the courtyard at her workplace in order to protect her employees. She has already emailed someone at work to accomplish that.

A couple weeks ago she had dinner to celebrate with her friends her 2-year anniversary having survived a cancer diagnosis. She had an open conversation with her friends about how hard it's been for her. For the first time, she was able to share this difficult journey and received lots of support from her friends. This is an example of her being more authentic, taking a risk and feeling connected to others.

She also said that she's planning to go to Italy with her husband. She has a much more positive outlook, feeling so much better being able to make these kinds of plans.

She thinks she would like one more medicine journey with just psilocybin. She's aware that it can be a more challenging experience. I asked her if I could share her journey with all of you and she said yes. It was such an honor to sit with Jill.

My Own Process as a Facilitator

As a facilitator, I feel strongly that you can't facilitate unless you have an embodied experience with the medicine. That doesn't prepare you for everything that can happen, but it familiarizes you with several different qualities of the medicine. Each journey is uniquely individual and singular.

I never thought that I could sit with someone who had eye shades on and a headset, listening to music for 5 to 6 hours. My poor body, I thought. What will I do, sitting for an interminable period of time?

I listen deeply to the client, to the beautiful music, I sit and ground myself with an attuned presence, and I can sense when the medicine is beginning to take effect. I meditate. I find myself checking in verbally every hour or so if there is no conversation to see how the journeyer is doing. It is a great lesson for me in being present, grounded, available, in my heart, and trusting the medicine. Trusting that it will show the journeyer exactly what they need to see to heal, to grow, and to blossom. Trusting that their inner healing intelligence is wiser and more tailored than anything I could come up with in my rational mind.

At the end of the session, I have taken notes of everything the journeyer has said while in the medicine. I type it up and send it to them the next day. They are also recording their experience on their phones so they can play it back and remember what they said and hear the music again, which can evoke emotions that may not be accessible otherwise.

As a facilitator, I have been able to witness and trust the unique and wise inner healing intelligence of each journeyer.

In my own journey, I have learned that my grief for my husband and the life we led will always be a part of me. Sometimes the grief comes in big waves and sometimes in small ripples. Now I can navigate those waters with more compassion and ease. I am more able to ask for what I need. I'm not sure if this is a result of psychedelics or just that time has passed. Probably both.

Journey work is not for everyone. There has been so much press and published research on how these medicines have helped clients with PTSD (especially for Veterans), depression, and end of life existential anxiety, potential journeyers can come with high expectations and be disappointed when they have difficult experiences. Also, there is a list of antidepressants (SSRIs, MAOIs), migraine medicines, herbal supplements, and over-the-counter cold medicines that people need to discontinue to be able to experience a full journey. Sometimes medicine reduction can take months under supervision of their psychiatrist before a client is ready. Serotonin syndrome, though rare, can be lethal. A family history of bipolar disorder, psychiatric hospitalizations, etc., are contra-indications.

The FDA will likely approve MDMA for PTSD in 2024 and psilocybin in 2026. This is a new world of clinical trials, treatment, and learning to support and facilitate non-ordinary states of consciousness in the service of healing. Being a part of it has been a profound journey for me.

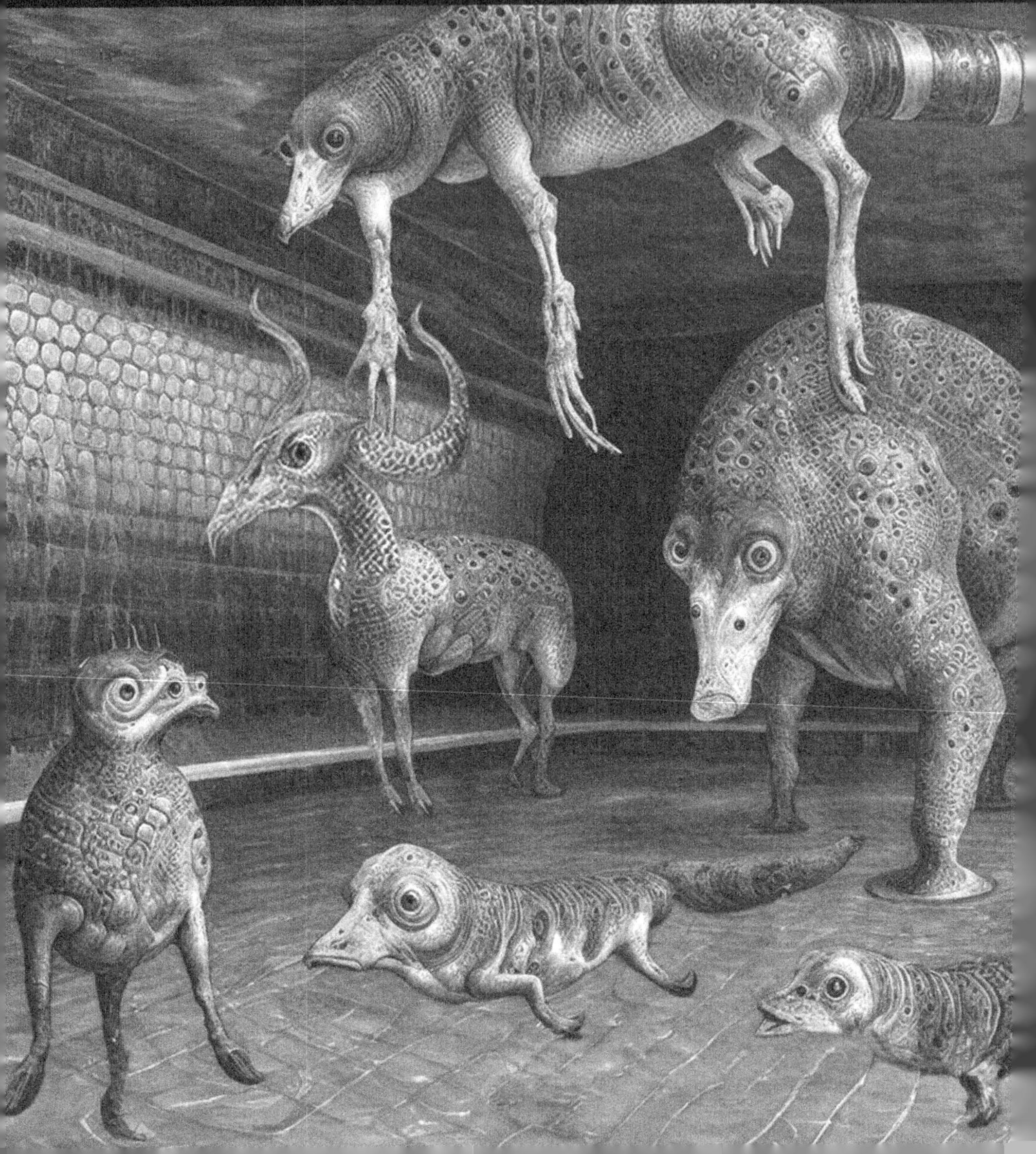

Deborah Servetnick

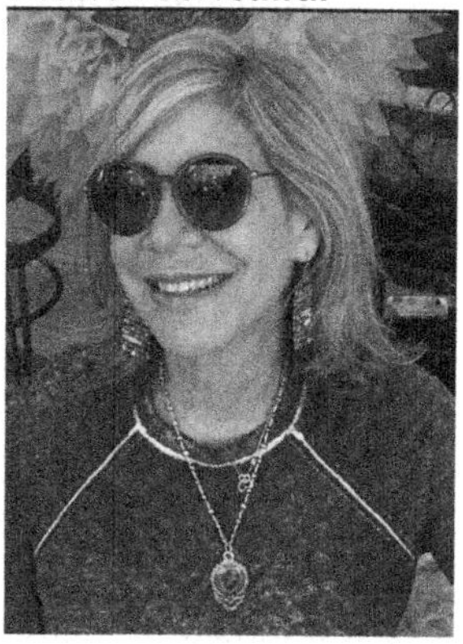

DEBORAH SERVETNICK is an international speaker and transformational coach committed to expanding safe and ethical psychedelic practices. A participant in the pioneering Johns Hopkins Psilocybin Cancer Study in 2012, Deborah has dedicated her life's work to integrating psychedelics into healing and personal growth. A best-selling author, death doula, bodyworker, and certified psychedelic-assisted therapist by Naropa University/MAPS, she is the founder of Serve-Medicine, a non-profit providing a free guided psychedelic journey for those with life-threatening illness or end-of-life diagnosis, and currently serves on the advisory board for EOLPC (End-Of-Life Psychedelic Care).
deb@gratefuldeb.com

Become the Ocean

THE FIRST TIME I WAS SCHEDULED TO JOURNEY as a participant in the Johns Hopkins University (JHU) psilocybin cancer study, I received a placebo.

This was 2012, and I had been diagnosed with Stage 3 breast cancer in 2011. I had chemotherapy, which nearly killed me, a bilateral mastectomy, and radiation that resulted in third degree burns. I didn't know what I'd done to get dealt such a terrible hand. I ate organic. I studied metaphysics and Chinese medicine; I was a breath worker and a bodyworker, and I had already been to over 100 Grateful Dead concerts and knew I loved LSD and psilocybin.

And I knew this wasn't a psychedelic experience.

I was pissed!

My disappointment and my victimhood were an excruciating combination. I was too sick to do my sourcing of psychedelics my usual way—in the Shakedown lot outside a Dead show. Side effects from chemo made it difficult to walk and nearly impossible to stand in one place. I couldn't walk in a crowd without falling down if someone stopped in front of me on the way to their grilled cheese, or anywhere, without warning. My balance was affected, and I couldn't dance because I couldn't feel my feet. My scars hurt all the time. I had constant stomach pain caused by the pain meds. Cancer was the worst thing that ever happened to me, and there were many times I wished I would die.

So, I prayed that I'd be accepted into the JHU study because I intuitively knew I needed psychedelics or I would die. I had a 12-year-old daughter, I deeply loved my husband, Donnie, and I knew my only hope of getting safe psychedelics was as a participant in this study. Because this was a study for depression and anxiety following a cancer diagnosis, I worried whether I would be depressed enough to qualify—and what if I was too depressed? What if I said the wrong thing? How much experience would be too much? Do I tell them I used ayahuasca in 1989? I didn't even know how to spell it, or anyone else who used it. The qualifying was so stressful. No matter what, I needed to get into this study. Looking back, if I wasn't a resident of Baltimore I would have never been able to participate; there were many, many hours and whole days of visits to fill out paperwork when I could barely hold a pencil. I had to have an EKG and other tests and meet with JHU psychedelics researcher Roland Griffiths—when I couldn't even find the words to finish a sentence.

And then, my initial trip, the trip I prayed for and desperately needed, was a pathetic disappointment.

"What did you give me? A placebo?!? Don't you know I have cancer? I might not even make it until you bring me back for the real thing. I might be dead."

I've always wondered why we make people argue for their limitations in order to get treatment. Insurance companies require patients to gain more weight before they can get bariatric surgery. Women spiraling into early menopause after chemotherapy don't receive follow-up care that will allow them to continue to live life uninterrupted—to work and sleep like they did before mood swings, headaches, and drenching sweats, or prevent their bones from thinning and shattering, while their marriages burn out in company with their vaginas. Bouncing from gynecologist to gynecologist, I have begged for hormone replacement therapy. Patients must receive a diagnosis of treatment-resistant depression before they qualify for a psilocybin or MDMA psychedelic study. Treatment is dragged out for decades, intimate relationships hit a wall, while patients continue into their 40s to take meds prescribed when they were in high school that they aren't even sure have made their lives better. What about these practices are good medicine? Shouldn't the desire to fully live be enough?

I thought about the lack of integrity, the damage a double-blind study could do to someone already suffering from the anxiety and depression of a diagnosis and the trauma of cancer treatment. Self-doubt, shame, and blame permeated my every thought during those days. What if I left my daughter motherless? What if I would never feel any better than this? I had psychedelic experience and awareness, and I knew I didn't receive a psychedelic. Why was there no help for me?

How long are we going to study the effectiveness of psychedelics at the expense of real people, with real side effects from treatment? Many people apply for studies, and myriad factors can make them ineligible. We know psychedelics can eliminate suicidal thoughts, alleviate PTSD, and expand our consciousness. Why was my suffering not important? Instead of breakthrough treatment, my suffering was left to oxycodone.

At my Naropa University MAPS Psychedelic-Assisted Therapies training more than a decade later, when I had already coached and guided hundreds of underground psychedelic clients, I secretly asked my courageous trainers how they felt about the use of a double-blind protocol in these psychedelics studies: if they thought that practice was out of integrity.

They told me exactly how they felt. They confessed they were unwilling to participate in this practice any longer.

I am confident that the people who have devoted their lives to the study and practice of psychedelic medicine irrefutably feel their connection to Infinite Intelligence. They recognize that we each have an inner-healer. Spirit has guided them to steward our wellness. I know there has been criticism of the JHU studies, saying they are biased in favor of a mystical experience. That was not my experience. And some, even those who are publicly recognized, those who are the face of cutting-edge leadership roles in psychedelic research, might not get it. They might not loosen up or let go until their own life-threatening diagnosis. I remember thinking as I was interviewed post-journey, "Roland doesn't get it." There was a gift in my life-threatening diagnosis that he couldn't understand until many years had passed and he had his own cancer diagnosis. A life-threatening illness or end-of-life diagnosis can create new awareness that we have a finite life, yet an infinite existence. I listened to his interviews and his keynotes as he embraced new words, noticing how he had begun to truly live and help others create and live a new life. We create with every word. We get what we think about, whether we want it or not. Psychedelics taught me that.

Doctors need to experience psychedelics to prescribe them. They need to have lots of experience.

Psychedelics have a way of revealing truth. We don't have to wait for an end-of-life diagnosis to meet God. Recalling my subsequent life-changing JHU journey continues to beckon my emotions, like the journey itself, to the ineffable. Since that trip, I've felt more connected to God and the Universe.

My second journey, my consolation prize, featured a special guest: Jesus. On the cross.

It was completely unexpected; I'm Jewish. When I saw Jesus, I told him, "I know you must have something really important to tell me."

He responded, "You're attached to your struggle."

What could that mean? I would never give myself cancer.

Immediately, I was whisked through lifetimes and lifetimes of crawling through the dirt: walking the Trail of Tears, lifetime after lifetime of struggle. Belief that life had to be hard for me to feel worthy.

Integration of this transformational journey took 10 years; it took me to Nederland, CO, Grass Valley and Nevada City, CA, the Donner Pass, Morrison and Boulder, CO... over and over again, in gold mines and coal mines...through mountains of red rocks, walking through forests of snow...believing a hard life made me worthy, right up to the chemo that almost killed me. I stopped trying to fix things; stopped seeing anything as broken. I let go of politics and protest and noticed my beliefs, the words I spoke, and the activities I engaged with. Contrast is essential on this life path. It is what keeps us asking for more. That's the message behind Alan Watts' (1965/1970) often quoted, "If you get the message [or answer], hang up the phone" (p. 26). It was a decision to look for the good inside everything. Everything in my life was of value. Everything was an expression of Infinite Intelligence. Not just the things I liked.

The integration of a psychedelic experience is a practice. It is why meditation accelerates the process of integration. Meditation is a practice of noticing every thought; integration is served by noticing every thought, then deciding for the best feeling thought. It was a brand-new idea for me to give thanks in all things, but I desired to master this. I had lots of encouragement from my husband, Donnie, a master meditator. I never wanted to experience the lessons cancer brought ever again. One of my mentors explained it like this: "How many times do you pick up a crying baby? Every time."

When we love that baby we don't say, "I picked you up this morning," or "I did that yesterday." We pick that baby up and let it know we shower it with love every single time.

We are vibrational beings, and love is the highest vibration.

I stopped chemo against my oncologist's recommendation. My family scheduled an intervention with my treatment team, pleading with me to continue. After my anger at this ambush ended, I understood that this effort was driven by their fear that cancer would kill me, but I knew the chemo would kill me first. Confidently, I told them that I was going to get better with the help of cannabis, ayahuasca, LSD, mushrooms, MDMA, and ketamine, and I told my oncologist it was OK with me if he took the credit.

I never regretted that decision to leave medical treatment behind to use plant medicine and other entheogens exclusively. My family told me I was easier to live with, chemo brain improved, and I felt joy. I stopped living with the fear of cancer.

Side effects from medical treatment lasted years, and I still have some. Chemo brain was discouraging, demoralizing, and affected everything. It limited spatial ability. I couldn't judge where I was. For months, I drove in the left lane at a top speed of 40 mph; I was too afraid to drive in the right lane. I missed recognizing my turn repeatedly at a familiar intersection near home. I walked into things. I couldn't type or text; my fingers couldn't do it, and it took so much concentration on the keys I would forget what I was writing. It took me years to finish a sentence if I was interrupted. Teaching required more time than ever; to prepare effectively I had to write everything down and read from the paper every lesson. Grading in a timely way was impossible. Post-it notes were everywhere. It was frustrating and I nearly gave up. But once I shifted my perception of seeing this as negative, it evolved into a sign of divine discontent. I decided I would leave school and instead teach what I loved and valued, what helped me to not only want to live but to help others live their best life, no matter how much time they had. I asked the Universe to line me up with LSD, and it showed up without me knowing much about microdosing protocol. I microdosed every day for four months. I actually felt it repairing my nervous system. This is similar to how I experienced chemo moving through every cell of my body. Walking got easier, and I danced 4 hours nonstop at a wedding. I felt better than I had in years, and I continued to use LSD in my recovery.

I asked the Universe for LSD, and it brought me not only the LSD but my job as a cannabis consultant in one of the first dispensaries to open in Baltimore. I testified in Annapolis in favor of medical cannabis, and when I heard a dispensary was opening in my neighborhood I knew this job was mine; I repeatedly visualized myself working there. At the interview I mentioned I was microdosing LSD, and the conversation grew to healing cancer with cannabis and psychedelics. It's possible I am the first person you know of who got a job because they use an illegal substance! I connected with extraordinary mentors training me to become a transformational life coach and psychedelic guide. Looking back now I see the many ways my intuition has always guided me and how this path chose me. I've been a Death Doula since the AIDS epidemic. This was in the Bay Area, and psychedelics were available and plentiful. My deeper personal relationship with psychedelics and with a life-threatening illness shifted my inner narrative, stopped me from punishing myself, and steered me in the direction of my inner guidance. I became a full-time psychedelic coach and guide, modeling to others the ability to be, do, and have whatever we love, in accordance with our values, living a life beyond circumstances and conditions.

I don't wait for anything anymore. There is no medal for how hard it was when this is all over. Nobody gets a prize for suffering the most.

Psychedelics helped me see the value of my life. They didn't give me the side effects I had from medical treatment, and they didn't require me to use them for an extended period of time. Anyone using medicine requiring a daily dose or multiple doses a day would be surprised to see how efficacious psychedelic medicine can be and how sustainable the results of treatment are. Yet they're still classified Schedule 1.

Medicalization is a distraction. It won't serve the underserved, and it won't keep psychedelics from those who won't use them safely. We can't summon our inner healing intelligence by arguing for our limitations. We create—and re-create—with every thought. The power of recreational psychedelics invited me to twirl to Grateful Dead music 50 years ago and helped me create ServeMedicine, a nonprofit providing a guided psychedelic journey to people with a life-threatening illness or end-of-life diagnosis. If psychedelics and Grateful Dead made your life better, I invite you to submit your psychedelic story to our book *Wake Up to Find Out.*

Donnie died suddenly in September, 2022. He was the kindest, most generous, funniest, most loving person I have ever known. He was a runner, a master meditator and yogi, my personal court jester, my cheerleader for all my psychedelic ideas, a man of integrity, an attorney who worked pro-bono more than any lawyer I've known. He was diagnosed with Stage 4 cancer when I returned from speaking at the Sisters in Psychedelics conference in Vancouver, and he was dead 2 weeks after his diagnosis. He loved psychedelics; he loved my daughter and me, our dog, and our cat. And he refused to do chemo saying, "I saw what chemo did to you, and I won't do it. I experienced more love with you than I ever expected." He ate an eighth of mushrooms the week before he died. I feel his presence all the time, and more than ever I don't wait for anything anymore.

Your conscious vibration makes ripples.

Psychedelics are Infinite Intelligence, and we were meant to bring it into our lives.

In the words of the poet:

> The river needs to take the risk
> of entering the ocean
> because only then will fear disappear,
> because that's where the river will know
> it's not about disappearing into the ocean,
> but of becoming the ocean.
>
> —Khalil Gibran, "Fear" (public domain)

References

Watts, A. (1965/1970). *The joyous cosmology: Adventures in the chemistry of consciousness.* Revised edition. Vintage Books.

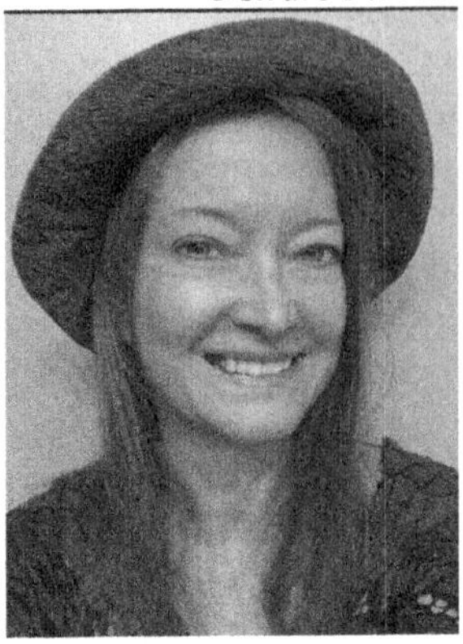

Deirdre Barrett, PhD, is on the faculty of Harvard where she teaches courses on dreaming. She has written five books, including *Pandemic Dreams* and *The Committee of Sleep*. She is past president of The Society for Psychological Hypnosis, president of the International Association for the Study of Dreams, and editor of the journal, *Dreaming*. Deirdre has lectured and led workshops at Esalen, the Smithsonian, and universities around the world.
deirdre_barrett@hms.harvard.edu

Interview with Deirdre Barrett

Steve Eichel: [Speaking with Deirdre Barrett, known for her work in the fields of dreams and hypnosis.] Deirdre, you're mostly known for your work on dreams, so tell me how you got interested in that.

Deidre Barrett: I just had very vivid dreams from as far back in childhood as I can recall. I remember dreams virtually every night, usually multiple ones, and they tended to be kind of long adventures. And I had vivid recall.

Eichel: How did you get interested in psychedelics?

Barrett: I'm 69 now, so I was just at the age that exactly as I was hitting puberty, they were becoming a thing, mostly with people 5 years older than me. There was a lot of very poor quality marijuana around when I was in high school. I was curious about [LSD] but definitely believing some of the scary or at least entertaining the possibility of some of the scary happening.

[In my small town] it was actually the kids who already had some degree of mental illness who did LSD... back then, I got exposed to like one person having a bad trip and no particularly good stories from the people I was close to about positive experiences with them. But I was reading the Timothy Leary stuff. I have a positive curiosity, but just like with anything, it's like you get curious a little bit before you get up the nerve to do something... When I got to college [Emory University in Atlanta] my group of friends were not initially doing LSD... But by then I was certainly reading the stuff that made it sound like an interesting experience, just as I was finding mainstream psychology so fascinating. I was finally getting to talk about dreams with PhD psychologists, not just informally.

I didn't like marijuana. I felt like my thinking was not very clear...I would feel it made me dumb...like I couldn't think, but I would be obsessively struggling to try to understand something that I felt impaired from understanding. Other drugs went the other way. They either didn't impair reasoning, or one didn't care while on [them].

I actually did all the other psychedelics before I did LSD. I was kind of hanging out with a crowd that was terribly into health foods and things being natural. So even [with] drugs, they were sort of more into [the view that] plant things were good, chemicals were bad. But that was not my bias.

So I think [my choices were influenced by] the people who I connected with intellectually. They were the ones reading the novels I wanted to read and talking interesting intellectual stuff. So I did peyote multiple times, and I didn't carefully choose it as the first hallucinogen to try. It was just the thing that came around.

Eichel: It sounds like peyote was the first hallucinogen that you ever tried. Do you remember that first time?

Barrett: I do. Someone had these peyote buds, and so we just chopped them up into small pieces because they were a little tough, and they did not taste very good, pretty bitter.

So we'd been somewhat instructed on how much to take. I remember it sort of being a very gradual onset like one of those "I'm feeling something; I'm not sure," like maybe it was coming on in subtle little waves. I was with several people part of the time, but then just with

Steve Eichel

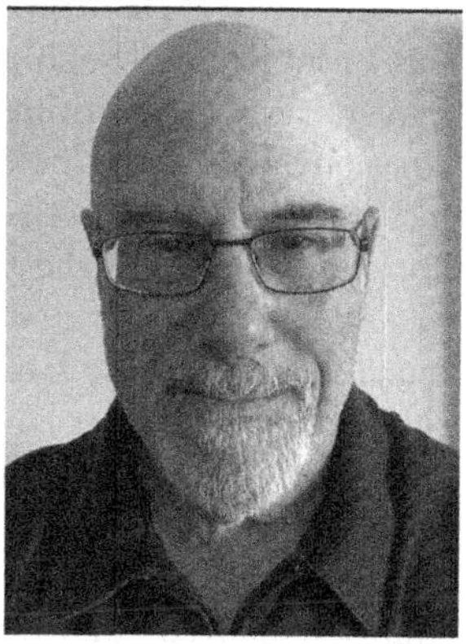

STEVE K. D. EICHEL, PhD, ABPP, CST is a licensed and board-certified counseling psychologist with a part-time independent practice. His subspecialties include clinical hypnosis (he is a former president of the Greater Philadelphia Society of Clinical Hypnosis), EMDR, and sex therapy. He lives in Newark, Delaware, with his wife Terri, stepson Tristan, five cats, and a mellotron.
steve@dreichel.com

my boyfriend at the time. We went off to one room, and I just remember having really sort of lovely, philosophical conversations, kind of about Eastern philosophy... And I remember that everything was very beautiful and sort of alive, but it wasn't vivid hallucinations. I mean the looking alive wasn't like faces were jumping out of the wall at me. It was more like subjectively everything felt like some living entity. And just like I was noticing more. So all the visual things were enhanced and distorted a little way, but that first time it was not full-on hallucinations. We had the lights on, maybe dim but on. I remember everything looking pretty, in the sense of the whole universe, but also every concrete object in it as having some kind of, if not consciousness, at least just life. But I remember the conversation as being the most interesting thing.

That was the first time, but then I did some from the same batch by myself within a week of that time. And I decided to do more because my experience had been fairly mild. I'd enjoyed it, nothing bad about it...so I went in my room, and the room looked really pretty in the dark, and it definitely looked sparkling and more like hallucinations. It was like there were just all these funny little light and texture effects that I think were partly because I was doing more, but partly because it was a really dark setting that didn't have bright lights on the real things there.

At first, it was just like the darkness was all alive and moving a little bit and had tiny hints of bits of changing light in it. And I do remember that when I first walked in the room, I was just really liking the visual effects. I began to see, as if on a projector, on the walls of my room, scenes from my childhood, especially. But then...they [the visions] were sort of all important interpersonal relationships...first with parents and then with some other people that might have played a more minor role in my life. As I was kind of reliving certain scenes...it was like watching a movie. I was very passive. It was half like I was living through it again and half like I was watching a film somebody had made for me about it. It was quite unlike the earlier experience.

I will tell you about my LSD experience next because I hallucinate dramatically with my eyes wide open in any sort of lighting when I'm on LSD. I hallucinate as vividly as anyone.

[LSD] is like the world around me just turns into some Disneyland fantasia, and I feel like the same person while watching it, mostly. I did it with people who had done it a number of times, and it wasn't a very big deal to them. They thought we should drop some acid and drive to this movie theater. If I'd had any experience with LSD I would not have been in the car with somebody driving. I would not have wanted to go to a movie as an LSD experience. But what did I know? I'd been wanting to try it for a while, and suddenly it turned up.

It was a Nicolas Roeg movie; it was very weird.[1] This couple lost their child, who probably drowned in the canal. She was wearing a little red riding hood as she disappeared. But then there's a midget walking around the town, in a red hood, but this may be the male character's hallucination. And it is intentionally meant to be visually confusing.

Anyway, so we go to the movie theater. So many other people are saying they're starting to feel it. I'm not feeling anything. We get into the movie theater as the previews are starting, and the other walls of the theatre begin looking more interesting than the screen. I'm feeling streaming sensations through my body. The white walls of the theatre

1 *Don't Look Now* (1973).

are just kind of lit up with very flat patterns...I thought I was just starting to get off. In the theatre, the walls were a sort of pastel...I just saw the classic trippy patterns, what all the LSD art looks like, happening all over the walls of the theater.

I turned around to look at the back wall of the theater. I do experience stronger visual effects than most people. So I was emphatically told by my friends that I had to sit facing forward. And I was having all these, like, electrical sensations through my body. I sort of wanted to ask them if this was normal...they weren't unpleasant, but I was still a little worried about whether electricity should be streaming through my body. That only happened early on, but I wasn't freaked out. It was more pleasant than not, but I was very frustrated that I couldn't look at the back walls and that everybody was fussing at me about being conspicuous and that I couldn't just talk or ask about the body sensations I was having.

But then I did sort of settle in as the actual film came on. And I couldn't figure that out. I definitely wanted to be asking people about this, and I couldn't. So I was having an interesting experience. And toward the end of the movie—for a while the movie was the most interesting thing—but then there were colored faces that were sort of popping out of the walls that just had this pastel flat pattern on them before, like just full-fledged, large surreal faces were stretching out... So, by the end of the movie, the walls were much more dramatic than the screen, but I knew none of this was real.

I wasn't considering that anybody was streaming electricity through my body. I just wanted to know if that was a normal part of the trip. And everybody's saying, "Wow, you are really tripping!" even though they are talking about seeing patterns and little figures, and odd body sensations, and somebody was talking about their teeth a lot. They were definitely tripping, but they were also somehow noticing that I was tripping more than they were tripping.

And we get back in the car, and we start driving. And it was summer, and I saw snow all over the ground. And I just knew it could not have snowed. It was June or something, in Atlanta. And I saw snow... Is this reflection? Is there something odd about? I was sure that it had to be sort of an illusion, but they were just like, "No..." But we were driving along, and there was like 4 inches of snow everywhere.

We pass this vacant lot and this pink marble. It was really as tall and skinny as the Neuschwanstein Castle in Germany, but this was like a pink marble Neuschwanstein. It was the tallest, skinniest castle I've ever seen, and it was made of pink marble with sort of the other colors.

And this deep crack happened in the middle of this large, vacant piece of property. And this castle came shooting up out of the ground very quickly. The earth split open. This [palace] crashed up until it was about the height of the Neuschwanstein. And it simply remained there. It's this flat open area—so I saw it as we were sort of approaching it and not right next to it when it happened Then we drove right past, and it realistically looked bigger as we got nearer. And I turned around and watched it behind the car as we drove on. And it just stayed there, and I knew it wasn't real. I knew that the ground could not have split and sprouted a huge, bizarre marble castle. But then there were castles everywhere. Like [the marble palace] was in one spot, then it was behind me. The ground still had snow on it. That was consistent as we drove past other things. And that the castle was maybe the single most dramatic thing [I saw], but I was seeing all kinds of architectural objects that could not have really [existed]...this was a familiar drive that we were on.

The hallucinations were very three-dimensional. And they tended to be very persistent. They weren't changing, and they'd go away as we drove past them. But snow was on the ground the whole time.

Once home, I stopped seeing these 3D, super realistic things. All the plain walls had 2D images that danced...not just dancing but lit up. They weren't just colors, but they were glowing patterns that mostly stayed on the walls and were two dimensional. But now, with [psychedelic rock group Spirit's] *Twelve Dreams of Dr. Sardonicus* album playing, they were timed with it like those flashing lights that respond to the beat and music. They were doing that, and they had been completely abstract and occasionally were forming...not even cartoonish doll-looking...but very simple, slightly humanoid entities would form and break up. And they seemed to match things the lyrics were saying. And I definitely knew this was all the trip. And I was really enjoying this. It was fascinating and beautiful. I was also noticing that I didn't feel any different, that I wasn't having profound, interesting, philosophical thoughts like on psilocybin, and that while I was enjoying it, I wasn't in a euphorically good mood like quaaludes... I wasn't ridiculously happy, and I didn't feel like a different entity. I wasn't having profound thoughts, but I'd just never seen anything like this.

I don't remember if I compared it to dreams at the time. I would now say that it's the only time I visually hallucinated as absolutely as in a dream, the content being much more sort of geometric and fast-moving. Maybe the pink castles shooting up through the ground was more like a dream, but all the little things that formed in response to lyrics and all were very different from a dream. But still, like just for a level of hallucination, I would now compare them as kind of the most visually dream-like experience.

I don't even remember what phrases in [the Spirit album] I thought were related to some of these kind of stylized entities I was seeing, but I at least thought that the music was triggering some of the specifics. But most of the time the patterns are just doing their thing, and it seems to be mostly a white or otherwise just lightly colored, unbroken wall. But the more the room is crowded with other fully-formed objects or the walls are colored, covered in other things, the more I'll just get some distortions...but not hallucinations; they don't develop as fully.

And I remember the walls constantly forming these 2D patterns that at times morphed into little humanoid things. I remember that just a few times I turned, and when I first looked in another direction there would be some of these flat kachina-like humanoids that would be waddling around the room like they couldn't walk in three dimensions. They were like cutouts that could move by wobbling side to side a little bit. And they looked just like the patterns as if you'd cut out the patterns on the wall, you know, cut out a piece of wall, and now the piece of wall was sort of waddling its two-dimensional self around.

Let me tell you one last LSD experience. I went to Burning Man [in 2005]. I hadn't been doing any drugs at Burning Man until the night of the burn, when another woman [Vivian] and I were hanging out a lot together. And so she wanted to do LSD for the night of the burn. Because I seem to visually trip so much harder than anyone I knew, I decided it would be really interesting to see what half a dose of acid was like.

So I went to the burn with Vivian. And I was not full-on hallucinating. I was just... the fire dancers with their flames looked sort of more magical, and the flames were shooting out further and more, you know, whatever. But I wasn't seeing any 3D things that completely weren't there. So it incredibly enhanced all this fire-dancing around the burning man before they set off fireworks, before they're actually lighting him. They've gotten very good at sort of starting the man burning slow enough that it takes quite a while for the flames to ascend and him to be fully on fire.

And then for him to finally fall over, it's a very protracted. The crowd is just like kind of screaming in these euphoric...just this nonverbal sort of rhythmic screams as this is happening. There's some drumming and some more intentional chanting, but then the crowd just sort of starts screaming. And they developed this kind of slow rhythm. So I'm convinced that part is a real perception, but it just sounded more perfectly in unison and more magical and whatever...

This was maybe my most memorable LSD experience, even though it was certainly the mildest sort of chemical effect.

I'm always a little on the fence about whether MDA (3,4-methylenedioxymethamphetamine) and MDMA (methylenedioxymethamphetamine) should be classified as hallucinogens. Everything usually looks pretty and enhanced, and I notice things. And I feel like my state of consciousness is the most changed on them, right? But it's not full-on visually hallucinatory. In dreams, the visual stuff is not necessarily surreal. The visual stuff can be realistic. But I am just a somewhat different me who thinks about things somewhat differently in some of my dreams, but not all. And I feel like I change and get into a different part of myself. I'm still me, but I'm a very different part of myself. Sometimes when I'm on Ecstasy—or again, I'm a subtly different, yet part of myself, on MDA—again, I'm not even sure if I would call those hallucinogens. But I do think of them as altered states of consciousness drugs that have something related to dream experience, even though it's a different aspect of dream experience than the visual hallucinatory. The secondary visual cortex is getting so much stimulation from both REM sleep and on most of the things we call hallucinogens.

MDA is different from MDMA. But I sort of in ways like both, just differently, I would say that I have more interesting intellectual thoughts and intellectual conversations on MDA, that I feel even more connected to people and empathic with people, sort of loving of both the people I'm with and humanity in general, on MDMA. But they each have a fair bit of what I'm saying I like best about the other one. It's something about the intensity of those two.

And also, I would say the kind of visual look that's just a kind of illusory beauty to everything...the visuals are almost identical for me on [MDA or MDMA], like everything's enhanced. Colors are more jewel-like, and anything with texture looks more kind of soft and beautiful. Everything looks beautiful...softer for shapes and textures, but more intense for any color that's already a bright color.

Eichel: What are your thoughts about how these chemicals can be used therapeutically, from your experience and from your research?

Barrett: Yeah, I'm very ambivalent about the medicalization of [psychedelics], because I do think of them as informally therapeutic—especially for some of the hallucinogens—[they can be a kind of] coming to terms with individual mortality. It sort of matches a lot of the informal experiences. And I think that marital therapy and PTSD are the two things that MDMA has gotten test runs on.

So it's not just that I think they're informally therapeutic, but I can definitely see immediately when hearing about it how they would be therapeutic in a formal situation. And now I have friends who have done the training for some of those trials. And I'm hearing positive things. But if psychiatrists and pharmaceutical companies control the access to these, and they are thought of as something that you should have a disorder to be using...those are the aspects [of medicalization] that are negative. I mean partly it's sticking them under big business to make them a prescription pharmaceutical. Partly it's medicalizing them, and I think of the things that the hallucinogens are most useful for as more in the psychological realm. So I don't like the idea that you need to have a disorder or even problem to have a positive growth-enhancing experience with these [chemicals]. I don't like the medical professional profession having control of them. And I even more don't like the pharmaceutical companies and this whole just clown show of so many companies trying to take the known hallucinations and find...not at all necessarily something that works better...but that just has one molecule changed to make it patentable. And so they can do the FDA trials on something they own the rights to, and [it's really a] substance that's been used for centuries.

I was on this cruise, a conference speaking tour where I was one of the speakers and Rick Doblin, PhD [a founder of MAPS, the Multidisciplinary Association for Psychedelic Studies] was one of the speakers. I was kind of sounding off about how glad I was psychedelics were more popular, but how much I didn't like the pharmaceutical companies and the prescription uses for them and that you could trip if you had a psychiatrist's [prescription]. I didn't like that from a financial standpoint or from just a psychological self-exploration standpoint. And Rick was saying that he saw the medical uses and legalization of medical uses as the best first step to getting drugs legalized. That was exactly what had happened with marijuana. Some states started legalizing it as a medical drug. That didn't mean the medical profession maintained control over cannabis for all time. It meant that it didn't seem as scary or bad.

Eichel: So, back to psychedelics and their connection to the two fields you are most renowned for: hypnosis and dreams.

Barrett: I see dreams and hypnosis as very related, as being altered states of consciousness that have something in common in visual imagery being enhanced, and verbal and logical/linear reasoning usually damps down (in the case of hypnosis, unless you're specifically trying to enhance it).

So I've always thought of dreams and hypnosis as somewhat related states of consciousness and thought a lot about how I think they're potentially useful in therapy. I think so many of our neuroses and character pathologies have to do with just ingrained patterns and defense mechanisms where we always respond to a certain kind of problem or stressor or situation. A sort of over-learned narrow set of responses that served us well in some childhood situation but no longer serve us that well. We have a lot of trouble breaking out of those patterns. In dreams, the prefrontal cortex and the verbal areas are a little less active, and the visualization areas are much more active.

Dreams and hypnosis, like psychedelics, make an end-run around our usual defenses and can allow us to have an experience kind of already being the other way. You can vividly experience being a non-smoker and hating the smell of cigarettes in a hypnotic state, and if you get lucky...I've definitely heard examples of people suddenly having completely different attitudes towards smoking in a dream; then after they woke up, they didn't want to smoke any more.

I used hypnosis and dreams in the therapeutic work I did. It's still you in your brain but in a very different biochemical state. It puts those standard characterological, over-learned patterns on hold. It gives you an experience of still thinking about your usual thoughts and concerns in this visual, intuitive, much less linear, and just less ingrained, over-learned, rigid...it lets you think outside the box, let's you more easily visualize things that haven't happened.

So I think of hallucinogens as having all those qualities of the two areas that I have researched and done therapy with. It's a different you; you get to experience being a different way, having a different attitude. You think outside the box and will try out behaviorally, or just in mental imagery, a different way of doing things. In your standard state of consciousness, you just censor yourself and don't let yourself do something new.

I think MDMA is the drug that fascinates me the most, at least for its therapeutic potential. Each time I do it, it's got the novelty of the first time.

Eichel: Well, Deirdre, we have come to the end of this interview. As one of the premier researchers and writers in the fields of dreams and hypnosis, your personal experiences and insights into the role psychedelics can play in personal growth as well as psychotherapy have been invaluable. Thank you for your time.

> But along with the feeling of ineffability, the conviction that some profound objective truth has been disclosed to you is a hallmark of the mystical experience, regardless of whether it has been occasioned by a drug, meditation, fasting, flagellation, or sensory deprivation. William James gave a name to this conviction: the noetic quality. People feel they have been let in on a deep secret of the universe, and they cannot be shaken from that conviction.
>
> —Michael Pollan

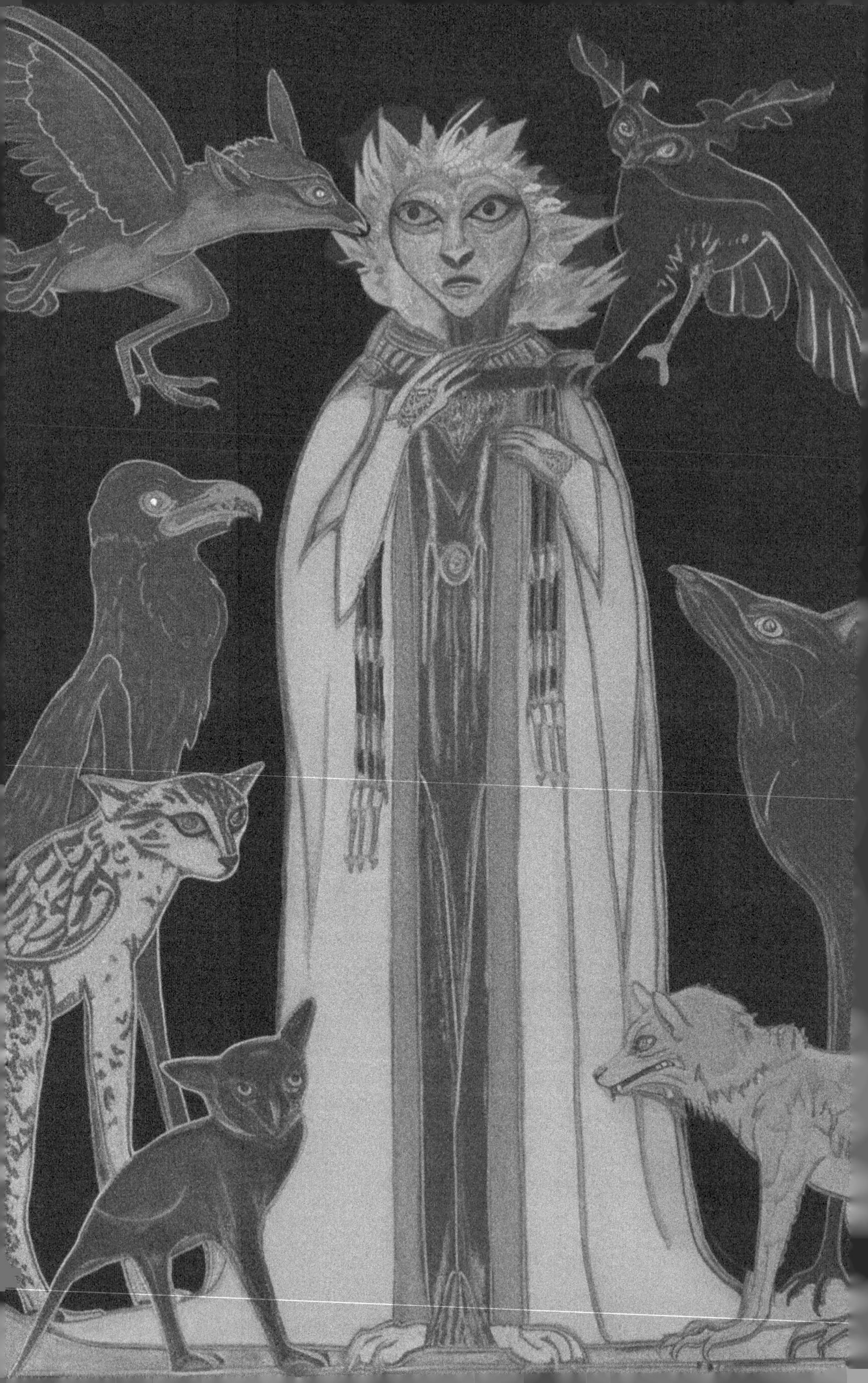

Ewa Tracz

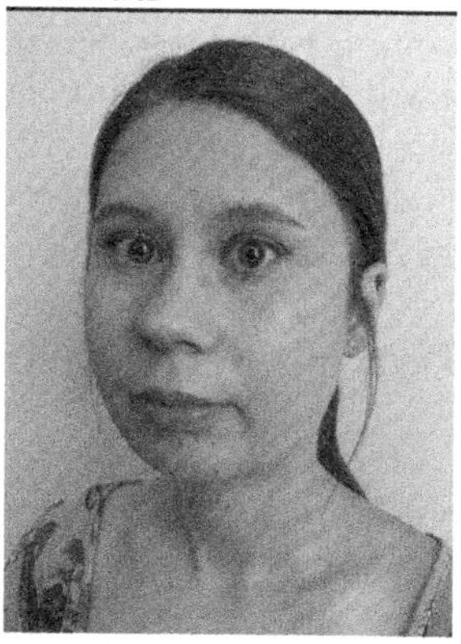

More-Than-Human World in Psychedelic Visions

Ewa Tracz, PhD candidate, is a Polish anthropologist. In 2022, she defended her master's thesis, "Altered States of Consciousness. A Study in the Field of Psychedelic Anthropology," in which she presented the concept of psychedelic anthropology and described the phenomenon of psychedelic spirituality. Currently her research focuses on the topic of practices and values among people creating the psychedelic community in Poland.
ewatra@amu.edu.pl

The psychedelic experience is difficult to describe in words. All learning is based on translating experience into language, and then most often into written text. This double filtering of experience makes the attempt to describe it shallow compared to what we feel. In the course of writing this paper, the inner feelings of my interviewees are also condensed and given a certain form.

The topic of human use of psychedelics can be studied from many perspectives. What can anthropology offer in this context? The ethnographic interview provides a tool through which we can learn about other people's beliefs and show their perspectives (including one unrelated to scientific/academic perceptions) on a given topic. I believe that such a description of the experiences of users of psychedelic substances can bring a new point of view to the current renaissance of research on psychedelics.

My premise is to present socio-cultural perceptions and practices regarding the use of psychedelic drugs in Poland. One of the most important goals I set for myself when I began the research for my thesis was to learn/understand what psychedelic spirituality was for my interviewees. I believe that the use of psychedelics for this purpose is just one possible path to spiritual development. What I find interesting, however, is the experiences of those who choose to follow such a path. So I believe that the psychedelic experience can be a tool for exploring spirituality.

Here I will focus on answering the question: How can we understand the concept of *psychedelic spirituality*? I will explore this through several shared trip reports, that is, descriptions of experiences under the influence of psychedelics. A person who experiences such inner insights may consider them a vision coming from his imagination or a real interaction with an otherworldly but real world. I will focus on accounts depicting encounters with non-human entities that appeared in the psychedelic visions of the people I interviewed. Their reported feelings, emotions, and thoughts triggered by such experiences show what meaning psychedelic users give to such experiences.

Psychedelic Spirituality

For the purposes of my ethnographic research, I have included all descriptions of visionary experiences while under the influence of psychedelic substances in the category of a phenomenon that can be described as *psychedelic spirituality*. I define spirituality as a person's desire to expand his or her own consciousness through self-development, which can be based on religious or meditative practices, among other things. All of these practices involve ritualized activities.

Psychedelics are another tool (besides religion or meditation) used in spiritual practices. An integral part of these practices is self-healing through experiencing altered states of consciousness. Spiritual practice based on the use of psychedelic experiences involves confronting our subconscious and thus bringing to the surface the inner states that show us our current psycho-spiritual condition. By noticing these states and becoming aware of them, we can work with them. People who enjoy such experiences treat them as the most important source of their spiritual experiences.

In his paper "Psychedelic Experience as a Cognitive Experience," Szymon Nowak (2015) points out that a description of a person's state after taking a psychedelic substance should additionally be based on philosophical reflection. He believes that the special interest in the effects of psychedelics is precisely due to the fact that the overtones of the psychedelic experience have a spiritual meaning for the individual. The author draws attention in his text to the fact that the concept of spirituality does not appear (or at least has not appeared until now) very often in scientific descriptions. Nowak believes that this situation has changed, firstly thanks to the invention of LSD by Albert Hofmann. The second reason he gives is the increased interest in the scientific world in Indigenous cultures, which often use plants and mushrooms with psychoactive properties in their rituals.

Furthermore, Nowak (2015) joins the debate widely taking place in scientific circles on the issue of naming psychedelic substances. One of the terms he uses is "mystico-mimetic." This word refers to the state caused by the ingestion of substances from the group of classic psychedelics, which is referred to as a "full mystical experience." Another term he uses is "entheogen," derived from a combination of the two Greek words *entheos* (inspired, full of God) and *genestai* (to become). We can translate the term as "discovering inner divinity." According to Nowak, the term was invented in 1979 by researchers studying the use of psychoactive substances in a ritual context. The modern meaning of the term refers to substances from the group of classic psychedelics. Nowak goes on to mention that entheogens taken while following a set of rules referred to as "set and setting" (the appropriate environment and setting of the person experiencing the altered state of consciousness) can induce a mystical experience that is phenomenologically indistinguishable from mystical experiences induced by other techniques, such as meditation. Nowak believes that the creation of this neologism introduced a new research perspective into scientific language, making it possible to study and describe the practice of taking psychedelic substances in a ceremonial context.

Trip Reports

The following excerpts from psychedelic trip reports contain descriptions of encounters with non-human entities. All of the narratives are from transcriptions of recordings I made after conducting ethnographic interviews (while preparing source material for my master's thesis).

The first interviewee told me about a vision she experienced during an ayahuasca ceremony. She related it as follows:

> I saw formations of birds. I saw each of these birds in a kind of bubble, and they were connected to each other. It was very interesting to me. And then I had this feeling as if I was at the end of a space-time tube. (...) I could see the tube, but it wasn't so tangible, because I could see beyond that there was the ocean, rocks, and other things [she was describing the actual environment in which she was taking her psychedelic trip—the beach by the ocean]. Through this tube, I began to have contact with beings from outer space. It was interesting, because I had this feeling as if these beings in me, in my body, were jumping into it, and I was consciously allowing it. These beings were lifting this body and looking around to see what it's like here. And they had this "*Wow*, how beautiful it is here, how wonderful it is!" I had this sense that there was a line of these beings there, and each one of them just wanted to see. It was amazing, because I felt with these beings, like I was somehow connected to them, like I was a little bit from their planet. And somehow it was like I was here for them a little bit. It was so beautiful. I saw them, but I can't say now...I mean I know they were hairy, they had long hair, they were very elongated. Then I was on their planet, and this planet was beautiful because it was very green, but it also had a lot of blue, basically like the vegetation was blue. There were plants everywhere, but they were scaled up; they were so big, like I was a worm, literally, but I felt safe in it all. At one point I reached a cave, and in the middle of it there was a round skylight and in the center under this skylight there was an islet, on this small lake. And on this islet, something was happening. Now, of course, I don't remember exactly what...on this islet as if some kind of ritual was taking place. I was part of a congregation that was watching this ritual and in some sense also participated in it as if energetically. (Personal communication, ethnographic interview, 2021).

After telling me this story, my interviewee added that she had always been a person with her feet firmly on the ground, trying to think and analyze things in a rational manner. On the one hand, she knew that "it's not like we are here alone." She never believed that we were just a shell, a body. She said she had always known that there was something beyond the known world, life. She believed it was possible to make contact with "energy" or "spirits," but at some point in her life she began to strongly question the rationality of her beliefs. She began to have doubts, on the principle that if what she believes in is not researched, it means it doesn't exist. She concluded that if belief in spiritual life is ridiculed by certain people, then it probably just isn't there. She then concluded that she may have been wrong in her previous beliefs. However, after the psychedelic trip described above, she realized that no one could tell her that something is or isn't real. She said that if she feels there can be a spiritual world, that means it is true for her. She concluded her statement with a rhetorical question: "Why did I even give anyone the power to tell me what is and isn't real?"

My second interviewee described his experience this way:

> It was the most intense mushroom experience and generally such a psychedelic experience in my life. (...) I prepared it all for myself. I had powdered two grams of mushrooms, and I threw them in juice squeezed from a lime. And I had this goblet. I prepared everything for myself in this goblet. I had never eaten that amount of mushrooms before, and I didn't know what would happen. I accepted this sacrament and lay down in bed. (...) Not 15 minutes had passed when I suddenly began to feel that my ability to relax through sleep yoga—yoga nidra—was somehow absurdly strong, reactive. I'm thinking to myself, my right leg is relaxing and my right leg is melting away. Suddenly I felt that my whole body was like cotton wool, like a sponge. I melted all over. I'm thinking to myself, this is quite interesting and at that moment...I felt a presence.
>
> This is also the answer to the question of whether I have ever felt the presence of any beings. Yes, then, this one time, it happened on substances other than changa [DMT-soaked herbal mixture], when I had the impression that there was some kind of feminine energy close to me. I felt that her hair was loose, and I felt that she was very lively. Also, this happened at a moment just when there was a void in my head, so it was as if there was space for anything that could happen there. Then I felt the presence of this being; well, I heard moans of pleasure as if someone was having an orgasm, and then the psychedelic journey exploded in my head. And suddenly an explosion of colors appeared before my eyes. With my eyes closed, I traveled through an ever-evolving fractal that was increasingly wrapping one way or the other. I was absolutely certain of this; it was so obvious to me that this space I was in, that I was traveling through, this was the essence. This was the energy. I was convinced that I was just getting to know this essence more and more.
>
> When I was looking at some visualizations of mathematically generated fractals for myself, I was shocked at how similar it was, because I kept seeing similar structures that sometimes looked like ferns, sometimes like shells, and various patterns. And I kept seeing as if different spaces in these fractals were connected to each other in a certain way. It suddenly became obvious to me that, aha, this is a network of connections between all sentient beings. In a sense, I had this presentation of what this network of interdependence of humans and other beings looks like, how they connect to each other and how they also diverge. I saw that there was one figure that was like a positive electrical charge and it literally attracts this other charge, but there's just nothing there. And by itself, it was as if this emptiness, next to this one being, was already causing something to be drawn to it; in other words, the very fact that there was space for this other being was already causing this emptiness to simply want to be filled. (...) Then very many other figures appeared during my visions. As I watched the evolution of this particular fractal of interdependence of sentient beings, I tried to understand it somehow. Theories appeared in my head about it, and in a way, my subconscious was sort of reconstructing some points of view in the form of my friends. They sort of visited me. I have one acquaintance who is a strong skeptic, sometimes even a cynic, and when I was trying to think of a theory, he sort of appeared in my head and said something along the lines of, "And how do you know this? Are you sure of what you are saying?" And so, I thought to myself, *hmm, actually, no.* I tried to put a more scientific bite on it because at some point I noticed some regularities. At that moment, my master's supervisor along with the assistant supervisor appeared in my head and they commented on my attempts to put it in scientific language. They were kind of trying to support me in this a little bit too, but they didn't give me any answers, so they were more on the sidelines and commenting on what I was saying. It's more along the lines of...not teasing, but more a kind of presence, that if I said something stupid, well, they wouldn't fail to laugh at it. (Personal communication, ethnographic interview, 2021).

As we can see, the world of extraterrestrial beings was intertwined in my interviewee's visions with real people from his life. In the end, he unexpectedly added this sentence: "These visions lasted for some time, and I realized that for a guy who talks so much about love, I don't have a clue what it is." In the above narrative, we can feel some tangled threads. I specifically brought up this longer description to show how chaotic the stream of thoughts can be during a psychedelic experience.

I present one last vision description. This third interviewee described her experience as follows:

> We went to the park. These were the first such warm days of the spring. I had this vision that the very photons that were falling from the sky, from the sun, made everyone suddenly kind of intoxicated with this first blush of spring. It was so intense, and it was a very spiritual experience, so I started exploring psychedelics for myself later. (...) And as for contacts with beings...you know, I'm not saying here that this is some kind of objective reality, that it's outside of me, and that there really is some kind of God or something. I would like it to be so. (...) It makes me sad when someone takes away this idea that this could be some objective reality outside of our minds. Indeed, if it were just a figment of our imagination...or if the fact that our brains are similar to each other, and usually these experiences are very archetypal, but they are untrue because they are artificial, because they are created by our brains...it would hurt me a lot if that were the case. I can't say that what I experienced was contact with some other beings, but yes, they appeared. Once in my life, on DMT, I had that. I definitely smoked less than 50 mg of DMT. ... And I'm prone to all kinds of mystical experiences like that; I go into a trance very quickly. I can even sit in a movie theater and feel myself floating above myself, because I just have that predisposition.
>
> First I was in a tunnel; there I had the impression that there were beings that were not exactly friendly to me. I think they might be those Santos Niños [holy children] they describe in South American legends, but Terence McKenna (1993) calls them "mechanical elves." (...) And then I come out of the tunnel; something connects to me. Later I realized that it was probably a face. Maybe I search for it...because we have something in our nature that we search for faces; we see a face everywhere. It plugged into me and it was like this: "Focus, here I am, focus." I say, "Well, I'm with you." And there were more of them there, and they asked how I communicate with them. I felt such a stir in that place as if it was...I'm a scientist, as if it was a scientific study. They had some kind of technology to communicate with beings from another world. I say, "through music and psychedelic substances." That's how I answered him, and then I moved on.
>
> Later I was in this bubbling substance, consisting of light. It was a substance of very dense matter suspended in nothingness. And it was feminine energy. Very friendly, good, just like Mom. That's how I talked to her. I felt that I was inside her, and I said, "It's cool that I'm already back, that I'm ready." She said, "No, it's not time for you yet." I said, "What do you mean? I don't want to go back there at all." I felt her pain; she didn't want to let me go at all. She said, "It's not time for you yet." And she let me go like that, like a lotus onto the water. I was such a ball of energy, so tiny, and I came back to Earth and saw other such balls of energy going to her. And you know, when I came back later, for a long time I... Because I was with a friend at the time, and he asked me, "Are you there yet?" I say, "I don't know who I am. I'm not a human being. That's not my name. I'm not a woman. I don't know who I am." And so it took me about 15 minutes to recover from that. (Personal communication, ethnographic interview, 2021).

In telling me about her experience, my interviewee got emotional. After this psychedelic experience, she began searching for information about what she might have experienced in her vision. After some time, she came across a similar description of an experience in Aleister Crowley's (1986) book *Little Essays Toward Truth*. Crowley was a British occultist and author of many books on mystical subjects. In this book, he described the concept of the Kabbalistic tree, which includes a description of the fact that there are different sephiroth or different forms of emanations of God. My interviewee explained to me that the five sephiroth are responsible for the elements that relate to our world. Then the abyss is depicted in this concept: "where language no longer exists, because what I felt there was not speech, it was simply empathy." The abyss is where you lose language; you don't use language. You don't use the concepts with which you as a human being consider reality. My interviewee then listed several more sephiroth, until she came to one she called Bina, meaning feminine energy, the place of disintegration and reintegration of the self. She told me about the experience, using the method of personification: "I was there, and she wouldn't let me pass on. And it was amazing."

Closing

I consider the research topic I have undertaken to be important because encounters with beings (substance spirits) are presented by psychedelic users as one of the most interesting and transformative experiences they have while in an altered state of consciousness, in this case under the influence of a psychedelic substance. I believe that attempting to describe and understand this type of experience should be important for psychedelic users themselves, as well as for professionals helping to integrate psychedelic experiences. When analyzing scholarly texts, I feel that they fail to sufficiently address the topic of psychedelic users' encounters with non-human beings during their psychedelic visions, which appeared in almost every one of the ethnographic interviews I conducted.

In 2018, a panel discussion on the topic of psychedelics took place at a conference organized by the American Anthropological Association. Among other aspects of the topic, the panel discussed the role of ethnography in reimagining psychedelic substances as drugs. The description of the content covered during this discussion indicates that despite the ban on the use of psychedelics introduced in 1971 by the United Nations, many people around the world use them as a means of psycho-spiritual therapy. These people reject the term "hallucinogen," because they believe it implies that the substance induces illusions, which in this case is not true. The second term, "psychedelic," is also rejected by some users, because of the negative connotations the word took on in the 1960s. According to the authors of the speech, most users of psychedelic substances prefer the term "entheogen," with its connotation of discovering inner divinity, as discussed above. The lecture goes on to give examples of psychoactive flora and fungi valued as sacred sacraments in some contexts. Mention was made of substances such as ayahuasca, which was and is still used in Indigenous communities, or cannabis species, which have long been used in some Hindu traditions and are a major hallmark of Rastafarianism. Twentieth-century Mazatec healers in Mexico engaged in the ritual use of mushrooms containing the entheogenic alkaloid psilocybin. Today, referring to the practice of Indigenous peoples of northern Mexico, there has been a syncretization of ancient beliefs with the Christian religion. Religious practices are merged with Indigenous practices through the use of a peyote decoction (containing mescaline) during ceremonies. This practice is used by the Native American Church, and their syncretic religion is called Peyotism. The last example mentioned in the speech was the followers of the Bwiti religion of West and Central Africa, who consume iboga root (containing ibogaine) during initiation rituals (American Anthropological Association, 2018).

Spiritual experiences induced by psychedelics are perceived by the person experiencing them most often through feelings of elation, overflowing with a state of joy, love, fulfillment, and understanding of the meaning of life. On the other hand, the person may experience feelings of deep sadness, grief, or anxiety. What a person will experience depends on his or her psycho-physical state when taking a psychedelic. All these feelings are difficult to translate into language because they are not related to the intellect but more to a person's emotional state. Just experiencing such a state is sufficient to feel spiritual elation; it is not necessary to understand this state with the help of reason. However, if we want to understand these experiences better, it is necessary to try to translate them into language.

References

American Anthropological Association. (2018, November 16). *Panel: Reimagining psychedelic drugs as medicines: Ethnography's role in assessing ritualized psychoactive therapies.* American Anthropological Association Annual Meeting 2018, San Jose, CA. Organizers: Blainey, M. & Labate, B. Retrieved from https://chacruna.net/psychedelic-panel-at-the-2018-american-anthropological-association-annual-meeting/

Crowley, A. (1986). *Little essays toward truth.* San Francisco: Stellar Visions.

McKenna, T. (1993). *True hallucinations: Being an account of the author's extraordinary adventures in the devil's paradise.* San Francisco: Harper San Francisco.

Nowak, S. (2015). *Doświadczenie psychodeliczne jako doświadczenie poznawcze.* Retrieved from http://hdl.handle.net/11089/20341

> The psilocybin experience is a way to connect with our own sense of spirituality and find meaning in our lives.
>
> —Rick Doblin

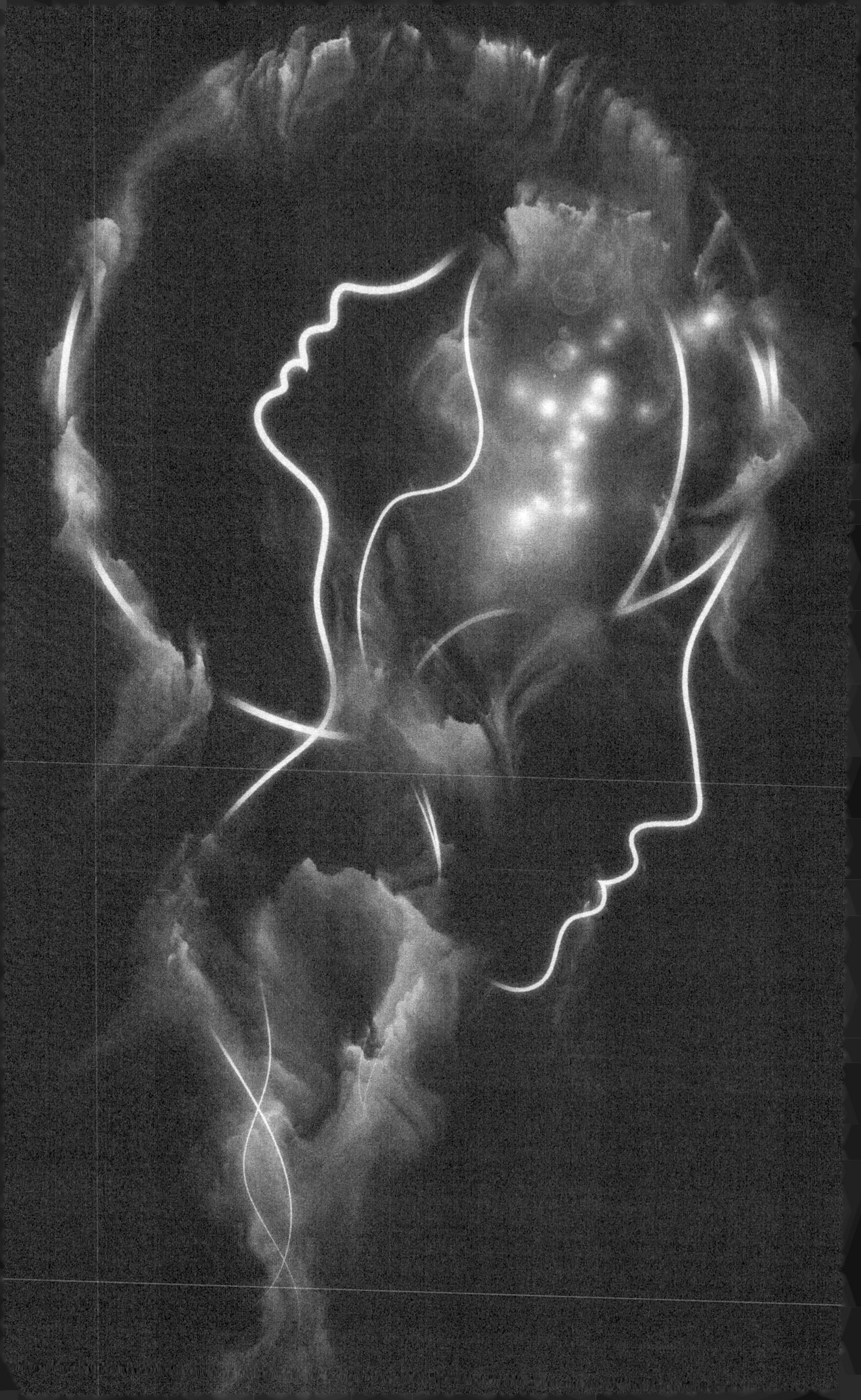

David Doane

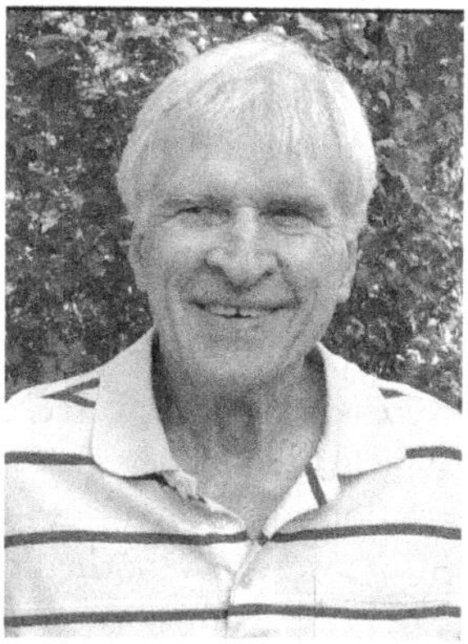

David Doane, PhD, was a psychologist in private practice for 46 years, his primary focus being experiential and relationship psychotherapy. Retiring has meant letting go of the professional role and having more time to turn inward and pay attention to the person within the role, which endeavors are essentially the core of both psychotherapy and the psychedelic experience. He appreciates *Voices* being a journal in which and through which to express one's voice.
dsdoane@hotmail.com

Psychedelic Experience:
Shaking And Waking

...what I have seen is unsurpassable...In this playhouse of infinite forms I have had my play and here have I caught sight of him that is formless.
—Rabindranath Tagore

Culture has defined psychedelic to be a drug that produces altered or abnormal states of consciousness including distorted perception, cognitive functioning, and mood, hallucinations, or states of awareness sometimes resembling psychosis. However, the meaning of psychedelic from the derivation of the word differs from the cultural definition.

The word *psychedelic* is composed of the two Greek words *psyche* and *deloum*. Psyche is the essence or core of a person, referred to in some traditions as the soul. Deloum, the root of -delic, means to manifest or reveal clearly and fully. Psychedelic means to manifest clearly or fully the essence or soul of existence.

My thoughts about psychedelics are based on my ontological view, that is, my view of existence. My view is that there is Ultimate Being that is infinite and eternal, the essence and source of all that is. It is the Ground of Being, to use theologian Paul Tillich's (1957) term. It is out of Ultimate Being that all that is appears, takes form, exists. Ultimate Being is Ultimate Consciousness, also referred to as Psyche or Soul, the human expression of which is human consciousness, psyche, or soul. Human consciousness is a finite stretch of the infinite bandwidth of Consciousness. Ultimate Being is one. All existence consists of innumerable different expressions of one existence, one whole, with no separation.

Human consciousness is also the result of conditioning that is provided by parents, family, teachers, religion, peers, and the entire culture from the time we are born, if not sooner. We are taught what reality is, what truth is, what to see and think, and what not to see and think. We function from a limited, conditioned stretch of human consciousness, not from our whole human consciousness which is significant but only a small stretch of Infinite Consciousness.

As we go through life, we have experiences that shake and expand our conditioned limited consciousness, sometimes resulting in our seeing reality differently than as we were conditioned to see. Many experiences shake us, some to a very small degree and some to a large degree. Experiences that shake us to a large degree may be an intimate relationship, a life-or-death experience, a deep meditation experience, a peak experience in nature, a psychotherapy experience, a spirituality experience, a shamanic retreat, a psychedelic substance. Each experience is an aperture into awakened and expanded consciousness.

Many believe that there is existence beyond finite material existence and say we are in the world but not of it. Many believe all existence is fundamentally one unified field. The psychedelic experience expands human consciousness to a glimpse of seeing self as a manifestation of Ultimate Existence, in this world but not of it. The psychedelic experience precipitates expanding consciousness beyond our usual conditioning to see that all is one, a one consisting of innumerable manifestations that are different but not separate, all of which are totally interconnected and interdependent expressions of one unified whole.

The psychedelic experience precipitated by a substance can alter body chemistry and consciousness, shaking a person to his or her roots. Psychedelic experiences that are not substance precipitated also occur, though typically less intense than those that are substance precipitated. I know that because I have had psychedelic nonsubstance experiences. I have had brief times of the 220-watt light going on and seeing the oneness of all that is and seeing myself as one tiny whirlpool in one ocean of existence. It's an ecstatic moment that subsides but doesn't go away entirely as I'm left with a 25-watt remnant of the experience, and as a result, I am different than I was.

I think my life experiences, definitely including my psychotherapy and spirituality experiences, set me up for the psychedelic experiences. An early and profound psychotherapy experience that precipitated psychedelic awareness for me was participation in my first marathon group therapy in the early 1970s. The marathon group therapy lasted 24 consecutive hours, a duration that fosters defenses dropping and intimate interaction increasing. Over the course of so many hours together, you sort of swallow in one another. During the marathon group, I felt oneness with myself and others, and I could see and understand people and interactions clearer than ever. I was at times in a different reality, my consciousness and perception altered. Following the marathon group, I got back into the ups and downs of life, but the psychedelic consciousness expanding experience, reinforced by additional experiences, remained part of me such that I could tap into it and the broader perspective it gave me. Another experience that precipitated psychedelic consciousness for me was a spirituality experience facilitated by 15 years participation in a study group that included and fostered in-depth reflection on spirituality from East and West, with especial focus on the Vedic tradition.

Our culture turns us outward, away from our essence or soul. It pushes us toward what is called material reality and separates us from self, others, and the universe. Psychotherapy and psychedelic experiences turn us inward, going beyond the ego self and separateness, and awakening consciousness of oneness with self, others, and the universe, opening a glimpse of the essence or soul of existence.

The psyche or soul is the territory of both psychedelic and psychotherapy experiences. The psychotherapy experience in its fullest is soul revealing, consciousness expanding, and soul healing. The psychedelic experience is primarily soul revealing and consciousness expanding and can also be healing, in that expansion of consciousness is healing in and of itself. By revealing and expanding consciousness, the psychedelic experience can be a valuable partner to psychotherapy. Persons asleep to their underlying psyche could be awakened to it by a psychedelic experience. Psychotherapy, by healing separations in consciousness, is a valuable partner to the psychedelic experience.

A psychedelic experience that is an intense revealing of the soul of reality or self can be positively life changing. It can also be overwhelming or even traumatic if more manifesting or altering of perception occurs than is tolerable. It is advisable for one to be adequately together and stable as a person when initiating a psychedelic substance experience. A psychedelic substance experience may be overwhelming for the individual in acute mental disturbance, such as acute disturbance of psychotic proportion. It is advised to have a trusted guide familiar with the psychedelic substance experience present during any such experience.

Psychotherapy and the psychedelic experience can both be profound and life changing. The harmony of the psychedelic and psychotherapy experiences is obvious. In our world of such limited vision and so many problems that are the result of limited consciousness, it is important that the harmony of psychotherapy and psychedelic experiences, including psychedelic substance experiences, continue to be explored and researched.

References

Tillich, P. (1957). *Dynamics of faith.* Harper Colophon.

While radical interventions like 500 mcg of LSD or 30 days of restricted diet in a silent meditation retreat can help us acquire and retain wisdom, so can a weekly psychotherapy session with a therapist who sees increasing wisdom as their own goal.

—John Rhead

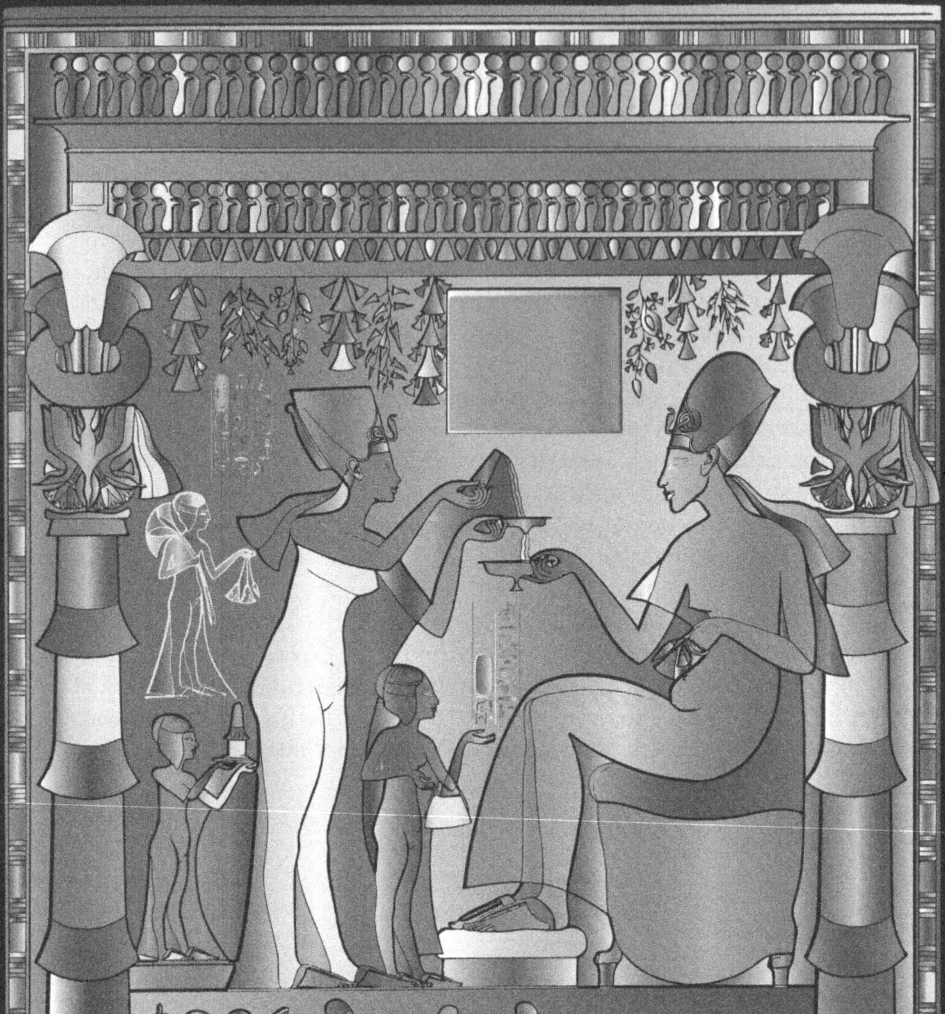

Mackenzie Amara

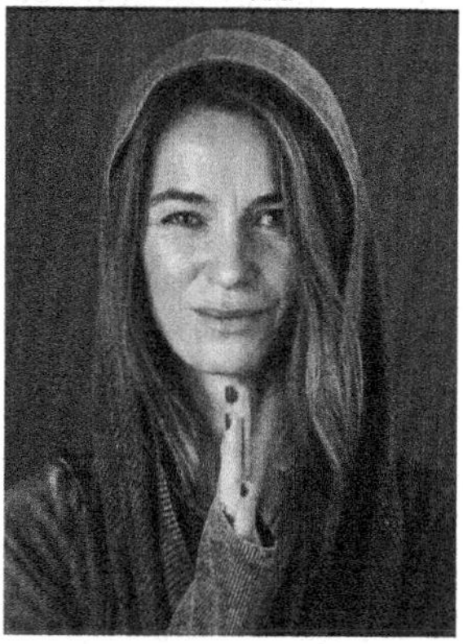

MACKENZIE AMARA is a Jungian analyst-in-training under the tutelage of the International School of Analytical Psychology in Zurich. She is a doctoral candidate at Saybrook University, where she researches the impact of dreaming on the psychedelic integration process. She holds a master's degree from Columbia University and is a certified 5Rhythms® teacher.
makenzie.amara@gmail.com

Psychedelic Insights for the Practice of Psychotherapy: Healing, Wisdom, & Devotion to Life

WRITING THIS ESSAY HAS BEEN A GODSEND—I truly did not know how much my work with entheogens has served me in my capacity as a psychotherapist. It has been a true privilege to reflect upon and give thanks to all of the psychedelic compounds and plant medicines that have graced my journey thus far.

In this essay you will find a mix of opinions, personal reflections, and academic evidence. I am a trained Jungian analyst and my doctoral studies have unfolded through the lens of the existential-humanistic perspective; both orientations are deeply embedded in my thinking. I argue that psychedelics can offer vital insights into the human condition and the change process of therapy. Namely, they can facilitate the removal of our enculturated defenses against healing and change, dissolve the boundaries between self and other, offer broader perspectives on relating to suffering, open up shamanic attunements, and bring us into right relationship with life and death.

Healing is an Inside Job

Our modern world has become overly reliant on the doctor's intervention in moments of illness, a symptom stemming in large part from our rift from the reality that healing is a natural process. A system—embodied, psychological, or ecological—will endogenously undergo a healing process if (a) the source of toxicity is removed, and (b) the conditions are reasonably optimized for systemic flow. In the body, this could look like cutting back on under-nourishing foods and engaging in simple physical activity. In a psyche, this could mean confessing shameful truths, confronting developmental traumas, and forming new ways of relating to negative inner voices or painful memories. In an ecosystem, removing burdensome poisons, ensuring water retention, and enriching the microbial layer of the soil can create enough alignment for the entire network to begin to right itself.

In our physical bodies, as in nature, when something is out of balance so much that there are deleterious effects, many processes self-initiate to return the system to homeostasis. Chemicals, hormones, and microbial beings all jump into action when signaled—and the actions of these autonomous systems naturally lead to our healing. But we have forgotten how to listen to our body's signals, programming our tastebuds to crave unhealthy foods through overstimulation with sugar and table salt, chemically numbing pain instead of treating it as a communication regarding where to focus healing attention, and overriding myriad pleas to rest in a world that demands our constant progress. Instead of taking care of our physical needs through movement, exposure to natural light, drinking plenty of pure water, resting enthusiastically, and eating nutrient-dense foods, we take our weakening, drained bodies to doctors, complain of poor health, and demand physical intervention. We have forgotten how to foster the conditions for healing that would allow our body to naturally, gracefully, and unequivocally right its own wrongs.

Unfortunately, this paradigm of projecting our healing onto the qualified other has metastasized to the psychological arts as well. Patients seek out known techniques and evidence-based interventions to address the seeming problems of their inner worlds, unconsciously submitting to the collective standard set by averages to address a pain that they uniquely carry, or else desiring a *DSM* diagnosis, some way to make sense of their inner turmoil. The result of such a codification of one's being, though, tends to mean a person moves further away from their authentic feeling, not closer. The negative consequences of applying systematized interventions and labels are many: firstly, a label becomes somehow indelible, offering no pathway of evolution or transformation; secondly, when tools that supposedly work for others don't work for a given individual, the failure is perceived as personal, as if it were the individual's own fault their cognitive-behavioral treatment didn't work; thirdly, and perhaps most importantly, when we use the outer world of quantities, statistical means, checklists, and quasi-arbitrary symptom groups to try to understand the individual, we inadvertently reduce the individual to a mere list of indications, an expression of certain trends, thus prohibiting them from gaining healing access to the depths that might be underneath their myriad complaints. This kind of psychological practice precludes the necessary conditions for healing, as it maintains the false belief that healing happens through external intervention. The reality, however, is that one can only heal by making direct contact with the aliveness inside of oneself—be it troubled or exalted—much the same way that a body or an ecosystem heals by revitalizing the natural life forms operating within it.

The word "therapist" has its etymological roots in words that mean care for, attend, and companion, the implication being that there is something healing in the act of paying attention. I am reminded of the poet Mary Oliver's (2008) words: "Instructions for living a life: Pay attention. Be astonished. Tell about it" (p. 37). We could equally name those as the instructions for true therapy. This means that my job as a therapist is not to offer solutions, advice, or teachings but simply to attend to someone's journey as they find their way back to themself. Within this gentle framework, I can endeavor to foster the optimal conditions for healing, such as the capacity for insight, emotional and relational safety, and the presence of genuine positive regard. Within the container of these conditions, a distraught psyche will heal itself, as all systems possess the evolutionary imperative to self-correct when the circumstances allow. Psychedelic literature speaks of contacting an "inner healing intelligence"—that is, that which automatically heals once given the green light (Mithoefer, 2013). In my experience, psychedelics play a vital role in my ability to create these conditions for another, as they allow me to maintain contact with my own inner healer, clear my own emotional debris from my heart, build bridges to disowned parts, and source ever-deeper wells of strength and integrity within my own bodymind. From this place of clarity and presence, I can attend to whatever a client brings me dispassionately, holding a clear enough space for them to begin the process of healing themselves.

Non-duality & Suffering

The psychedelic experience also continually teaches me that there are no others. As a longtime student of advaita vedanta, this teaching expands well beyond my psychedelic experience; however, I find psychedelics to be a reliable reminder of this core mystical principle. For me, it shows up again and again in my consulting room in the visceral, sometimes shattering, experience of being deeply mirrored by my client. Every psychotherapist knows the importance of mirroring our clients, but we rarely speak of the confounding phenomenon of them inadvertently mirroring us. Regularly, I will experience synchronicities such as having an argument with my partner wherein I discover some deeply held assumption based on some minor childhood trauma, and the very next day, a client will speak to me about their discovery of the self-same pattern. Or, while journeying with medicine, I will contact a deceased relative that sheds light on my relationship with abundance, and my next client conversation will center around the generational stories of scarcity passed down through parental communications. There have been such inexplicable things as dreaming of certain events that come true within the analytical container, dreaming fragments of the same dream as a client on the same night, and experiencing a personal synchronicity involving the same content (e.g., a specific number, animal, or song coming on the radio). I take no credit for the arrival of these phenomena, for the undeniable sense is that something so much larger than me, we, us orchestrates them, nor do I wish to make the mistake of reducing all of life's distinctions and healthy discernments into one amorphous, collapsible monad. That does not serve, nor does it articulate the profundity of what seems to be happening. The sense is that the one which has no other, the nondual ineffable isness which permeates all, the Self of which Jung (1980) writes, which is both the center and the circumference, comes alive in the healing relationship between two people and shows itself through uncanny connections. By being willing to look at myself in the mirror of my client—not dissociate from their human experience as something separate from my own—I settle into a profound trust, one which transcends the smallness of our simple biographical stories.

This trust is also what empowers me to suffer with my clients, without falling prey to that all-too-human impulse to somehow alleviate another's suffering by offering solutions, advice, or suggestions about how to fix it. When I reside in the truth of *there are no others*, not only am I not separate from the seeming other sitting in front of me, but I am not inclined to offer some contrived way out—for that contrivance will necessarily be limited by my own egoic separateness. It is as if, instead of relating to the separate entity of the qualitatively autonomous person sitting before me, I am relating to the weaver of the web which manifests such bizarrely connected experiences as those aforementioned. When I am in contact with that intrinsic force, the web that contains all of life's apparent parts, I am in contact with the rightness, the necessity of my clients' suffering, like the necessity of the forge to fashion the blade or the destruction of the seedshell to sprout the flower. In this place, there is no need to take suffering away, but only to support the other to engage in what Jung (1970) refers to as "legitimate suffering" (§129)—that is, the capacity to experience one's authentic feelings without ego defenses, spiritual bypasses, or egoic narratives. To feel precisely what one feels without telling a story about it, misconstruing it, or avoiding it.

Psychedelics have proved instrumental in teaching me how to sit with suffering. Specifically, I am able to sit and calmly watch as another suffers because I have been shown countless times how what I perceived as suffering in one season of my life was ultimately a boon, the experiential antidote I needed to forge a new tool for battle, craft a new magic potion for spiritual immunity, or shed another layer of false self. In other words, as trite as it may be, I have learned that we never get more than we can handle, and learning to handle what we have been given is the process of *becoming* whereby we step into our deepest most gifts, align with our most radiant service, and show up with treasures for our communities. Thanks to psychedelics, I know never to rob my patients of their suffering but, instead, help them suffer legitimately so that they may forge themselves in the alembic of their personalized trials.

The analytical philosopher Bernardo Kastrup (2018) frames this profound, yet mind-boggling mystical truth of nondual awareness in terms of ontology in his paper "The Universe in Consciousness." He offers a philosophically sound explanation of *cosmopsychism*, or the ontology which attributes all phenomenological experience to an ultimate cosmic consciousness. He asserts that each discreet entity that operates as a seemingly autonomous subjective consciousness—i.e., each lifeform—is akin to a dissociated part of a larger whole, in the same way that someone suffering from dissociative identity disorder (DID) is in possession of multiple co-conscious personalities inside their singular, integral psyche. In a lecture given at the 2022 Interdisciplinary Conference on Psychedelic Research (ICPR) in Haarlem, The Netherlands, Kastrup (2022) expanded upon this point with the argument that by decreasing the inner mechanism that contributes to a perceived separateness between physical entities, psychedelics enhance our ability to see the truth of cosmic consciousness which rests behind our so-called dissociation. This theory of the mechanism of psychedelics was made popular by Aldous Huxley's (2009) account of a mescaline journey in *The Doors of Perception*, wherein he speaks of the "reducing valve" of consciousness. Neurological research has confirmed that while psychedelics increase intraneurological connections—that is, connections amongst various cortices of the brain—they also decrease the dominance of certain networks within the brain overall (Carhart-Harris et al., 2012). Kastrup (2022) suggests that this decrease in brain activity correlates to the diminishment of the parts of human consciousness that keep us stuck in a false belief of separation from the cosmic consciousness, the web of life that flows through us all.

The Rainmaker

In *Mysterium Coniunctionis*, Jung (1976) shares a story about the miracle of the rainmaker, who was asked to bring rain to a village suffering from drought. Unlike the other clergy and spiritual leaders who had been asked to make pleas to the gods on behalf of the desperate villagers, the rainmaker merely asked for a quiet house in which he could remain undisturbed for as long as he needed. Three days passed without a word from this mysterious man. On the fourth day, large storm clouds gathered, and the small town was bathed in an unseasonable snow—enough to adequately refill the diminished groundwater supply. No one knew whether to attribute this freak weather to the rainmaker or chance; however, when asked, the rainmaker offered a curious explanation, saying "I did not make the rain. I am not responsible." He went on to explain that in the land from whence he came, things are in order, in the *Tao*; that in this village, they were not. For 3 days he sat with the disorder present in the land, all the while allowing his inner landscape to turn toward his original state of order. After these 3 days, he said, he had returned to *Tao*, and then naturally, the rains came. After sharing this parable, Jung reflects on the psychological significance, noting the almost mystical power of attitude in perceiving life's circumstances. He writes:

> If one has the right attitude, then the right things happen. One doesn't make it right, it is just right, and one feels it has to happen this way. It is just as if one were inside of things. If one feels right, that thing must turn up, it fits in. (§420)

In my work as an analyst, I am often confronted with neuroses, destructive personality traits, and psychological dysfunctions that seem immune to insight. Recalcitrant complexes do not shift through consciousness alone, for awareness is only the first part of a change process. Beyond creating the conditions for self-healing, something deeper is often needed, something akin to the balancing act of the rainmaker. To truly be of service in healing intractable soul droughts, I must make of my psyche a rainmaker; that is, I must let the disorder of the other fully in and allow myself to settle back into order from that place. If it were not for the depths of ecstasy, remembrance, and homecoming by which I have been graced with the aid of psychedelics, I would be at a loss as to the path back to order from disorder. Were it not for the fact that I've—through no personal will (I take no credit)—touched the majesty of truth again and again, I would be utterly unable to quietly invite the untruth of the other to obscure my soul and then patiently carve a path back to the light on both our behalfs.

As a servant of soul and a steward of Self, the highest offering I can make is to imbibe the spiritual desiccation wreaking havoc on my client's heart and assimilate it within myself to such a degree that it returns to wholeness by its own accord. To do this fully, it is imperative that I have a deep knowing of said wholeness—otherwise, the moment I drink from their inner dearth, we are both lost. Which is not to say that such a co-disappearance does not happen; there are myriad landscapes that have proven too barren, isolated, hellish, or incomprehensible to find my way back from. And were it not for my psychedelic experiences, there would surely be many multiples more. Truth is like a lighthouse, and the greater the depth of access to truth, the more powerful the light becomes. In the storm of severance from one's soul, orienting toward the lighthouse of truth within is sometimes the only thing we can do. Working with psychedelics has given me something very close to ready access to that lighthouse; and when I forget, as I often do (for ultimately realization is a game of hide-and-seek, as Alan Watts (1966) so aptly writes about in *The Book*), I am so grateful to have a trustworthy relationship to various plant medicines and entheogenic compounds that can help me remember. This remembrance inevitably proves to do more good for my clients than all of the advice, listening, mirroring, and practical intervention combined.

Life & Death in the Consulting Room

Perhaps one of the most poignant paradoxes played upon by psychedelics is that of life and death. Ancient Greek mystery cults employed the use of psychedelics to intentionally court the mysteries of death (Muraresku, 2020). The Indigenous peoples of the Amazon rainforest have named their main psychedelic sacrament *ayahuasca*, which means "the vine of death." The Bwiti of Western Africa, whose sacrament is called *iboga*, speak of the initiatory experience of this medicine as the experience of reviewing one's life at the moment of death. In the *Rig Veda*, the ancient religious text of Hinduism, we hear of the profound heavenly realization—a state of self-transcendence wherein all illusion dies—brought about by *soma*, a brew believed to contain the psychedelic mushroom *Amanita muscaria* (Wasson et al., 1986). Even modern neuroscience has begun to formulate theories about the phenomenology of ego-death and study the mechanism of mystical experience (e.g., Griffiths et al., 2006; Nur et al., 2016; Millière, 2017). Paradoxically, each of these traditions reveals that as individuals gain greater insight into the mystery of death—and more specifically, as one learns to relate to one's own inevitable death—a lot more vitality becomes available to the system.

In Jungian terms, we refer to this vitality as *anima* or *animus* (henceforth referred to as *animx*). Often anthropomorphized as a humanesque entity, psychologically speaking, the animx is the animating principle within oneself—that is, it is the spark of life that ignites through participation with the world. Experiences of deep aliveness—passion, play, creativity, intimacy, purpose, and emotionality, to name a few—indicate that we've contacted the animating principle within. And as we draw nearer toward the things in life that are meant for us, our animx lights up. Oftentimes, however, the power and vitality in these kinds of encounters proves intolerable for one reason or another, and so we defend against them.

There are many reasons a psyche contorts to keep out the vital lifeforce within: shame, perfectionism, fear of the unknown, fear of abandonment, over-identification with a particular role, developmental traumas, and insufficient emotional attunement, among others. The process of self-development, referred to by Jungians as *individuation*, is a process of facing these resistances to life, thus creating space for more of one's unique vitality to flow. Paradoxically, as the Indigenous wisdom traditions aforementioned suggest, to truly move beyond a well-defended stance against life, one must fully accept one's inevitable death. Without this acceptance, one unconsciously lives in fear of life, playing at immortality by never really sinking one's teeth into what is alive inside them, almost as if to say *if I never live, I'll never die.*

This apprehension of lifeforce, the denial of death, and subsequent fear of life have proved invaluable to my practice as a therapist. Just this week, a client shared that, while on a medium-sized dose of LSD, he had made contact with a deeply uncomfortable feeling within himself, one that might be described as coming up empty. He was beset by a kind of life review and, upon reflection while in this psychedelically-expanded state, noticed the presence of a deep despair. "What have I done with my life? I feel I've got nothing to show for it; I've not made anything of myself," he lamented. I named my own experience of his words—that of something decaying, a kind of deadening—and he immediately responded with a longing to make contact with the spark of life. But, he admitted, he did not really know how. Upon further exploration, he became aware of how he had spent his life following the supposed trajectory—get a lucrative job, have a family, send your kids to the right schools—to such a degree that he now felt completely cut off from any other impulses toward life. He remarked that any contact with what was soulful or vital inside himself felt blocked by a compulsive need for order. Internally, I noted the presence of our modern Western enculturation which privileges rationality and material objects over what is irrational and experiential. We deny the life force inside ourselves simply because it cannot be neatly ordered. In our conversation, I offered that there may be something beyond his biography that holds meaning—that perhaps his despairing life-retrospective was an invitation to meet that part of himself that is not purely factual.

By relating me to the mystery of death and the finitude of my own existence, psychedelics have given me my life back. Contact with my own vital spark within is what allows me to recognize that spark in another—and, grace willing, ignite it when it has gone out. Without this orientation to life and death, I genuinely believe I could not practice Jungian analysis; the whole ordeal would be washed away in the meaningless expanse of forever. Furthermore, without an orientation to the animating principle of life which draws one into the deepest, most personal participation with what is theirs and theirs alone to do, I might make the mistake of using the therapy technology to satisfy clients' egoic desires to be more well-adapted to society. Adaptation to society often requires severing quirks and singular callings, so to overly adapt necessarily means deadening one's unique life force. If I were to support my clients in this process of severing psychological limbs and inflicting mortal wounds on their souls, I would be making a grave mistake indeed.

Conclusion

Suffice it to say that my experiences with psychedelics have proved invaluable to my work as a Jungian analyst. I have been blessed with deep insight into myself and the human condition that binds me to all beings. I have felt the suffering that is required for true transformation to such a depth that not only do I no longer fear it, I welcome it. I have built a securely attached relationship to that which is in me that heals, and I trust this intelligence implicitly. I have pierced the veil of illusion to see the reality of selfhood that exists just behind the seeming separation of me and you. I have learned how to walk along the *via obscura*—the path of darkness—until I find the light of life again and again. And I have learned the poignancy of the life that flows through us all, a lesson that has repeatedly brought me to my knees in reverence and devotion. Ultimately, I have seen that it is this devotion to life and the mystery that contains it that facilitates true therapy.

References:

Carhart-Harris, R., Erritzoe, D., Williams, T., & Nutt, D. (2012). Neural correlates of the psychedelic state as determined by fMRI studies with psilocybin. *Proceedings of the National Academy of Sciences, 109*(6), pp. 2138-2143.

Griffiths, R. R., Richards, W. A., McCann, U., & Jesse, R. (2006). Psilocybin can occasion mystical-type experiences having substantial and sustained personal meaning and spiritual significance. *Psychopharmacology, 187*(3), pp. 268-83.

Huxley, A. (2009). *The doors of perception.* Harper Collins.

Jung, C. G. (1970). *Collected works of C. G. Jung, Vol. 11: Psychology and religion* (R. F. C. Hull, Trans.). Bolligen/Princeton University.

Jung, C. G. (1976). *Collected works of C. G. Jung, Vol. 14: Mysterium coniunctionis* (R. F. C. Hull, Trans.). Bolligen/Princeton University.

Jung, C. G. (1980). *Collected works of C. G. Jung, Vol. 12: Psychology and alchemy* (R. F. C. Hull, Trans.). Bolligen/Princeton University.

Kastrup, B. (2018). The universe in consciousness. *Journal of Consciousness Studies, 25*(5-6), pp. 125-55.

Kastrup, B. (2022, Sep 24). *Psychedelic experience is one piece of a much larger puzzle* [Conference lecture]. Interdisciplinary Conference on Psychedelic Research, Philharmonie, Haarlem, The Netherlands.

Millière, R. (2017). Looking for the self: phenomenology, neurophysiology and philosophical significance of drug-induced ego dissolution. *Frontiers of Human Neuroscience, 11*(245), pp. 1-22.

Mithoefer, M. (2013). MDMA-assisted psychotherapy: How different is it from other psychotherapy? *MAPS Bulletin 23*(1):10–14.

Muraresku, B. C. (2020). *The immortality key: The secret history of the religion with no name.* St. Martin's Griffin.

Nur, M. M., Evans, L., Nutt, D., & Carhart-Harris, R. L. (2016). Ego-dissolution and psychedelics: Validation of the ego-dissolution inventory (EDI). *Frontiers in Human Neuroscience, 10*(269), pp. 1-14.

Oliver, M. (2008). Sometimes. In *Red bird.* Beacon Press.

Wasson, R. G., Kramrisch, S., Ott, J., & Ruck, C. P. (1986). *Persephone's quest: Entheogens and the origins of religion.* Yale University Press.

Watts, A. (1966). *The book: On the taboo against knowing who you are.* Vintage Books.

If the doors of perception were cleansed, everything would appear to man as it is, infinite.

—William Blake

Leor Roseman

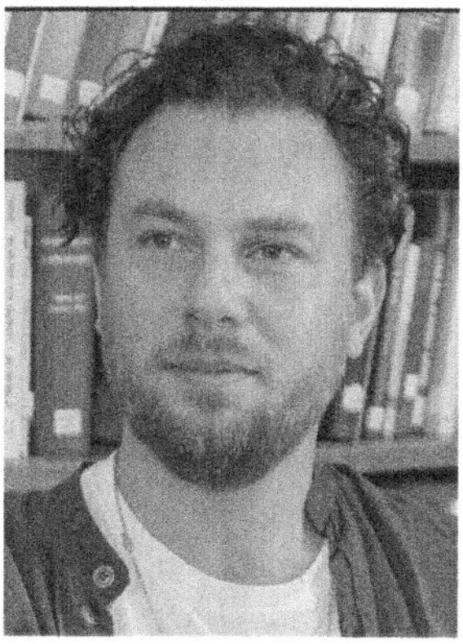

LEOR ROSEMAN, PHD, is a senior lecturer and psychedelic researcher at the University of Exeter, Department of Psychology. He previously worked at the Centre for Psychedelic Research, Imperial College London, under the mentorship of Prof. Robin Carhart-Harris and Prof. David Nutt, supporting the foundational work of a re-emerging research field. His interdisciplinary research covers neuroscience, psychology, phenomenology, anthropology and conflict resolution.
l.roseman@exeter.ac.uk

An Imaginary Interview with Martin Buber About Psychedelics

I PRESENT HERE AN IMAGINARY INTERVIEW WITH MARTIN BUBER ABOUT PSYCHEDELICS, using excerpts from his *I and Thou*, translated from German by Walter Kaufmann (Buber, 1923/1970). Through this interview, I hope to share a framework for psychedelic work that contemplates the spirituality of the between. I and You. Relation.

But before that, I share a bit about myself and my work.

In the past decade, I have enjoyed belonging to the re-emerging field of psychedelic research. As part of my work at Imperial College London, I have conducted some pioneering neuroimaging and clinical research in this field (Roseman et al., 2014; Roseman et al., 2017)—a source of much pride. Yet, as an enthusiast psychonaut, I felt that a vital component in my journeys was missing from my science: relations. Whether it was trips with friends in the desert or rituals in the jungle, other people with me were vital to the journey. So, I decided to move my research outside of the lab to study relational aspects of psychedelics in rituals and groups. The main sentiment behind this transition was that our decline in mental health is a socio-political problem, and solutions should also address societal causes as a trajectory of healing.

My first research in this direction was to show that psychedelic ceremonies enhance *communitas* (group bonding), and that this peak magical moment of a group can contribute to long-term changes in well-being (Kettner et al., 2021). Later, I supported the development of the Watts Connectedness Scale (Watts et al., 2022), arguing that psychedelics enhance a general sense of connectedness even after the journey. In that paper, we argued that enhanced connectedness—within the self and to others and the world—is one of the reasons why psychedelics work for different diagnoses, helping with some of the root causes of mental suffering: alienation and disconnection.

This is a psychopolitical statement.

To dive even deeper into psychedelic relationality, I needed a conflict to fix. Being an Israeli who lives in London, I continued to feel the pain of my homeland. Being a psychedelic researcher in the midst of the Psychedelic Renaissance, I was excited to examine the potentialities of these magical medicines on the intractable conflict of which I am part.

I teamed up with the Multidisciplinary Association for Psychedelic Studies (MAPS) and Palestinian activists and went on an adventure. During a month-long road trip, we interviewed Israelis and Palestinians who drink ayahuasca (a plant-based psychedelic brew) together, not necessarily with an explicit political intention. In this ethnographic-phenomenological study, we showed enhanced relationality during ceremonies—this was seen as enhanced intersubjective and intercultural connections. Ayahuasca intensified acts of communion and acts of recognition of the other and promoted visions of collective traumas (Roseman et al., 2021). From the same study, we also noticed the critique and limitations of such endeavour—harmony and oneness can sometimes serve the status quo by silencing conflictual voices. Yet revelatory-revolutionary moments can also occur, activating people towards change (Roseman & Karkabi, 2021).

To continue this line of research and bring it into practice, with a group of brilliant activists and facilitators (Awad & Roseman, 2023), we created an intentional peace-building retreat with ayahuasca. Such retreats led to strong bonds between group members, but the intense psychopolitical processes that took place within the ceremonies were even more interesting to me. Participants strongly affected each other in that space, and sometimes their visions interwove in a dialogical way. Insights, narratives, histories, collective traumas, music, fear, rage, fantasies, joy, and hope were amplified in the space between participants, coming together with this collective intention. This was revitalising for many, igniting a wish to act together. Yet now, when the cannons are heard and the muses are silent, those who attended those retreats and found inspiration and connection in them can suffer when returning to the madness of war, to the architecture of separation, or simply to the normalised oppression.

So, I summon Martin Buber for some more inspiration. I learned about *I and Thou* while starting to work on this project. A friend named Gon, with whom I very much enjoyed chatting about drugs, recognised my resonance with Buber and recommended a read. Buber immediately became my teacher and muse. I want to share this with you. May peace be upon us.

Oh, and one more thing: The translation to English uses the word "man" to describe any human. In German, Buber used the word "Mensch" (person, human) and not the word "Mann" (man, male). The translation into English as "man" was a conventional English term for person/humanity in that period.

Leor Roseman: Martin Buber, it is a great pleasure to have this interview with you. For a long time, I was fascinated by your work and felt very close to it. As you are not among us anymore, I took the liberty of conducting this interview with you based on excerpts from *I and Thou* (Buber, 1923/1970). Your book was written a century ago, but I find it very relevant to psychedelic research, so I created this imaginary interview with you. If you were alive today, you would probably be fascinated by psychedelic research and comment on it (as you briefly critiqued Huxley's writings on psychedelics). I suspect that you would have been initially critical towards this field of research based on misconceptions about what they do, but you would have eventually learned to appreciate them through a dialogical lens.

So, let's begin this interview with something at the heart of psychedelic research and culture—the experience. Many psychonauts, including myself, are very passionate about the experience—we see ourselves as experts in experience. Psychedelics teach us to be very sensitive to any experience and to explore the antipodes of the mind. I wonder what you think about the potentialities of the mind to create such mesmerising experiences.

Martin Buber: "The improvement of the ability to experience and use generally involves a decrease in man's power to relate." (Buber, 1923/1970, p. 91)

Roseman: Yes, I understand. I hear many people nowadays speak about the commodification of experiences. In that sense, people don't just consume things but also consume experiences. So, do you think this also applies to our inner experiences?

Buber: "All this is not changed by adding 'inner' experiences to the 'external' ones, in line with the non-eternal distinction that is born of mankind's craving to take the edge off the mystery of death. Inner things like external things, things among things!" (p. 51)

Roseman: Yes, I get what you are saying—but I do think that there are some qualities to some experiences that might make them more important and unique. For example, the mystical experience seems very meaningful to people.

Buber: "All this is not changed by adding 'mysterious' experiences to 'manifest' ones, self-confident in the wisdom that recognizes a secret compartment in things, reserved for the initiated, and holds the key. O mysteriousness without mystery, O piling up of information! It, it, it!

Those who experience do not participate in the world. The experience is 'in them' and not between them and the world." (p. 55)

Roseman: Strong words. In a way, you seem to oppose one of the main tenets of psychedelic therapy—which is the importance of the mystical experience (Roseman et al., 2017). I am aware that in your youth, you used to identify as a mystic and that your later shift to dialogue is related to ethical-political reasons (Buber, 1929/2003). But still, don't you think some unitive ego-dissolution is healthy for the self?

Buber: "All doctrines of immersion are based on the gigantic delusion of a human spirit bent back into itself—the delusion that spirit occurs in man. In truth it occurs from man—between man and what he is not." (p. 131)

"What has to be given up is not the I, as most mystics suppose: the I is indispensable for any relationship, including the highest, which always presupposes an I and You. What has to be given up is not the I but that false drive for self-affirmation which impels man to flee from the unreliable, unsolid, unlasting, unpredictable, dangerous world of relation into the having of things." (p. 125)

Roseman: So, how can you explain the well-replicated results showing that such experiences are crucial in psychedelic therapy?

Buber: "When man is for once overcome by the horror of alienation and the world fills him with anxiety, he looks up (right or left, as the case may be) and sees a picture. Then he sees that the I is contained in the world, and that there really is no I, and thus the world cannot harm the I, and he calms down; or he sees that the world is contained in the I, and that there really is no world, and thus the world cannot harm the I, and he calms down. And when man is overcome again by the horror of alienation and the I fills him with anxiety, he looks up and sees a picture; and whichever he sees, it does not matter, either the empty I is stuffed full of world or it is submerged in the flood of the world, and he calms down." (p. 120)

Roseman: I see. You say that such experiences are simply a temporary release from the anxieties of alienation. But, here, we can already contemplate that there may be another element in these experiences: a relation. After all, many—including myself—consider psychedelics as substances which increase connectedness. It may be wrong to say a psychedelic experience in the individualistic sense, and we should reflect on them also as enhancers of relationality as well. If that is the case, what is the mystical union? Can you help me reframe it?

Buber: "Mysticism? It relates how unity within duality feels. Have we any right to doubt the faithfulness of this testimony?

I know not only of one but of two kinds of events in which one is no longer aware of any duality. Mysticism sometimes confounds them, as I, too, did at one time.

First, the soul may become one. This event occurs not between man and God but in man. All forces are concentrated into the core, everything that would distract them is pulled in, and the being stands alone in itself and jubilates, as Paracelsus put it, in its exaltation. This is a man's decisive moment. Without this he is not fit for the work of the spirit. With this—it is decided deep down whether this means preparation or sufficient satisfaction. Concentrated into a unity, a human being can proceed to his encounter—wholly successful only now—with mystery and perfection. But he can also savor the bliss of his unity and, without incurring the supreme duty, return into distraction. Everything along our way is decision—intentional, dimly sensed, or altogether secret—but this one, deep down, is the primally secret decision, pregnant with the most powerful destiny.

The other event is that unfathomable kind of relational act itself in which one has the feeling that Two have become One: "one and one made one, bare shineth in bare." I and You drown; humanity that but now confronted the deity is absorbed into it; glorification, deification, universal unity have appeared. But when one returns into the wretchedness of daily turmoil, transfigured and exhausted, and with a knowing heart reflects on both, is one not bound to feel that Being is split, with one part abandoned to hopelessness? What help is it to my soul that it can be transported again from this world into that unity, when this world itself has, of necessity, no share whatever in that unity—what does all 'enjoyment of God' profit a life rent in two? If that extravagantly rich heavenly Moment has nothing to do with my poor earthly moment—what is it to me as long as I still have to live on earth—must in all seriousness still live on earth? That is the way to understand those masters who renounced the raptures of the ecstasy of 'unification.'

Which was no unification. Those human beings may serve as a metaphor who in the passion of erotic fulfillment are so carried away by the miracle of the embrace that all knowledge of I and You drowns in the feeling of a unity that neither exists nor can exist. What the ecstatic calls unification is the rapturous dynamics of the relationship; not a unity that has come into being at this moment in world time, fusing I and You, but the dynamics of the relationship itself which can stand before the two carriers of this relationship, although they confront each other immovably, and cover the eyes of the enraptured. What we find here is a marginal exorbitance of the act of relation: the relationship itself in its vital unity is felt so vehemently that its members pale in the process: its life predominates so much that the I and the You between whom it is established are forgotten. This is one of the phenomena that we find on the margins where actuality becomes blurred. But what is greater for us than all enigmatic webs at the margins of being is the central actuality of an everyday hour on earth, with a streak of sunshine on a maple twig and an intimation of the eternal You." (p. 134)

Roseman: Brilliant. This resonates well with my own personal experiences and with some phenomenological data I am collecting with students. When asking people to describe their psychedelic experience of unity, most answers actually describe some form of interconnection. It is rare to find experiences of a complete fusion between self and world. So maybe ego-dissolution and connectedness are related—the stronger the act of relation, the stronger the feeling of the dissolution of self. In that case, the complete unitive experience is simply on the spectrum of connectedness. It is a very intense connection—so strong that it feels like one, but still a connection.

So maybe there is something in the psychedelic experience after all, if you agree to see that they can also enhance connections—potentially enhancing I-Thou relation. I have observed this in my research on therapy and rituals and in my peacebuilding research with Israelis and Palestinians. I also know it through my own psychedelic encounters. Do you think that psychedelics might enhance I-Thou relations?

Buber: Yes.

Roseman: Thanks, I am very pleased you agree with me here. I thought it would be much harder to convince you, and I am happy you showed some flexibility, even if it was out of politeness. Where can we usually find I-You relations?

Buber: "Three are the spheres in which the world of relation arises:

The first: life with nature. Here the relation vibrates in the dark and remains below language. The creatures stir across from us, but they are unable to come to us, and the You we say to them sticks to the threshold of language.

The second: life with men. Here the relation is manifest and enters language. We can give and receive the You.

The third: life with spiritual beings. Here the relation is wrapped in a cloud but reveals itself, it lacks but creates language. We hear no You and yet feel addressed; we answer—creating, thinking, acting: with our being we speak the basic word, unable to say You with our mouth." (p. 55)

Roseman: Some people are also talking about connection to self. Do you understand what this means?

Buber: "When man does not test the a priori of relation in the world, working out and actualizing the innate You in what he encounters, it turns inside. Then it unfolds through the unnatural, impossible object, the I—which is to say that it unfolds where there is no room for it to unfold. Thus the confrontation within the self comes into being, and this cannot be relation, presence, the current of reciprocity, but only self-contradiction. Some men may try to interpret this as a relation, perhaps one that is religious, in order to extricate themselves from the horror of their Doppelgänger: they are bound to keep rediscovering the deception of any such interpretation. Here is the edge of life. What is unfulfilled has here escaped into the mad delusion of some fulfillment; now it gropes around in the labyrinth and gets lost ever more profoundly." (p. 119)

Roseman: Sounds like a spiritual bypassing of sorts. Yet, I think when people speak about connection to self, they often mean connection within self—between different aspects of the self. A certain wholeness. Anyway, yes, I very much resonate with the three spheres of relation, and my psychedelic use and practice usually enhance the relations in these three spheres. However, it is important to recognise that they can do the opposite as well sometimes. What impacted me when I first read you was to see the relation between those spheres. I learned to see spirituality in everyday relations. I think that psychedelically- intensified connections and your interpretive framework clarified it for me. Weirdly, there is some similarity between a fun chat with a person and being in nature or even with the so-called unitive experience. Isn't there?

Buber: "In every sphere, through everything that becomes present to us, we gaze toward the train of the eternal You; in each we perceive a breath of it; in every You we address the eternal You, in every sphere according to its manner." (p. 56)

Roseman: Exactly; when I'm in nature by myself or enter the flow of dialogue with people, I find some qualities that I also find in psychedelic experiences, and they seem to nourish me in the same way. Why would such relations nourish me so much?

Buber: "Whoever stands in relation, participates in an actuality; that is, in a being that is neither merely a part of him nor merely outside him. All actuality is an activity in which I participate without being able to appropriate it. Where there is no participation, there is no actuality. Where there is self-appropriation, there is no actuality. The more directly the You is touched, the more perfect is the participation.

The I is actual through its participation in actuality. The more perfect the participation is, the more actual the I becomes.

But the I that steps out of the event of the relation into detachment and the self-consciousness accompanying that, does not lose its actuality. Participation remains in it as a living potentiality. To use words that originally refer to the highest relation but may also be applied to all others: the seed remains in him." (p. 113)

Roseman: Yes, indeed, but I must admit that I am sometimes disappointed that this actuality—which comes with the act of relation—cannot be constantly felt.

Buber: "This is the realm of subjectivity in which I apprehends simultaneously its association and its detachment. Genuine subjectivity can be understood only dynamically, as the vibration of the I in its lonely truth. This is also the place where the desire for ever higher and more unconditional relation and for perfect participation in being arises and keeps rising. In subjectivity the spiritual substance of the person matures." (p. 113)

Roseman: You know, there is also another quality of psychedelic experiences which attracts me—this is liberation. I really enjoy the feeling of freedom that psychedelics can bring and the insights that can arise from it. And again, I find the same feelings when I am in nature, or when I am having a pure moment of relation. Or on the dancefloor. Do you think there is some relationship between I-Thou relations and liberation?

Buber: "Yes, in the pure relationship you felt altogether dependent, as you could never possibly feel in any other—and yet also altogether free as never and nowhere else; created—and creative. You no longer felt the one, limited by the other; you felt both without bounds, both at once." (p. 130)

Roseman: Thanks, Martin, for these great insights. Before concluding, do you have anything to say about the current state of the world? We spoke about alienation, and it does seem that alienation is a societal sickness which is the source of many of our mental health problems. Where does it all go?

Buber: "In sick ages it happens that the It-world, no longer irrigated and fertilized by the living currents of the You-world, severed and stagnant, becomes a gigantic swamp phantom and overpowers man. As he accommodates himself to a world of objects that no longer achieve any presence for him, he succumbs to it. Then common causality grows into an oppressive and crushing doom." (p. 101)

"But the path is not a circle. It is the way. Doom becomes more oppressive in every new eon, and the return more explosive. And the theophany comes ever closer, it comes ever closer to the sphere between beings - comes closer to the realm that hides in our midst, in the between. History is a mysterious approach to closeness. Every spiral of its path leads us into deeper corruption and at the same time into more fundamental return." (p. 168)

Roseman: Thanks, Martin. Prophetic indeed. Walter Kaufmann, who translated you, wrote that your work has "the central commandment to make the secular sacred." As a non-religious person, I can attest to that. You helped me see the spirit in everyday relations. Thank you. To end, can you please provide our psychedelic readers with one tip on how to nourish our world of relations?

Buber: "One does not have to strip away the world of the senses as a world of appearance. There is no world of appearance, there is only the world—which, to be sure, appears twofold to us in accordance with our twofold attitude. Only the spell of separation needs to be broken. Nor is there any need to "go beyond sense experience"; any experience, no matter how spiritual, could only yield us an It. Nor need we turn to a world of ideas and values—that cannot become present for us. All this is not needed. Can one say what is needed? Not by way of a prescription. All the prescriptions that have been excogitated and invented in the ages of the human spirit, all the preparations, exercises, and meditations that have been suggested have nothing to do with the primally simple fact of encounter. All the advantages for knowledge or power that one may owe to one or another exercise do not approach that of which we are speaking here. All this has its place in the It-world and does not take us one step—does not take the decisive step—out of it. Going forth is unteachable in the sense of prescriptions. It can only be indicated—by drawing a circle that excludes everything else. Then the one thing needful becomes visible: the total acceptance of the present." (p. 125)

Acknowledgments

I am grateful to Sam Shonkoff for constructive feedback and for sharing this passion, and to Gon Ben Ari for inspiring dialogues and directing me to Buber.

References

Awad, S., & Roseman, L. (2023). *From personal to collective: Ayahuasca as a peace-making tool among Palestinians and Israelis* [Keynote Address]. Psychedelic Science 2023, Denver, USA. https://www.youtube.com/watch?v=bynaa_UpLSU&ab_channel=Ripples

Buber, M. (1923/1970). *I and thou* (W. Kaufmann, Trans.). New York: Charles Scribner's Sons.

Buber, M. (1929/2003). *Between man and man (Zwiesprache)*. Milton Park, UK: Routledge.

Kettner, H., Rosas, F., Timmermann, C., Kärtner, L., Carhart-Harris, R., & Roseman, L. (2021). Psychedelic Communitas: Intersubjective experience during psychedelic group sessions predicts enduring changes in psychological wellbeing and social connectedness. *Frontiers in Pharmacology, 12*, 234. https://doi.org /10.3389/fphar.2021.623985

Roseman, L., & Karkabi, N. (2021). On revelations and revolutions: Drinking ayahuasca among Palestinians under Israeli occupation. *Frontiers in Psychology, 12*, 3668. https://doi.org /10.3389/fpsyg.2021.78934

Roseman, L., Leech, R., Feilding, A., Nutt, D. J., & Carhart-Harris, R. L. (2014). The effects of psilocybin and MDMA on between-network resting state functional connectivity in healthy volunteers. *Frontiers in Human Neuroscience, 8*, 204. https://doi.org/10.3389/fnhum.2014.00204

Roseman, L., Nutt, D. J., & Carhart-Harris, R. L. (2017). Quality of acute psychedelic experience predicts therapeutic efficacy of psilocybin for treatment-resistant depression. *Frontiers in Pharmacology, 8*, 974. https://doi.org /10.3389/fphar.2017.00974

Roseman, L., Ron, Y., Saca, A., Ginsberg, N., Luan, L., Karkabi, N., Doblin, R., & Carhart-Harris, R. (2021). Relational processes in ayahuasca groups of Palestinians and Israelis. *Frontiers in Pharmacology, 12*, 607529. https://doi.org/10.3389/fphar.2021.607529

Watts, R., Kettner, H., Geerts, D., Gandy, S., Kartner, L., Mertens, L., Timmermann, C., Nour, M. M., Kaelen, M., Nutt, D., Carhart-Harris, R., & Roseman, L. (2022). The Watts Connectedness Scale: A new scale for measuring a sense of connectedness to self, others, and world. *Psychopharmacology, 239*(11), 3461-3483. https://doi.org/10.1007/s00213-022-06187-5

Marilyn Clark

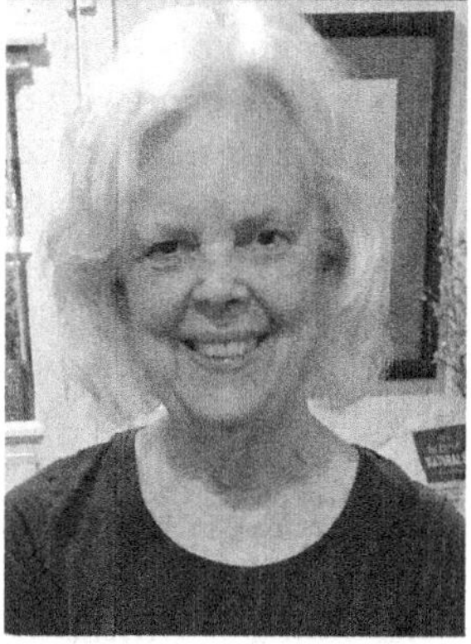

MARILYN CLARK IS AN LCPC and Fellow of the Association for Music and Imagery. She has advanced the Bonny Method of Guided Imagery & Music (GIM) by providing personal sessions, training colleagues, and publishing articles. Also, she has assisted volunteers participating in psilocybin research at Hopkins Center for Psychedelic and Consciousness Research. She enjoys facilitating individual GIM sessions and mentoring students studying GIM and a related process: creating mandalas for insight, healing, and self-expression. For more information: https://www.invitedbymusic.com and https://www.creating-mandalas.com

Music and Psychedelics

IN THE LATE '60S, when I came to Maryland after graduating from college in Texas, I had no idea what would be in my future. My move to Baltimore was challenging and confusing. I was searching for something, but I did not know what. A progression of events unfolded out of that spontaneous decision that led me to meet and work beside Helen Bonny, music therapist, LSD researcher, and mystic.

Working for a short time as a secretary at Koinonia Foundation, in the countryside outside of Baltimore, I met several people working for peace and justice at the American Friends Service Committee. They were forming a commune and wanted to have an equal number of men and women, and I was invited to join them. Toad Hall came into being with three men and three women. I knew that joining them would bring me right into the antiwar movement, to the People's Free Medical Clinic, and to women's liberation groups. I knew they were political activists and soon would learn that they were also seekers of consciousness expansion. Their perspectives were radically new to me, and I was excited and open to all that they were passionate about.

The Toad Hall Days

I was introduced to marijuana, mescaline, and LSD gradually. There was no pressure to join with those who were exploring altered states experiences. But I was curious and open to the possibilities, so I joined with others in the evenings to smoke marijuana. My first mescaline experience was at the beach where we had gone for a weekend adventure. Back at Toad Hall, my experiences were always with people I knew and trusted. Music was played on the record player, chosen randomly by preferences of those who were present. I enjoyed the music of the Moody Blues band with their interesting lyrics and musical effects that sometimes deepened and expanded my consciousness state. There was no guide to support me in my experience. There were those who were more experienced with the use of these substances who could be supportive. And there was usually someone in the group who, for personal reasons, had not dropped acid or smoked marijuana, who could attend to any obvious problems someone might have.

When I read through the journals I kept of these times, I have a picture of a confused, slightly depressed, and somewhat lost young woman. The altered-state experiences ushered me into a different way of looking at my life. I was gradually freed of scripts from middle class America's expectations for a young adult woman, and I expanded my understanding of spirituality, beyond or separate from, organized religion.

Helen Bonny and Guided Imagery and Music (GIM)

I began to explore the spirituality of Quakers, attending their meetings close to Toad Hall. Helen Bonny attended there, and I had been drawn to her due to her occasional messages [1] delivered in Meeting for Worship. She seemed often to attain a spiritual experience in the silence and could share the experience with those gathered. This ability impressed me, and I hoped to learn how to have those experiences someday. Perhaps I could find a way to make this possible by learning about spirituality from her. I also knew that she was involved in research with psychedelics at the Maryland Psychiatric Research Center on the grounds of the Spring Grove State Hospital.

I approached her one Sunday after Meeting for Worship with the hope of finding a way to connect with her. At the time I was not working, and I was willing to volunteer to do anything she might need of a secretary. She quickly took me up on this offer and gave me two cassette tapes to transcribe. One was an experience she and her sister had with elders in a Native American tribe her father had ministered to. The other was a minister's peak experience during a music therapy session with Helen. Both transcription tasks were enlightening, but I was particularly impressed by the minister's experience.

I had found in my own inner search that the psychedelic experience, while opening into amazing and sometimes challenging spaces, was difficult to integrate into my life. I wrote about these experiences in my journal but otherwise kept them to myself. I had tasted states of consciousness that indicated there might be more to my understanding of deep states than what I usually considered consensus reality, but there was no witness who could help me integrate what I experienced. The minister's peak experience was evidence that there were safer ways to reach expanded states of consciousness than obtaining and ingesting illegal psychedelics. And furthermore, that Helen was onto something very important: the power of music to affect human consciousness. [2]

After a few weeks of working for her, I gathered the courage to ask if I might have

1 Messages in a Quaker meeting come from seeking divine guidance and sharing that with those gathered.

2 In 2000, Helen Bonny was honored by the World Congress of Music Therapists for her life work and the Bonny Method of Guided Imagery and Music was recognized as one of five major international models of music therapy.

such an experience with her as the one I had transcribed. Her face lit up, and she said, "Of course!" The date was arranged, and I came to her apartment in Baltimore for my first Guided Imagery and Music (GIM) experience. She explained the process: relaxation of the body, quieting the mind, listening to a music program of her design, and reporting aloud my images and feelings. She encouraged me to respond verbally as well as to be open to emotions and physical responses. She chose to play her all-Brahms program titled "Emotional Expression." [3]

My initial imagery experience when the music began was of a barren landscape empty of humans. She encouraged me to explore this landscape and then suggested that I look up. Most likely it was Helen's intuition that led to this suggestion. When I looked up, I saw a whole new landscape. It was all white—trees, rocks, soil, etc. When I began to explore this white landscape, I was joined by a presence. It seemed to be male and was wearing a long white robe. Kindness, acceptance, and love flowed from this presence. I was flabbergasted. Nothing like this had ever happened in my inner world before or in my altered-state experiences. The presence stayed in my imagery experience for a while. Helen encouraged me to speak to him. What I wanted to know was "Who are you?" and "What is my life's purpose?" He did not tell me. He was not speaking, but I felt there was communication between us. He pointed away from me, and I understood this to mean "Continue on your path. You will know." I felt totally accepted, understood, and even loved by this figure.

Throughout this experience, the beautiful music of the all-Brahms program was playing. Helen's presence was nearby, and her gentle comments furthered the experience. For several days after this GIM session, I remembered the figure in white and longed for his presence in my waking life. I knew I had had a very important experience with Helen, music, and my inner world. It differed in important ways from the psychedelic experiences I had in the settings at Toad Hall. Helen was with me every step of the way, and her guiding helped me to focus and deepen into the experience. The music program was beautiful and invited my images to unfold before me. Afterwards, I was able to talk with her to begin to integrate what had happened and what that might mean in my life. This way of entering non-ordinary states of consciousness was safer and more applicable to my ordinary waking life. And it was entirely legal!

Helen also had a life-changing experience with music in her 20s, which became a milestone towards her later work with consciousness and music. At a churchwomen's meeting, she was asked by the minister to play her violin as part of an evening service. Midway through a short piece, a radical and inexplicable event occurred. Suddenly the tone quality issuing from her violin changed; it was of incredible beauty. The tones soared with an ease and purity beyond the boundaries of what she knew she could do. The marvelous flow of music continued despite her efforts to control it. The minister and congregation also experienced this wonder.

With a new commitment to bringing the possibility of transcendence to others through music, Helen pursued a degree in music therapy. She was hired in 1970 as a music therapist to work at the Maryland Psychiatric Research Center where her colleagues were Stan Grof, Walter Pahnke, William Richards, John Rhead, and others. These pio-

3 Emotional Expression Program: Brahms Piano Concerto #2 (Allegro); Brahms German Requiem Part1, 5; Brahms 4th Symphony (Andante moderato).

neers provided treatment with psychedelics in a carefully controlled setting for patients with terminal cancer, alcoholism, and other serious conditions. Music was regarded as an essential element of the research as it provided a structure for the patients in their explorations of inner mind states. Helen's particular genius was combining her musical and intuitive knowledge in the selection, structure, and sequence of music that would maximize desired therapeutic outcomes.

In their 1972 article, "The Use of Music in Psychedelic (LSD) Psychotherapy," Helen Bonny and Walter Pahnke, director of the Research Center Program, delineated their findings on how music can enhance the LSD experience. Their conclusions found the use of music to be a very important part of the deep altered states made available in LSD sessions. Music directed and structured the experience: facilitating a release of intense emotion and a sense of continuity in the experience of timelessness and enabling the traveler to enter more fully into their inner experience and reach a peak experience (Bonny & Pahnke, 1972). Music accompanies psychedelic experiences and is a presence for the traveler as well as for the guide. Early psychedelic researchers emphasized the importance of *set,* meaning mindset, and *setting,* meaning social and physical environment where the psychedelic experience is had. Careful music selection is an important component of optimal set and setting. Dr. Kenneth Bruscia's (2019) chapter in *Guided Imagery and Music: The Bonny Method and Beyond, Second Edition* captures more of Helen's guidelines for music selection, discussing how the right music helps one relinquish control and overcome resistance, allowing a deeper exploration of the unconscious and stimulating associations as memories, images, and fantasies arise is the psychedelic experience.

Early 21st Century Music and Psychedelic Use

The re-emergence of the use of psychedelics shows a very different picture now than in the hippie communes of the 1970s. Research is supporting the positive outcomes of the use of psychedelics. State laws are easing. There are training programs for persons who want to be guides for travelers. Many of the guides are also psychotherapists.

In today's world, music is very accessible to the psychedelic guide. World music, ambient sounds, chanting, sound baths, etc. are easily available to all of us who have a computer or smart phone. Careful music choice is an imperative consideration for the traveler's safety and successful experience. The psychedelic guide may interview the traveler ahead of the session and explain how music will support the experience. They can explore together what the musical preferences of the traveler are and whether there is openness to hearing music that they might not ordinarily listen to. The guide should carefully listen to and become familiar with any music they plan to use in the psychedelic settings. Using their knowledge of music, dimensions of consciousness, and in vivo intuition, the guide will be better equipped to offer music to the traveler.

How to choose the music for a psychedelic session should be a well thought out and tested process. Knowledge of the traveler's psychological process, including history of trauma, is important. The client's prior psychedelic sessions and hopes for the upcoming experience should be noted. Progression in real time of the psychedelic's onset, build to climax, and return to normal consciousness should be understood by the guide. About how long each of these levels last is useful to know and affects music choice. Some psychedelic guides will suggest that the client bring music that they choose to their own psychedelic session. For some clients, familiar music can be grounding and supportive. For others, it could be limiting or otherwise inappropriate to the set and setting. Some guides will thus encourage the client to trust the guide's music choices, tested over time. Sometimes playing our favorites can only take us to our memories of when we heard this music before. Letting go of the need to control the process and trusting in the guide's experience and training can result in a music selection that takes the traveler where they need to go.

It is important that the guide be cautious about using music for which they have a strong personal affinity or dislike. The traveler can be affected by their guide's emotional and spiritual responses to music even when nothing is said about the music by the guide. Using a ready-made playlist is an option as well. These could be made available through training programs or networking with other guides. This programmed playlist approach is often used by GIM guides. Due to the nuances of a psychedelic traveler's unfolding experience, the guide may need to change the music to suit the direction and flow of the traveler's process.

Recently I engaged the help of a psychedelic guide to have a psilocybin experience. As my guide, she also provided the mushrooms. I had decided what music I would like to have support the process. She would use my CDs and CD player. However, problems arose when she was not able to easily use my player. The tracks that played were not what I expected, and I began to feel uncomfortable. By then, the psilocybin was effecting a change in my consciousness, and for a while I felt paranoid about her. Even so, we were able to figure out together that the music was not what I had expected. We agreed that I would release my agenda, and she would use music that she had brought with her. As I let go of the need to control the music, I found that the music she provided was gentle and easy to take inside. Soon it was possible to get back into the state of mind made available by the psilocybin mushrooms. What followed in the experience was a profound sense of the pain of Mother Earth...the dismay that humanity is harming its mother. Sobs came from deep within me. After this expression of grief, I moved into a space that felt quite profound. There was a discussion of sorts, although the one with whom I was in discussion was more like an idea than another person or being. What was communicated to me was this: It is very simple to move into the experience of unity rather than to live in the world of duality. Many live in the unity dimension all the time. It is right next to where you are now. This realization has stayed with me. I have tried to sketch it and to put it into words of explanation. Neither have given justice to the insight, which as I write it down, sounds mundane and obvious. Yet I know it is a profound lesson to continue to contemplate and maybe someday to actualize.

Why I wrote this article

I turned off my Zoom call, sat back, and looked up the word "frisson." My online dictionary told me it is "a sudden sensation of excitement, a shudder of emotion, a thrill..." (Dictionary.com, 2024). The presenter on a Zoom workshop sponsored by a training program for psychedelic therapy had used the word to describe how to choose music for a psychedelic therapy session. He suggested that the listener's experience of frisson was an indication that the music was just right for that psychedelic experience. Having worked with dozens of people experiencing altered states of consciousness while listening to music, I know that music choice for altered states involves so much more than a shudder.

Reference

Bonny, H. & Pahnke, W. (1972). The use of music in psychedelic (LSD) psychotherapy. *Journal of Music Therapy 9*(2), pp. 64-87.

Bruscia, K. (2019). Helen Bonny's foundational theories of guided imagery and music (GIM). In D. E. Grocke, (Ed.), *Guided imagery and music (GIM): The Bonny method and beyond*, (Second edition, pp. 41-48). Barcelona Publishers.

Dictionary.com (n.d.). Frisson. In *Dictionary.com.* Retrieved 01/28/24 from https://www.dictionary.com/browse/frisson

---

Wonders of a lifetime, right there before your eyes
Searching with this life of ours, you gotta make the journey out and in.

—Michael Pinder (from the Moody Blues song, "Out and In")

Sian Seligman

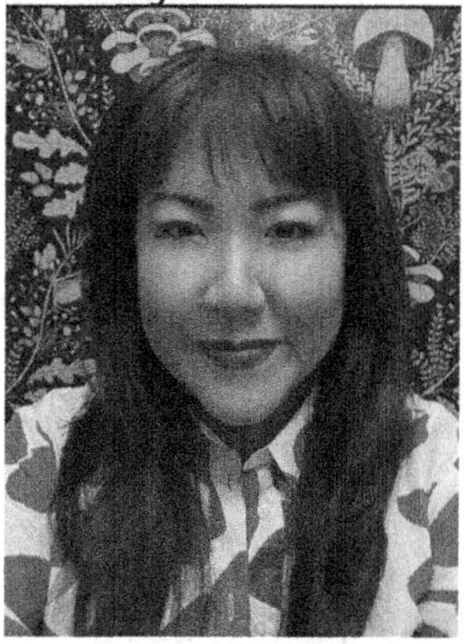

Sian Seligman, MS, is an herbalist, researcher, and strategist. Ms. Seligman was chief marketing officer in the cannabis industry, winning a Clio award in 2021. Prior to herbal medicine, she was a strategic consultant for brands like Nestle, Burger King, Audi, and Coca-Cola. She was chairperson of the board at City Club Los Angeles, as the first Asian female chairperson. She sits on the board of trustees at The Chicago School. She is a certified master gardner.
sian.seligman@achs.edu

Psychedelics as Treatment for Race-based Trauma

As a psychedelics researcher of color, I am often invited to community discussions centered around how psychedelics may aid in healing racial trauma. Racial trauma is defined as an emotional and psychological injury caused by discrimination based on one's race, ethnicity, or skin color (Ching et al., 2022). The cumulative effect of chronic exposure to discrimination may lead to internalized racism, resulting in negative self-perception and self-destructive behavior (Williams et al., 2018). Racial trauma attacks a victim's core identity, and because this cannot be altered, it can lead to shame, guilt, and unhealthy coping mechanisms that hinder emotional processing and exacerbate PTSD symptoms (Bannister et al., 2019). Shame may also contribute to social stigma, making it harder for survivors to seek care. The community discussions I participate in often lead to dialogue about the dehumanizing and isolating nature of racism. Finding healing can be difficult within communities of color due to the cultural stigmas toward both mental health treatment and illicit drug use. The FDA's breakthrough therapy designation carries substantial implications for developing MDMA and/or psilocybin-based treatments, particularly for racial trauma-related conditions, potentially destigmatizing psychedelics and enhancing public acceptance of psychedelic-assisted therapy.

Growing up, my family never discussed racism, let alone how to deal with it once I encountered it. The Pew Research Center (Ruiz et al., 2023) reports that 68% of Asian adults who grew up in the United States say they rarely or never talked with family about the challenges they might face because of their race or ethnicity when growing up. My parents always encouraged obedience, and following the rules became a means of survival for me. I distinctly remember the first time I recognized my race. I was in preschool, and a girl on the playground told me that my eyes were funny because I was Chinese, and that she didn't want to play with me, and that boys didn't like me because of it. Incidentally, my family is from Thailand. This was certainly not the last nor the only time I would be othered. According to the Pew Research Center (Ruiz et al., 2023), 78% of Asian adults have been treated as a foreigner in some way, even if they are U.S.-born. My maiden name is Ankhasirisan, and with a name like Sian Ankhasirisan you can only imagine what roll call was like on the first day of school. There was a time in elementary school when a White male teacher wouldn't even try to pronounce my name and said, "Let's just call you Smith," and the entire class laughed. I shrugged and joined them, because who was I to challenge an adult authority figure? Then upon entering high school and college with multiple classes, and on into my work life, the issue followed me constantly. I've had many teachers, acquaintances, bosses, and work colleagues who've never learned to pronounce my name accurately, nor did they ever ask how to pronounce it correctly. Ultimately, I became resigned to having my name pronounced incorrectly, even to this day. I've had grown adults yell across a parking lot, "Ching Chong, Ching Chong." I have been bullied, called terrible names, and harassed. I've been told to go back to the country where I came from, and I've been asked if I speak English many times throughout my life. Having been born and raised in the United States, this was extremely confusing, especially when I was young, because when I would visit my family in Thailand I was called a foreigner and an American. So I was never quite fully accepted in either country. While I have never experienced extreme violence, nor have I ever been physically attacked because of my race, discriminatory micro and macro aggressions have had lifelong cumulative and pernicious effects that have manifested in negative ways, such as generalized anxiety, shame, doubts of self-worth, and an inability to expose my vulnerability.

Psychedelics have been a profound tool in helping me find the capacity and empathy to cope and find healing with racism and beyond. They have significantly softened me as a human being. I've released the need to keep my edge. When it comes to seeing and hearing another human, I would rather use tools like kindness and gentleness as opposed to the skepticism and sarcasm that steeled me throughout my life. I have found that the use of psilocybin and MDMA has improved my own psychological flexibility, feeling seen and heard, reducing reactivity, as well as developing empathy for myself and my aggressors. And isn't empathy at the heart of it all? Without empathy, we cannot see the humanity in each other and healing cannot begin.

Mounting research on psychedelics has shown promising results across a broad spectrum of mental health disorders including treatment-resistant depression, anxiety, alcohol and tobacco use disorders, cancer-related existential fears, and PTSD. According to Williams et al. (2020), two clinical trials using psilocybin found decreased symptoms of depression and anxiety. Benefits from a single session lasted for 6 months. While trials have been positive, they remain small and lack Black, Indigenous, and people of color (BIPOC) inclusion. Williams and colleagues (2020) go on to state that across 18 global studies on psychedelic-assisted therapy, a disproportionate number of participants were White (82%), and BIPOC participants made up a very small, combined total: Black 3%, Latinx 2%, Asian 2%, Indigenous 5%, mixed race 5%, other 2%, and unknown 8%. Low to no BIPOC representation in psychedelic studies creates equity gaps in accessibility and benefits for BIPOC treatment.

Despite positive outcomes, there is a notable lack of empirical data regarding the influence of race and ethnicity on psychedelics in treatment, primarily because research participants and the researchers involved in the design of these studies are predominantly White. If one has not experienced racism as a lived experience, designing a study or reporting on racism becomes challenging. Race-based trauma is often underreported and undiagnosed due to low awareness or recognition by clinicians, discomfort with race-related dialogue, and lack of tools to assess race-based trauma (Williams et al., 2018). Experiences of racism are an important indicator of trauma (Williams et al., 2018). Everyday discriminatory experiences, including microaggressions, have been linked to anxiety, substance abuse, and depression (Williams, 2020). However, racial trauma is rarely caused by a singular or discrete event but instead by the cumulative effect of multiple discriminatory experiences over time (Ching et al., 2022). Fewer studies tend to focus on racial trauma, and racial trauma survivors also experience greater systemic disparities and are less likely to have access to mental health care (Williams et al., 2021). Cultural stigma of mental illness and attitudes towards psychedelic use further compound the issue.

Barriers to Racial Diversity in Research

BIPOC communities have been historically marginalized in the United States by being associated with illicit drug use. In the 1950s and 1960s, psychedelics were associated with the White-dominant hippie counterculture, which devalued the collective BIPOC contributions to psychedelics, and they were ultimately vilified by being associated with illicit drug use, violence, and civil disorder. This period saw the appropriation of many aspects of Black, Asian, and Indigenous cultures, including language, philosophy, music, fashion, and religion. While the hippie movement is credited with introducing psychedelics and influencing American values, the association with illicit drugs and stigma for Black Americans remains today (George et al., 2020).

The U.S. opioid crisis disproportionately affected White Americans, leading to a national public health emergency, and programs emerged to avoid incarceration. In contrast, the crack epidemic of the '80s mainly affected poor Black Americans and was largely neglected, leading to stigma and incarceration. This segmentation of drugs by race has associated psychedelics with White culture, as studies show that only 4% of psychedelic users are Black, compared to 20% who are White (George et al., 2020).

Current trends in psychedelic use among BIPOC millennials and older Gen Z individuals may be changing perceptions. These newer generations of BIPOC individuals are receptive to recreational psychedelic use, but lingering skepticism of clinical research remains. Seventeen psychedelic studies between 2000 and 2017 revealed that only 2.2% of participants were Black, 2.2% were Latino, 1.5% were Asian, and 4.7% were Indigenous (George et al., 2020).

Traditional screening methods do not account for race-related trauma and leave many BIPOC excluded from potential benefits. More inclusive recruitment is needed across different racial groups and ethnic diasporas. To ensure that BIPOC populations are represented in clinical trials, researchers must employ methods that are culturally sensitive, counteract negative views BIPOC may have about treatment, and promote trust within medical environments (George et al., 2020).

Distinct Characteristics of Race-based Mental Disorders

Smith and colleagues (2022) suggest that sustained isolation and dehumanization based on race fatigues the brain and body, resulting in deep and lasting trauma at the molecular level, which can be passed down generationally. Colonization may also contribute to generational trauma experienced by BIPOC. Despite this, few studies have investigated the prevalence or treatment to address generational trauma (Williams et al., 2021). Individuals experiencing racial trauma commonly report a range of psychological and physical symptoms linked with PTSD, including heightened emotional arousal and reactivity to trauma (e.g., hyper-vigilance, irritability), unstable mood, intrusive thoughts, heightened startle response, flashbacks, and disruptions in sleep patterns such as insomnia and nightmares. These symptoms are associated with abnormal levels of hormones and neurotransmitters (e.g., serotonin, GABA, dopamine, cortisol), as well as irregularities in brain wave patterns. Such disruptions in brain and body regulation contribute to adverse physical and mental health outcomes (Smith et al., 2022).

Another study examined the origins of race-related trauma leading to PTSD in communities of color. This type of trauma inflicts severe psychological and physical damage on BIPOC populations. What makes it particularly harmful is that it is linked to an inherent aspect of one's identity, like race, which can exacerbate its effects over time, potentially leading to PTSD symptoms and various other mental health issues. Importantly, traumatic events and PTSD can trigger a series of subsequent psychological, physiological, and epigenetic impacts on the body (Williams et al., 2021).

Ongoing stress triggered by daily systemic racism activates the hypothalamic-pituitary-adrenal axis (HPA-axis), a feedback loop system. This system initiates the release of cortisol, epinephrine (adrenaline), and norepinephrine, regulating the body's fight, flight, or freeze response. This physiological reaction often leads to increased heart rate, shallow breathing, and fatigue, making the body susceptible to illness and disease, particularly with repeated exposure over time. Consequently, individuals exposed to racial trauma consistently have elevated levels of stress hormones like cortisol, which are associated with gastrointestinal issues, hypertension, diabetes, heart disease, stroke, and a weakened immune response (Smith et al., 2022).

Similarly, the brain's response to stress disrupts neurotransmitters, neural connections, and communication pathways, akin to the negative effects of prolonged stress on the body (Smith et al., 2022; Conrad, et al., 2017). Studies revealed that racial stressors can result in physical effects such as elevated blood pressure, increased susceptibility to heart disease, and heightened vulnerability to various adverse health consequences. These physical outcomes can exacerbate psychological and emotional distress (Carter, 2007). Symptoms of racial trauma can lead to severe anxiety, nightmares, avoidance behaviors, embarrassment, dysphoria, isolation, and changes in mood and cognition. Due to its cumulative nature, it does not meet standard definitions as defined by the DSM-5 for PTSD and can result in comorbid disorders such as major depressive disorder, substance abuse, social anxiety, and psychosis. The DSM-5 does not include racial trauma within the context or criteria for PTSD, and cultural implications as an influence in psychopathology are also excluded (APA, 2022; Michaels et al., 2018; Carter, 2007). Many mental health professionals are not well-trained to recognize or treat race-based trauma, and racial inequity is often linked to PTSD. Trauma manifests diverse influences on the cortical structure of the brain, impeding one's capacity to feel emotions, maintain clear thinking, and establish connections with others. Importantly, numerous individuals diagnosed with trauma-related disorders express reduced pleasure, detachment from their surroundings, as well as symptoms of depression and challenges in cognitive functions like planning, thinking, and memory (Carter, 2007).

Racial trauma affects Black Americans (63%), Latin Americans (47%), Asian Americans (6%), American Indians/Alaska Natives (5%), and multiracial individuals (4%) (Williams et al., 2021). However, other studies suggest low reported rates among Asian Americans may be driven by a combination of underdiagnosis, cultural stigma, lack of service use, and unmet needs (Jang et al., 2019; Iwamasa, n.d.) and may be indicative of social desirability bias among Asian American cohorts. Michaels et al. (2018) suggest that Asian Americans and Black Americans have similar rates of obsessive-compulsive disorder (OCD), and the lifetime occurrence of severe depressive episodes is also comparable between the two groups.

Michaels et al. (2018) suggest that renewed study into psychedelic-assisted therapy and the second wave of research renaissance (2000-present) has shown the effectiveness of psilocybin, LSD, ayahuasca, and MDMA in treating depression, addiction, OCD, anxiety, and trauma symptoms. Mostly White samples limit the generalizability of findings or exclude BIPOC entirely, which conflicts with U.S. laws requiring varied clinical trial samples. To guarantee sufficient representation of ethnic and racial minorities in research conducted in the United States, Congress enacted the NIH Revitalization Act of 1993. This legislation requires that minorities and women are included in proportional numbers in all studies conducted or funded by the NIH.

BIPOC experience similar or greater levels of psychological distress than Whites, yet disparities in diagnosis and treatment can lead to poorer long-term outcomes (Williams et al., 2018; Michaels et al., 2018). For many disorders, including PTSD, substance abuse, generalized anxiety disorder (GAD), and major depressive episodes, Black Americans have comparable or higher prevalence rates than other ethnic groups. Hispanic Americans tend to have similar rates of substance abuse but higher rates of GAD than any other ethnic group. For example, 8.03% of Black Americans have PTSD in their lifetime, which is higher than the percentages of Hispanic/Latino Americans (5.59%), Asian Americans (1.84%), or Non-Hispanic Whites (6.45%). Asian Americans typically report lower lifetime prevalence rates for most disorders (Williams et al., 2018; Michaels et al., 2018). Further research and treatment paradigms must consider BIPOC populations in all research stages to better understand the efficacy of treatment and improve the chances of success (Williams et al., 2018). While the prevalence of mental illness in BIPOC populations is likely underestimated due to differences in age, socio-economic status, and how people were selected for studies, data shows that BIPOC experience psychological distress at equal or higher rates than Whites (Williams et al., 2018; Michaels et al., 2018). Discrepancies in accurate diagnosis among Black Americans make treatment access difficult. While the lifetime occurrence of major depressive episodes is also similar between Black and White Americans, fewer Black Americans stay in treatment (Michaels et al., 2018).

Psychedelics as Treatment for Race-based Trauma Findings

Classic psychedelics bind to serotonin receptors, particularly 5-HT2A, inducing altered states of consciousness and profound shifts in mood, cognition, and perception. Studies on the potential psychedelics have in treating PTSD show a reduction in anxiety, depression, and avoidance behaviors, common in those experiencing racial trauma. Psilocybin, for example, enhances psychological flexibility, emotional processing, and fosters connection, counteracting feelings of disconnection from discrimination (Williams et al., 2021; Ching et al., 2022; Davis et al., 2021). Different dosages may target various aspects of racial trauma—high doses may induce mystical experiences and feelings of unity deepening connections and reducing shame; lower doses may bolster trust between patient and therapist and enhance emotional processing.

Psychological flexibility involves being present, open to experiences, and acting on values-directed behavior. Psychedelics may strengthen psychological flexibility and can be a useful tool in coping with racism. Individuals can better manage distressing emotions, thoughts, and sensations that arise from discrimination. They are less likely to avoid or suppress these experiences, which can exacerbate mental health symptoms and internalized racism. Instead, individuals are more likely to engage in activities that promote well-being and connectedness, such as social support, self-care, and advocacy. Psychological flexibility can also help individuals maintain their sense of identity and values, which are often threatened by racism and discrimination. By remaining connected to their values and beliefs, individuals can counteract the negative messaging often associated with racism.

Williams et al. (2021) conducted a cross-sectional study of BIPOC participants aged 18 or older (U.S. and Canada). The study examined the effects of classic psychedelic use on mental health symptoms resulting from racial trauma. Participants reported past experiences of racial trauma and psychedelic use, memorable psychedelic experiences, and immediate and lasting effects. Participants reported a lasting decrease in depression, anxiety, and traumatic stress symptoms after using psychedelics. Notably, 58% of participants reported an experience occurring at least 3 years ago, indicating lasting effects; 75% of participants reported using a moderate to moderately high dose, and 19% reported a high dose. Psilocybin was the most commonly used among participants, accounting for 37%. This suggests that psychedelics may effectively treat racial trauma and mental health disorders in BIPOC, which can be exacerbated by discrimination and racism and not speaking up about it. Many BIPOC do not take action, and around 50% have never resorted to extreme measures (lawsuits, leaving a job, or relocating) to address racism (Williams et al., 2021). The study also found that systemic disparities make it harder to find solutions for race-based PTSD.

Williams and colleagues (2021) found that acute psychedelic effects, particularly acute insight, and challenging experiences had positive effects on trauma symptoms. Davis et al. (2021) support these findings, suggesting that psychedelics cause brain connectivity changes and induce awe and ego dissolution, leading to therapeutic success. Acute psychedelic effects are effective in reducing racial trauma symptoms and are a major element of psychedelics as a treatment for racial trauma.

Younger Asians (18-40 years old) commonly engage in recreational psychedelic use, specific to coping with racial discrimination. Asians were overrepresented in a trial of

MDMA-assisted psychotherapy for PTSD. Further research is needed to understand how psychedelics can help alleviate the symptoms of racial trauma among Asians who are using psychedelics (Ching et al., 2022).

Psychedelics produced a notable decrease in racial trauma symptoms (such as hyperarousal, feeling alienated/isolated, and worries about potential racial negative events) and psychological distress at moderate doses. The study found that greater acute mystical and insightful experiences (unity/oneness, sacredness, and ineffability) and lowered challenging experiences (extreme fear, feelings of loss of control or sanity, and physical discomfort) were associated with greater declines in symptoms. However, the study's findings were not separated by ethnicity or race, and there is a need for more research to investigate the effects of psychedelic use on the aftereffects of racial discrimination. Empirical data on the effects of psychedelics on ethnic identity is lacking, despite evidence suggesting that stronger ethnic identity may lead to improvements in racial trauma symptoms. Strengthening ethnic identity may protect against the negative effects of ongoing discrimination, according to the rejection-identification model (Ching et al., 2022). The rejection-identification model (RIM) suggests that the adverse effects of stigma, like reduced self-esteem, could be lessened if individuals from the stigmatized group opt to identify more with each other rather than with the dominant culture (Bogart et al., 2018).

Ching and colleagues (2022) found that 40.2% indicated psilocybin as their most meaningful psychedelic experience in Asian American cohorts; 78% reported moderate to moderately high doses. The study examined whether ethnic identity was mediated by psychedelics, which had not been previously tested. In Asian participants, racial trauma symptoms decreased after their most meaningful psychedelic experience. This finding is the first of its kind to show the potential benefits of psychedelics to reduce racial trauma symptoms among Asian Americans. Additionally, a correlation was found between dose and intense personally and spiritually significant experiences. Analyses revealed that improvements in symptoms mediate the connection between insightful experiences and ethnic identity, suggesting the potential for psychedelics to heal racial trauma among Asians.

Jones and Nock (2022) discovered that lifetime psilocybin use is linked to decreased odds of experiencing psychological distress for Hispanic and Asian participants but not for Black, Indigenous, and multiracial participants. The study investigated whether race and ethnicity affected the relationship between lifetime psilocybin use and psychological distress and suicidality, and significant interactions were discovered across all relevant outcomes. Relationships between psilocybin use, distress, and suicidality differed significantly among different identity groups, with White participants experiencing the most beneficial effects.

Davis et al. (2021) found that mystical effects or higher doses were not significantly linked to changes in racial trauma symptoms. Greater acute insight effects and lower challenging effects were directly related to changes in psychological flexibility. A direct relationship between psychological flexibility and changes in racial trauma symptoms suggests potential as a contributor to positive mental health outcomes. These findings support psychological flexibility as a target for treating race-based trauma.

From a biological and physiological standpoint, humans are identical, regardless of race. However, our individual experiences shape the trauma we endure. In the United

States, race significantly impacts the experiences of BIPOC, resulting in trauma that can be particularly challenging, harrowing, and potentially life-threatening. Generalizing findings across the entire population from psychedelic research is crucial for uncovering effective treatments for mental illness. However, without fully understanding how racism and trauma manifest into PTSD and other psychopathology in the bodies and minds of BIPOC, the therapeutic potential of psychedelics remains unknown.

While studies continue to support positive outcomes in psychedelic-assisted therapy for the treatment of race-based trauma, the bigger issue is one of awareness. My goal is to continue to encourage open dialogue and raise awareness of the lack of diversity and inclusion in psychedelics research. BIPOC are already using psychedelics as a tool to find healing from racial trauma on their own (Williams et al., 2021; Ching et al., 2022). How might outcomes improve with the guidance and intervention of a mental-health professional? More research is needed to understand manifestation similarities and differences among various ethnicities and how treatments may vary. Communities of color are also likely unaware of the potential psychedelics may have for healing. The development of culturally-sensitive treatment modalities and holding space for open and safe discussions are also needed.

References

American Psychiatric Association. (2022). *Diagnostic and statistical manual of mental disorders* (5th ed., text revision).

Bannister, J., Colvonen, P., Angkaw, A., & Norman, S. (2019). Differential relationships of guilt and shame on posttraumatic stress disorder among veterans. *Psychological Trauma, 11*(1), 35-42. doi:10.1037/tra0000392

Carter, R. T. (2007). Racism and psychological and emotional injury: Recognizing and assessing race-based traumatic stress. *The Counseling Psychologist, 35*(1), 13-105.

Ching, T. H., Davis, A. K., Xin, Y., & Williams, M. T. (2022). Effects of psychedelic use on racial trauma symptoms and ethnic identity among Asians in North America. *Journal of Psychoactive Drugs, 55*(1), 19-29. https://www.tandfonline.com/doi/abs/10.1080/02791072.2022.2025960

Conrad, C. D., Ortiz, J. B., & Judd, J. M. (2017). Chronic stress and hippocampal dendritic complexity: Methodological and functional considerations. *Physiology & behavior, 178,* 66-81.

Davis, A. K., Xin, Y., Sepeda, N. D., Garcia-Romeu, A., & Williams, M. T. (2021). Increases in psychological flexibility mediate relationship between acute psychedelic effects and decreases in racial trauma symptoms among people of color. *Chronic Stress, 5,* 24705470211035607. https://journals.sagepub.com/doi/full/10.1177/24705470211035607

George, J. R., Michaels, T. I., Sevelius, J., & Williams, M. T. (2020). The psychedelic renaissance and the limitations of a white-dominant medical framework: A call for indigenous and ethnic minority inclusion. *Journal of Psychedelic Studies, 4*(1), 4-15.

Iwamasa, G.Y., (n.d.) *Recommendations for the treatment of Asian American Pacific Islander populations.* American Psychology Association. https://www.apa.org/pi/oema/resources/ethnicity-health/asian-american/psychological-treatment

Jang, Y., Yoon, H., Park, N. S., Rhee, M. K., & Chiriboga, D. A. (2019). Mental health service use and perceived unmet needs for mental health care in Asian Americans. *Community Mental Health Journal, 55,* 241-248.

Jones, G. M., & Nock, M. K. (2022). Race and ethnicity moderate the associations between lifetime psychedelic use (MDMA and psilocybin) and psychological distress and suicidality. *Scientific Reports, 12*(1), 16976.

Michaels, T. I., Purdon, J., Collins, A., & Williams, M. T. (2018). Inclusion of people of color in psychedelic-assisted psychotherapy: A review of the literature. *BMC psychiatry, 18*(1), 1-14.

Ruiz, N., Tian, Z., & Klein, H. (2023). *Discrimination experiences shape most Asian Americans' lives.* Pew Research Center. https://www.pewresearch.org/wp-content/uploads/sites/20/2023/11/

RE_2023.11.30_Asian-American-Discrimination_Report.pdf

Smith, D. T., Faber, S. C., Buchanan, N. T., Foster, D., & Green, L. (2022). The need for psychedelic-assisted therapy in the black community and the burdens of its provision. *Frontiers in Psychiatry, 12,* 774736.

Williams, M. T., Printz, D., Ching, T., & Wetterneck, C. T. (2018). Assessing PTSD in ethnic and racial minorities: Trauma and racial trauma. *Directions in Psychiatry, 38*(3), 179-196.

Williams, M. T. (2020). Microaggressions: Clarification, evidence, and impact. *Perspectives on Psychological Science, 15*(1), 3-26. https://doi.org/10.1177/1745691619827499

Williams, M. T., & Labate, B. C. (2020). Diversity, equity, and access in psychedelic medicine. *Journal of Psychedelic Studies, 4*(1), 1-3.

Williams, M. T., Davis, A. K., Xin, Y., Sepeda, N. D., Grigas, P. C., Sinnott, S., & Haeny, A. M. (2021). People of color in North America report improvements in racial trauma and mental health symptoms following psychedelic experiences. *Drugs: Education, Prevention and Policy, 28*(3), 215-226.

Psilocybin can help us break down the barriers between ourselves and others and foster a sense of empathy and compassion.

—Katherine MacLean

Shaina Fawn

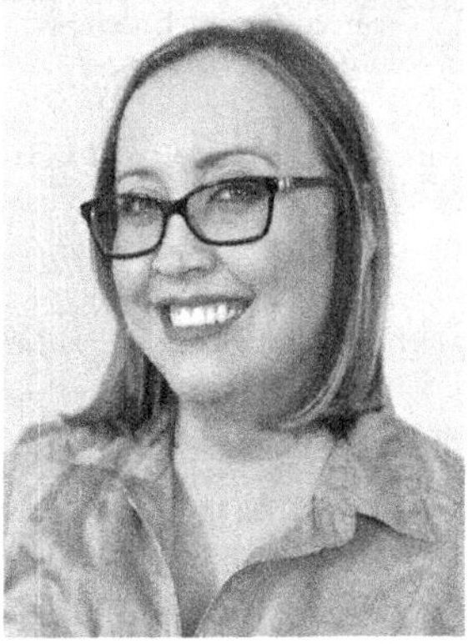

Shaina Fawn is a licensed clinical social worker and PhD candidate. She is trained to provide psychedelic-assisted therapy (PAT) services under Oregon's Measure 109. She was born and raised in New Mexico, adjacent to Mexican and Pueblo Native communities. Her young life experiences inspired her to pursue a career in social work. She has 20+ years of experience supporting individuals and communities and views decolonial practice as essential to her work.
shaina@therapeuticbridges.com

Decolonial Praxis During the Third "Psychedelic Renaissance"

The story of the therapeutic use of psychedelics in the United States is one filled with cultural appropriation and attempts to exert power and control over Black and Indigenous people of color (BIPOC) populations. Long before modern psychotherapy, Indigenous communities used hallucinogenic agents to promote healing and to assist in religious ceremonies. An article published by *National Geographic* last year reported that archeologists recently tested remains of human hair found at burial sites in a cave in Menorca, Spain, and confirmed the use of psychedelics by these pre-historic Europeans nearly 3,000 years ago as part of shamanic rituals. Archeologists have further confirmed that ancient hallucinogenic drug use has been found on almost every continent, with the oldest direct evidence being from Asia, roughly 4,600 years ago (Metcalfe, 2023; Gonzales, 2023). Psychedelics were also an essential component of Mayan and Incan civilizations in that they were used for political, social, and economic purposes (Labate & Rodrigues, 2023). When European colonizers arrived in Latin America, however, they deliberately attempted to control and eliminate the use of psychedelics by Indigenous communities, as they considered the practices to be barbaric (Gonzales, 2023).

In a time known to many as the third "psychedelic renaissance," [1] we now see modern medicine taking an increased interest in the healing potential of psychedelic agents, spurring a rapidly rising interest in psychedelic-as-

1 Author's note: It is important to acknowledge that the term "psychedelic renaissance" can be considered problematic, given that Indigenous communities have been using psychedelics as a healing practice for thousands of years, and it is only revolutionary because it is making its way into the mainstream. The term is used in this piece as a colloquialism and to provide historical context.

sisted therapy (PAT). Ballot Measure 109 passed in Oregon in November of 2020, allowing the Oregon Health Authority to now regulate the manufacturing, sale, and use of psilocybin as a therapeutic intervention. PAT facilitators are now being trained, and a plan for the rollout is underway (Oregon Ballot Measure 109, 2020; Gonzales, 2023). In 2022, Colorado also passed a measure decriminalizing the possession of psilocybin, further paving the way for the expansion of PAT (Colorado Proposition 122, 2022; Gonzales, 2023). Psilocybin currently has over 138 Food and Drug Administration (FDA) clinical trials showing statistically significant results for treating post-traumatic stress disorder, major depressive disorder, alcohol use disorder, and end-of-life anxiety for terminally ill cancer patients (Gonzales, 2023).

In addition to its potential therapeutic benefits, the psychedelic drug market presents a significant economic opportunity. Presently, psychedelic drugs generate a global revenue of $3.8 million and are on track to make upwards of $11.2 million by 2029. While PAT has incredible potential to help reframe the healing process for individuals and communities, the unfortunate reality is that the same system providing therapeutic services is built on colonial and capitalistic ideals. This means the majority of the financial gain in this budding industry will likely not serve nor uplift the very communities from which these practices came unless intentional, decolonial methods are taken. A literature search on the topic generates a mountain of articles containing a common cautionary tale: Sacred psychedelic plant medicines are in danger of extinction or exploitation during the present wave of the psychedelic renaissance.

At the same time, PAT has the potential to bring powerful healing to a world in considerable need. The COVID-19 pandemic has created a mental health crisis unlike any we have ever seen. Coupled with the uncertainty created by global warming, geopolitical turmoil, and the social reckoning of systemic and racial oppression, it is clear that our collective mental health is suffering. By carefully utilizing decolonial practices to ensure that BIPOC populations are protected from further exploitation, we can also begin to amplify their voices as an essential source of knowledge from which these powerful healing practices are rooted.

Three Waves of the Psychedelic Interest and Resurgence

According to some scholars, the first wave of the psychedelic renaissance occurred in 1938 when chemist Albert Hoffman accidentally created lysergic acid diethylamide (LSD) in his lab, sparking an interest in psychiatry and psychotherapy of the time about its ability to mimic mental illness to be better able to research and treat symptoms (Lowe et al., 2021). The second wave occurred in 1957 when the same chemist received a sample of dried mushrooms containing psilocybin from a shaman in Oaxaca, Mexico, furthering the interest in the potential benefits of utilizing the substances to support the development of new mental health treatments. This second wave continued into the 1970s; however, it ended promptly with the passage of the Controlled Substances Act in 1971, with the formation of the Drug Enforcement Agency (DEA) occurring 2 years later in 1973.

The third wave did not pick up again until 2004 when researchers in clinical trials at the University of California in Los Angeles began exploring the use of psilocybin to treat pain and anxiety in end-stage, terminally ill cancer patients. Since then, PAT has gained strong popularity as a potential mechanism for healing. However, psychedelic agents such as psilocybin and LSD continue to be listed as Schedule One substances, along with substances such as heroin and crack cocaine. Nonetheless, the interest in psychedelic research for neuroscience and therapeutic purposes is greater now than at any other time in history (Doblin, 2019).

The War on Drugs: A Brief Historical Overview

Scholars interested in decolonization and history have extensively researched the War on Drugs (WoD) as it relates to our current society, stratification, oppressive policies, and prison industrial complex. The term *War on Drugs* reflects the policy action taken by the Nixon Administration during the 1970s with the passage of the Controlled Substances Act in 1970. A top Nixon aid was interviewed about policies implemented during this period and stated the following:

> The Nixon campaign in 1968, and the Nixon White House after that, had two enemies: the antiwar left and black people....We knew we couldn't make it illegal to be either against the war or black, but by getting the public to associate the hippies with marijuana and blacks with heroin, and then criminalizing both heavily, we could disrupt those communities. We could arrest their leaders, raid their homes, break up their meetings, and vilify them night after night on the evening news. Did we know we were lying about the drugs? Of course, we did (Lockie, 2019).

It was also during this time that the United States began exerting control over countries in Latin America in an attempt to quell any socialist revolution attempts. A direct link exists between the suppression of these revolutions and the attempt to exert control over the growth, sales, and distribution of substances targeted by the WoD and the Controlled Substances Act of 1970. Cruz (2017) explores the complexities of U.S. foreign policy at the time and states, "researchers have argued that the policies of the WoD in Latin America are a renewed expression of American neo-colonialism" (p 638). Cruz also explains that the WoD helped position the United States as a key figure in the creation of a global drug prohibition movement. Governments in countries where drugs were grown, including Colombia, Peru, and Bolivia, also worked in tandem with the United States to create policies that attempted to address the impact that the drug market was having on their own soils. The WoD had devastating effects on Latin America that reverberate well into our present day. Presently, for example, the country of Honduras is experiencing high rates of violence and political instability due to the failure of the WoD and the country occupying one of the main drug trafficking routes between Latin America and the United States.

The WoD has also devastated communities of color within the United States. Research has consistently shown that people of color are 4 to 5 times more likely to be arrested and convicted of drug-related charges than their White counterparts (POCPC, 2023). The incarceration of people due to drug-related charges tears apart communities and families, creating a painful lineage of generational trauma. This generational trauma often manifests as social determinants of health. For example, according to the Adverse Childhood Experiences survey, the incarceration of a parent is considered one of the 10 adverse life experiences known to be linked to diminished health outcomes later in life (Gjelsvik et al., 2014).

Psychedelic Tourism

The colonial mindset is dangerous when it comes to the potential for exploitation of BIPOC communities with the rising interest in psychedelics. As such, "psychedelic tourism" is a phenomenon that requires careful scrutiny. The story of the Mexican curandera Maria Sabina highlights the devastating and heartbreaking effects of psychedelic tourism in Oaxaca, Mexico, that sparked the second wave of the psychedelic renaissance. Maria Sabina was a local healer who used sacred mushrooms to heal her community members during shamanic rituals and ceremonies. In 1955, author and banking executive Gordon Wasson became the first White foreigner to enter the small Mazatecan community where Sabina lived. She graciously introduced Wasson to her healing mushrooms. Wasson sent samples to Swiss chemist Albert Hoffman, who began scientifically studying the substance's use in psychiatry at the time. In 1957, Wasson published a wildly popular article in *Time Magazine* called "Seeking the Magic Mushroom." The article also spurred a lot of interest in these healing mushrooms in the cultural consciousness of the United States and the counterculture of the time. A relentless wave of White psychedelic tourism ensued in Sabina's community. This put enormous pressure on the social fabric of her community. After the Mexican government started surveilling the town, her fellow community members turned on her, burning her house to the ground and murdering her son. Sabina, a woman once revered as a community healer, died poor and alone (Gonzalez Romero, 2021). Sabina's story persists in the psychedelic community as a cautionary tale of what can occur when issues related to privilege, economic interest, and capitalism are left unchecked.

During the third wave of the psychedelic renaissance, we see psychedelic tourism persisting, with the potential for a similarly devastating impact. Dr. Andrea Pennington (2022) explores the challenges of using an Indigenous healing method without properly acknowledging or honoring its history or the harm committed. She openly discusses the dangers of psychedelic tourism. She argues that it is a social justice issue that exploits Indigenous communities and harms people and the environment, with one of the most prominent examples being ayahuasca tourism in South America, which is contributing to the destruction of the Amazon rainforest and has the ability to cause the potential extinction of tribal communities residing there (Pennington, 2022; Gonzales, 2023).

Re-classification and Decriminalization

One of the most enduring and harmful components to come out of the Controlled Substances Act and the WoD is drug scheduling. Under current drug scheduling criteria, psilocybin and mescaline are classified as Schedule One drugs, the highest of all of the scheduling. Other drugs in this category include heroin and crack cocaine. Drug scheduling was initially developed on the assumption that Schedule One drugs had the highest health risk, the highest risk for abuse and dependence, and no medicinal value. However, FDA clinical trials are now proving that, based on this categorization, many substances are grossly misclassified. For example, studies have consistently proven that psilocybin has one of the highest safety profiles of all classified substances and is proven to be non-addictive, as it does not work on the dopamine neurotransmitter receptor in the same way that other substances do. In fact, psilocybin is even showing promise in

FDA clinical trials for the treatment of addiction, specifically for alcohol use disorder and tobacco use disorder. Furthermore, psilocybin and other drugs such as ketamine, a Schedule Three substance, and 3,4-methylenedioxymethamphetamine (MDMA), another Schedule One substance, are showing statistically solid significance in clinical trials for the treatment of major depressive disorder, post-traumatic stress disorder, and end-of-life anxiety associated with terminal illness.

Drug reclassification is something that has already been underway with regard to marijuana. Marijuana is now legal in 38 states and the District of Colombia, and the DEA recently announced that it would be reclassifying marijuana from a Schedule One to a Schedule Three drug. While this is promising in terms of paving the way for other drug reclassification, it is important to highlight that prisons continue to be filled with individuals convicted of possessing and distributing marijuana (National Conference of State Legislatures, 2023). These imbalances and contradictions highlight how the colonial mindset continues to influence drug policy in the United States. As psychedelic substances are used more and more for therapeutic benefit, the PAT community has an ethical obligation to join criminal justice reform and reclassification efforts.

Social Justice, Representation, and Access to PAT Treatment

In addition to understanding the harm caused by the WoD, drug scheduling, and psychedelic tourism, it is essential to acknowledge the potential harm that can be done to Indigenous communities and other communities of color as it relates to ongoing research and PAT. As it stands, racial disparities are pervasive in psychedelic spaces involving research, academia, and treatment. For example, a literature review of 17 psychedelic studies between the years 2000-2017 found that 82.5% of study participants were of Caucasian descent and that recruitment of BIPOC participants was extremely low (George et al., 2020, p. 9). From a sampling perspective, this is problematic as the results of these studies can only be generalizable to White populations. Further research is needed to understand the efficacy of psychedelics for BIPOC communities. Furthermore, the current medical model that dominates much of the psychedelic space is led by White, cisgender male doctors and researchers. George et al. (2020) argue that this "Western medical hierarchy" privileges medical doctors while largely ignoring the voices of Indigenous healers who have valuable cultural and historical expertise (p. 10).

Culturally Responsive PAT Practice

Another area of advocacy with regard to PAT concerns the ethics of treating vulnerable communities and people of color, as these communities tend to experience high rates of trauma and marginalization and have been the most affected by racist and classist drug enforcement policies. PAT practitioners must ensure that BIPOC and indigenous individuals have a strong safety net of support when undergoing psychedelic experiences (Pennington, 2022). An example of this would be to ensure proper evaluation of an individual's social support prior to undergoing a psychedelic experience and ensure that a proper plan for connecting with support (family, friends, community groups, affirming therapists, etc.) exists during the integration phase of treatment. Additionally, cost and access must be considered when working with marginalized communities that may not have access to monetary resources. Lastly, practitioners must be mindful of the ways in which systems, particularly the medical system, have harmed BIPOC and Indigenous people and be prepared to assess for and address any traumatic triggers that may be present. This is particularly concerning regarding Indigenous communities, who may be unable to access the medicine their ancestors used for healing (Pennington, 2022; Gonzales, 2023).

The People of Color Psychedelic Collective (POCPC) is a non-profit founded in 2017 to help advocate for people of color within both the context of treatment and the context of psychedelic policy reform efforts. POCPC's mission statement reads:

> The POCPC brings psychedelic education to people of color. Our organization creates spaces for people of color to learn about the harms of the war on drugs and the healing properties of psychedelics. We are committed to helping build a healing infrastructure that centers care, affordability, and accessibility for communities of color while reducing harm. We provide outreach, events, and educational content created by and for people of color to further our collective knowledge. We aim to build our table instead of asking for a seat at another. (POCPC, 2023)

The POCPC is a powerful example of decolonial praxis. It seeks to empower and elevate people of color, advocates for criminal justice reform, and is home to a coalition called The Psychedelic Alliance for Healing and Justice, by which they seek to engage in discussion around psychedelics that addresses social justice, research the needs of communities of color, shift practitioners' standards of care, develop "culturally attuned healing-based models," and promote education and skill building in the psychedelic community (POCPC, 2023). Furthermore, programs such as the Psychedelic Assistance Fund are attempting to increase access for affected communities by offering scholarships for PAT services for individuals who were formally incarcerated and who are struggling with post-traumatic stress disorder (Psychedelic Assistance Fund, 2023).

Ethical Principles of Decolonial Practice

Researchers Celidwen et al. (2023) explore decolonial praxis as it relates to psychedelics and Indigenous communities. They discuss concerns with regard to the budding multibillion-dollar psychedelic industry and the fact that Indigenous communities make up only 6% of the world's population but represent 30% of people living in extreme poverty (p.2). In exploring the harm and potential for ongoing harm to Indigenous communities, they have proposed eight ethical principles to guide practitioners and researchers who are engaged in the movement. They state, "Indigenous voices can be a powerful and beneficial solutions-orientated force for well-being derived from ancestral wisdom and insight from the heart of Mother Earth" (p. 8). These authors propose the following eight ethical guidelines: (1) reverence for mother nature, (2) respect for Indigenous ways of knowing and being, (3) responsible use, (4) relevance of Indigenous knowledge, (5) regulation of traditional Indigenous use, (6) restoration of Indigenous authority, (7) reparation of sharing of benefits, and (8) reconciliation of Indigenous-Western relations. Non-Indigenous researchers and practitioners who are committed to ethical and decolonial practices should be careful to implement these guiding principles in their practices.

Actionable Steps to Implement Decolonial Practice Immediately

Decolonial practices are concepts that are not new for BIPOC communities; however, more often than not, they are new concepts for individuals belonging to privileged social locations such as those with cisgender, heterosexual, and Caucasian identities. Unfortunately, most individuals involved in PAT are not intentionally examining their role in decolonial practice. In fact, many of the PAT programs that currently exist in the United States devote little time to this type of dialogue and exploration. Given the delicate history of the WoD, drug scheduling, and the history of exploitation of psychedelics, it is incumbent upon researchers and practitioners interested in the healing power of psychedelics to dedicate themselves to decolonial practices that uplift Indigenous knowledge and acknowledge the harm that has been caused to marginalized communities. Actionable ways to do this include: (1) writing a decolonial and equity statement and plan prior to providing PAT services and publishing it on websites and other literature, (2) creating a system of providing sliding scale rates for BIPOC clients, (3) educating themselves on the ways in which the WoD has harmed marginalized communities and the impact this has on our present society, (4) joining advocacy efforts that call for the reclassification or delisting of psychedelics like psilocybin, (5) becoming knowledgeable about Indigenous healing practices using psychedelic substances and be able to uplift these voices when appropriate. Additionally, privileged PAT practitioners must be committed to (6) holding other non-BIPOC clinicians accountable to these standards of practice, especially when they occupy spaces where there is potential for further harm and exploitation to be committed.

References

Colorado Proposition 122. (2022). *Colorado proposition 122: Decriminalization and regulated access program for certain psychedelic plants and fungi initiative.* Ballotpedia. (n.d.). Retrieved April 9, 2023, from https://ballotpedia.org/Colorado_Proposition_122,_Decriminalization_and_Regulated_Access_Program_for_Certain_Psychedelic_Plants_and_Fungi_Initiative_(2022)

Celidwen, Y., Redvers, N., Githaiga, C., Calambás, J., Añaños, K., Chindoy, M. E., ... & Sacbajá, A. (2023). Ethical principles of traditional Indigenous medicine to guide western psychedelic research and practice. *The Lancet Regional Health-Americas, 18*, 100410.

Cruz, G. M. (2017). A view from the South: The global creation of the war on drugs. *Contexto Internacional, 39*(3), 633–653. https://doi.org/10.1590/S0102-8529.2017390300009

Doblin, R., Merete Christiansen, L. & Burge, B. (2019). The past and future of psychedelic science: An introduction to this issue. *Journal of Psychoactive Drugs, 51*(2), 93-97, DOI: 10.1080/02791072.2019.1606472

George, J. R., Michaels, T. I., Sevelius, J., & Williams, M. T. (2020). The psychedelic renaissance and the limitations of a White-dominant medical framework: A call for Indigenous and ethnic minority inclusion. *Journal of Psychedelic Studies, 4*(1), 4-15.

González Romero, O. S. (2021, May 27). María Sabina, mushrooms, and colonial extractivism. *Chacruna*. Retrieved April 7, 2023, from https://chacruna.net/maria-sabina-mushrooms-and-colonial-extractivism/

Gonzales, S. F. (2023). *Psychedelic assisted therapy: An innovative approach to the treatment of addiction* [Unpublished Paper]. Integrative Social Work Department, Saybrook University.

Gjelsvik, A., Dumont, D. M., Nunn, A., & Rosen, D. L. (2014). Adverse childhood events: Incarceration of household members and health-related quality of life in adulthood. *Journal of health care for the poor and underserved, 25*(3), 1169–1182. https://doi.org/10.1353/hpu.2014.0112

Labate, B. C., & Rodrigues, T. (2023). The impacts of the drug war on Indigenous peoples in Latin America: An overview. *Journal of Psychedelic Studies* (published online ahead of print 2023). doi:

https://doi.org/10.1556/2054.2023.00239

Lockie, A. (2019, July 31). Top Nixon adviser reveals the racist reason he started the "War on Drugs" decades ago. *Business Insider.* https://www.businessinsider.com/nixon-adviser-ehrlichman-anti-left-anti-black-war-on-drugs-2019-7

Lowe, H., Toyang, N., Steele, B., Valentine, H., Grant, J., Ali, A., Ngwa, W., & Gordon, L. (2021, May 15). The therapeutic potential of psilocybin. *Molecules, 26*(10), 2948. doi: 10.3390/molecules26102948. PMID: 34063505; PMCID: PMC8156539.

Metcalfe, T. (2023, April 6). European 'shamans' took psychedelic drugs 3,000 years ago. *National Geographic.*

National Conference of State Legislatures. (2023, April 17). Report: State Medical Cannabis Laws. https://www.ncsl.org/health/state-medical-cannabis-laws

Oregon Ballot Measure 109. (2020). *Oregon measure 109, psilocybin mushroom services program initiative.* Ballotpedia. (n.d.). Retrieved April 9, 2023, from https://ballotpedia.org/Oregon_Measure_109,_Psilocybin_Mushroom_Services_Program_Initiative_(2020)

Pennington, A. (2022). When trauma resurfaces: How shadow experiences can be transformed by psychedelic-assisted therapy without re-traumatization. *Psychedelic Assisted Therapy Global Summit.*

People of Color Psychedelic Collective. (n.d.). [Website]. https://www.pocpc.org/aboutpocpc. Accessed 30, May 2023.

Psychedelic Access Fund. (n.d.). Psychedelic therapy access nonprofit: New York, NY. [Website.]. https://www.psychedelicaccess.fund/

A radical inner transformation and rise to a new level of consciousness might be the only real hope we have in the current global crisis brought on by the dominance of the Western mechanistic paradigm.

—Stan Grof

Adriana Kertzer

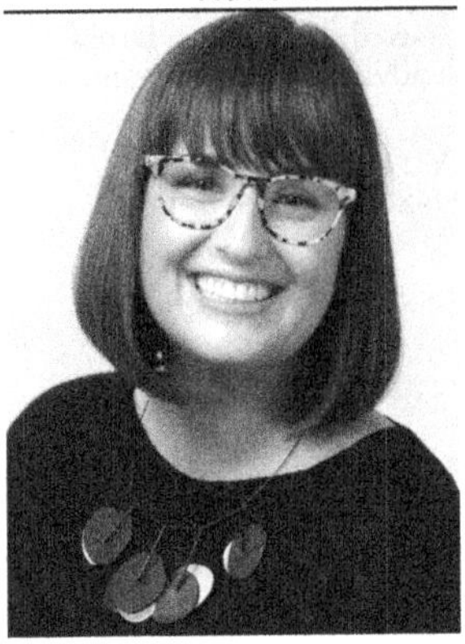

ADRIANA KERTZER is a NY-based Brazilian-Texan Jewish activist, psychedelic lawyer, and cultural producer. She is co-founder of Plant Medicine Law Group, a law firm specialized in psychedelic infrastructure, and the Jewish Healing Society, an organization committed to fostering a supportive environment for Jews in psychedelic medicine and science, born out of her Instagram account, JewWhoTokes. JWT began as a collection of profiles on Jewish individuals involved in the psychedelic and cannabis industries. After the October 7 attacks, it became a community for Jews confronting antisemitism in these industries or needing community. Adriana sits on the board of advisors of the Shine Collective, a nonprofit dedicated to addressing abuse in the psychedelic industry.

Psychedelic Community Mobilization in the Wake of the October 7th Attacks in Israel

IN AN UNPRECEDENTED GROUND INVASION THAT BEGAN ON THE MORNING OF OCTOBER 7, 2023, during the Jewish holiday of Simchat Torah, Hamas terrorists entered Israel and murdered over 1,200 civilians, kidnapping 240 more to Gaza. This massacre—and the glee with which Hamas committed and publicized the murder, torture, and rape of civilians including women, children, and the elderly—is unprecedented in modern-day warfare. It also represents the single deadliest day for Jews in modern history since the Holocaust. At the time of this writing, 120 civilians remain in captivity (Reuters, 2024). By the end of 2023, Hamas had fired at least 12,000 rockets into Israel, as the Israeli Defense Forces (IDF) continued their counter-offensive in Gaza aimed at eliminating Hamas leaders, members, weapons, and infrastructure (Gavrielov, 2023).

The massacre that unfolded was a devastating intrusion on the euphoria synonymous with rave culture. Terrorists killed, raped, tortured, injured, and traumatized rave attendees at the Nova Festival in the south of Israel, where a significant majority of more than 3,000 attendees were under the influence of substances that distort perception, delay responses, and heighten emotional sensitivity.[1] This fact adds an important dimension to how we consider the needs of the survivors and the place this attack now holds in psychedelic history as the worst

1 There were actually three gatherings in the south of Israel where the attacks took place: Nova Festival (3,882 people attended, 364 murdered, 44 kidnapped (5 returned)), PsyDuck Rave (100 people attended, 17 murdered), and Midburn preparatory weekend (120 people attended, 1 murdered) (Tadmor, N., 2024), for purposes of this article referred to collectively as the Nova Festival, the largest of the attacks, which has received more news coverage.

"trip" known to history.[2]

Little news coverage has been dedicated to the fact that the massacre at the Supernova Sukkot Gathering (now more commonly known as the Nova Festival) was not only the largest terror attack in Israel's history, and the worst Israeli civilian massacre ever, it was also the largest psychedelics-related act of violence or massacre at a music festival in history (Gifford, 2023; Ghermezian, 2024).

The Nova Festival was an open-air psytrance music festival near kibbutz Re'im organized by the Tribe of Nova together with the Brazilian psytrance festival group Universo Paralello (Supernova, 2023).[3] It was scheduled to coincide with the final day of the Jewish holidays of Sukkot and Simchat Torah. The rave was billed as a celebration of "friends, love and infinite freedom" but as the sun rose on October 7th, amid the pulsing beats and vibrant atmosphere of the open-air rave, Hamas invaded (Morris et al., 2023). Sunrise was also the moment at which many rave participants had just begun to experience the full psychoactive effects of the psychedelic substances they had taken. At the same moment, Hamas

Pinchas Baumol

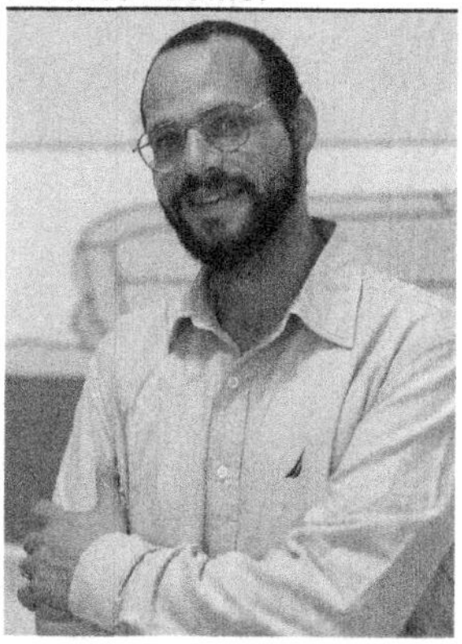

PINCHAS "PINNI" BAUMOL is an Israeli social worker dedicated to harm reduction, integration, access to psychedelic-assisted therapy, drug policy reform, and education. Pinni is currently launching the Shaarei Nefesh Resilience Center and has co-founded several initiatives, including the Access Center for Psychedelic Therapy (ACPT), Oxygen Harm Reduction Education, and the Keter Ketamine Clinic in Jerusalem. Pinni shares his extensive knowledge of the recreational, spiritual, and therapeutic use of psychedelics as a volunteer with the Israeli government's drug committee research team, a community leader in Medabrim Psychedelia (Israel's largest online psychedelic community), and through Anashim Tovim (Israel's leading safe space festival crew).

2 One question that exceeds the scope of this article but hopefully will be addressed in the near future is whether the way trauma was imprinted on the survivors was exacerbated by the use of these substances at the time of the attack. It is also worth exploring whether the rapid response to survivors' needs translated into a reduction of harm.

3 The Israeli rave scene (aka "nature parties," "psytrance," or "trance" subcultures) has evolved since its inception in the late 1980s into a dynamic cultural force, marked by distinctive values, rituals, and, notably, substance use patterns (including common use of hallucinogenic substances), attracting attention from researchers (Bonny-Noach, H. et al., 2023).

Madison Margolin

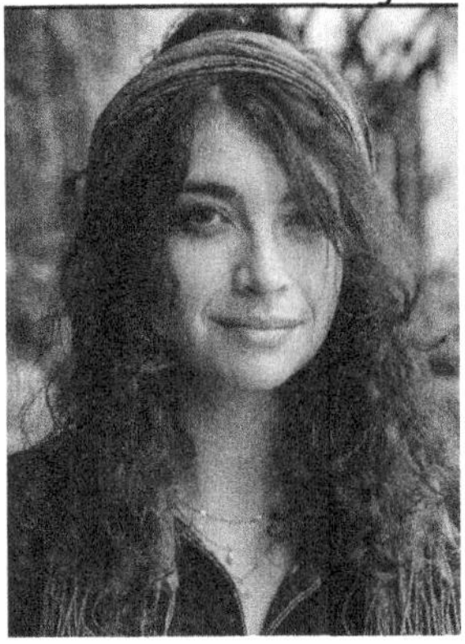

Madison Margolin is an author, journalist, and educator focused on covering the intersection of psychedelics and Judaism. She is the co-founder of psychedelic media startup and magazine *DoubleBlind*, as well as co-founder of the Jewish Psychedelic Summit. Currently a contributing editor to Ayin Press, as well as the host of the *Set & Setting* podcast on the Be Here Now Network, she has written for outlets like *Rolling Stone, Playboy, Vice, Tablet Magazine.* Her first book *Exile & Ecstasy: Growing Up with Ram Dass & Coming of Age in the Jewish Psychedelic Underground* was published by Hay House in November, 2023, and she has two more forthcoming. Originally from Los Angeles, she now splits her time between New York and Israel.

invaded the festival premises and began shooting at participants, chasing them down in the surrounding fields, raping them, kidnapping them, and killing them (Gettleman et al., 2023; Rubin, 2023; Tabachnick, 2023; Gillet et al., 2023). Festival goers were under the acute effects of drugs like 3,4-methylenedioxymethamphetamine (MDMA) and lysergic acid diethylamide (LSD) as they fled for their lives.

The attack on the Nova Festival resulted in 364 civilians killed, at least 40 hostages taken, and many more assaulted and injured (*The Times of Israel*, 2023). It also led to a significant number of festival goers arriving at the emergency room still under the influence of psychedelics, presenting medical teams with additional mental health needs. In the United States psychedelic community's only published account of the Nova massacre to date, author Mary-Elizabeth Gifford described the reaction of Dr. Roy Salomon who was among the first to be notified about the hundreds of patients who were arriving "tripping and distraught":

> "When I saw that request for two helpers I said, well there were over 3,000 kids at this festival, we don't just need two people to get over to an emergency room—we're going to need hundreds of people to help," said Salomon, who has received training by MAPS (Multidisciplinary Association for Psychedelic Studies) to provide MDMA-assisted psychotherapy during clinical trials. He said he reached out to the leaders of SafeZone and SafeShore, organizations that provide psychedelic harm reduction services. "I called two of my friends who are leaders of the harm reduction groups here who actually go to festivals." It was immediately clear that clinicians and mental health practitioners were needed, and that it was essential "they understand psychedelics and trauma." (Gifford, 2023)

It quickly became clear to those tending to survivors of the attack that care had to reflect the reality that participants had consumed psychedelics and that their trauma might be exacerbated as a result.

Hadas Alterman

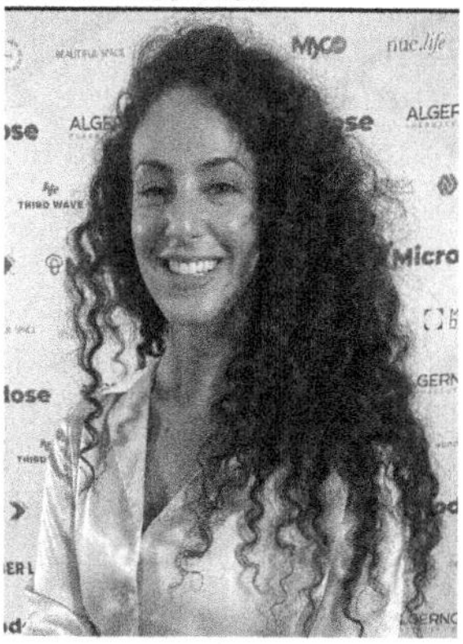

Hadas Alterman´ is an Israeli-American New York-based lawyer and activist. She is a real estate director at AIPAC. Prior to joining AIPAC, Hadas was the director of communications & policy for the American Psychedelic Practitioners Association and co-founder of Plant Medicine Law Group, a boutique law firm specialized in psychedelic infrastructure. She was a board member of the American Psychedelic Practitioners Association, founding board member of the Psychedelic Bar Association, member of the Equity Subcommittee of the Oregon Psilocybin Advisory Board, and policy director and co-founder of New Yorkers for Mental Health Alternatives, which successfully lobbied for the introduction of a New York bill to decriminalize psilocybin by statute.

This article offers an overview of therapeutic initiatives that have become beacons of hope in the aftermath of the Nova Festival tragedy. The projects summarized herein extend beyond conventional harm reduction—a term that refers to a range of intentional practices to lessen the negative consequences associated with drug use—and therapeutic practices. These projects encompass broader types of psychological aid, resource dissemination, opportunities for expressive integration, and physical places that foster a sense of solidarity. The rapid and sophisticated response to the needs of the Nova Festival victims was possible due to a confluence of factors which, when considered in combination, are unique to Israel. First, there is psychedelic-assisted therapy in Israel using ketamine, esketamine, and cannabis, and Israel has been one of the clinical trial sites for psilocybin and MDMA. This means that the country has a significant number of mental health professionals trained in psychedelic-assisted therapy. Second, the Israeli rave scene dates back to the 1980s and is now considered a mainstream aspect of the country's contemporary society. The psytrance "tribes" are community oriented and have developed a robust harm reduction infrastructure staffed by harm reductionists that have an understanding of substance use patterns among the psytrance community (Shapira et al., 2023).[4] Third, for the past decade, Israeli harm reduction

4 The Israeli psytrance culture, known for its outdoor rave events, has cultivated a unique fusion of music, spirituality, and community. A research study by Bonny-Noach et al. (2023), conducted through a cross-sectional online survey of 1,206 participants, highlighted the prevalence of illicit substances such as cannabis, LSD, MDMA, mushrooms/psilocybin, ketamine, and cocaine at Israeli nature rave parties. Contrary to global trends observed in studies from Australia and New York, Israeli rave attendees exhibited distinctive substance use patterns, notably the dominance of hallucinogenic substances, particularly LSD and mushrooms/psilocybin. This shift in perception and usage of psychedelics underscores the need for nuanced harm reduction strategies tailored to the specific substances prevalent in the Israeli context.

volunteers have paved the path in addressing issues of substance use, rave culture, and mental health, from the dance floor to the parliament and academic circles. Progressive attitudes towards harm reduction in the Israeli mental health community and a track record of advocacy meant there was expertise to draw on in a time of crisis.[5] Lastly, virtual communities that predated the October 7 attacks and technology allowed Israelis to rapidly mobilize in response to the rave attacks.

The October 7 attacks prompted an unprecedented mobilization of activations that range from harm reduction efforts providing crucial support, information, and safe spaces for survivors; community safe spaces and artistic projects, both physical and virtual, to facilitate healing, share resources, and commemorate the victims; and psychedelic-assisted therapy initiatives. While the terrorist attack on the Nova Festival cast a profound shadow over Israeli society and global Jewry, the activations described below were driven by a collective sense of resilience and may in the future inform how the larger psychedelic community discusses the risks of psychedelic use, the role of harm reduction, and psychedelic culture.

I. Harm Reduction Activations

To meet the immediate needs of the survivors of the Nova Festival attack, the Israeli psytrance community quickly began to mobilize resources.[6] Harm reduction volunteers from within the rave community became instrumental in providing support. The harm reduction community is guided by the principles of the global rave culture—peace, love, unity, and respect —and rallied to support survivors, hostages, and the families of victims. Volunteers embodying these values have played a pivotal role in the treatment of survivors, offering solace, creating memorials to honor the lives lost, offering resource dissemination, and fostering a sense of solidarity. The range of responses highlighted the resilience ingrained in the community, transcending the traditional boundaries of harm reduction.

Anashim Tovim

Among the notable groups responding to the October 7th tragedy was Anashim Tovim ("Good People"), which served as the harm reduction team at the Nova Festival. Anashim Tovim is run by Maayan Shenkar and Moshe Elad, both of whom survived the attack. Their on-the-ground experience offers poignant insight into the challenges faced and the compassion exhibited in such dire moments. Operating in the midst of chaos, Anashim Tovim navigated the intersection of harm reduction principles and immediate crisis response. The crew's efforts extended beyond traditional harm reduction protocols, engaging with survivors, providing emotional support, and facilitating access

5 Harm reduction attitudes within the Israeli rave scene are complex, with a recent study (Bonny-Noach et al., 2023) revealing higher positive attitudes but challenges in implementation. The discourse around harm reduction, particularly concerning substances like MDMA and LSD, is relatively new in Israel. The negative perception of law enforcement further complicates harm reduction efforts, necessitating a nuanced approach to reconcile community values with safety measures.

6 Harm reduction in Israel includes several distinct projects based mostly in the psychedelic scene, led by Anashim Tovim, Safe Shore, and the Israeli Burning Man community. Other harm reduction initiatives include Yizhar, a needle exchange pilot program, and opiate management programs (Bonny-Noach, 2019).

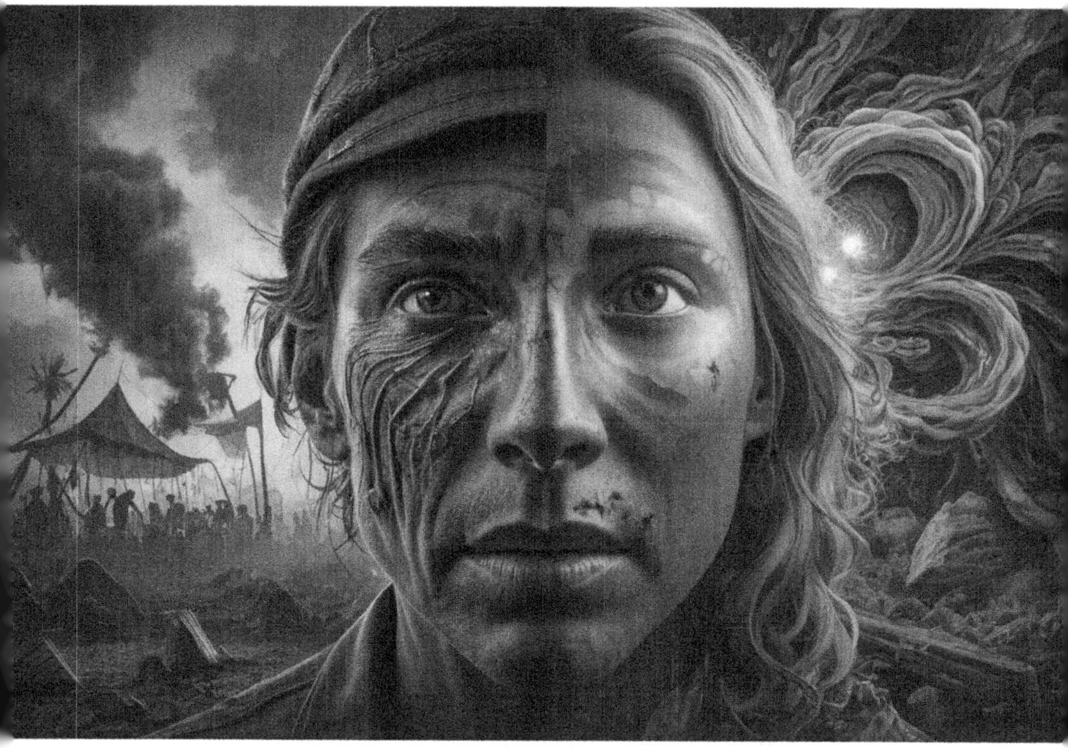

Pinni Baumol, *Splintergration*, AI-generated art, Aug 1, 2024

to essential resources.

Anashim Tovim was initiated by ELEM/Youth in Distress in Israel, Israel's leading nonprofit organization, founded in 1982 and dedicated to treating and transforming the lives of troubled and at-risk youth (ELEM, 2024). Anashim Tovim volunteers identify young people in crisis due to psychoactive substances at popular events like raves and then stay with the individual to provide psychological aid and support (Bonny-Noach, 2019).

Anashim Tovim's safe space at the Nova Festival and two vans were destroyed, and three of their nine-person team members were killed during the attack, representing the first harm reductionists killed doing their job (Y. Polizer, CEO of IsraAID, personal communication, February 19, 2024). As such, their own trauma made it harder for them to mobilize in the aftermath of the attack as quickly as other organizations. But after a 6-month break, Anashim Tovim returned to work both in the field (conducting training courses and running on average two safe zones at parties each month since March 2024) and through advocacy work with the Knesset's drug committee.

SafeHeart

Israeli mental health providers and harm reduction organization volunteers created the SafeHeart initiative to support the survivors of the Nova Festival massacre. Within hours of the attack, SafeHeart was established by eight therapists to support Nova survivors in need of mental and emotional assistance. After posting a request for psychedelic-informed therapists on Facebook on October 7th and launching a website on October 8th, SafeHeart mobilized a nation-wide network of clinical providers within days of the attack. During the project's first week, over 1,200 inquiries were addressed by therapists, safe space leaders, and harm reduction specialists, bringing together expertise in psychedelic harm reduction, trauma work, and clinical practice on an emergency scale (SafeHeart newsletter, May 6, 2024).

For the following month, SafeHeart coordinated with the Israeli Ministry of Health to ensure expanded mental health coverage for survivors. As SafeHeart's head of psychedelic education, Nir Tadmor, M.Sc., a certified transpersonal psychotherapist, described it in an interview in early 2024, "I had to translate the need for a mass psychedelic-informed trauma response by trained practitioners to the government-run healthcare system" (personal communication, February 13, 2024). The effort was successful, and SafeHeart is now recognized by the Israeli Ministry of Health and the National Social Security Service (Bituach Leumi) as an official mental health services provider for the survivors of the Nova Festival attack and as an official member of the Israeli Trauma Coalition as a National Resilience Center. Because of SafeHeart's official recognition, it is able to offer therapy to survivors free of charge, with therapists compensated at the rate of $100 per session.

By October 14th, SafeHeart had established a network of over 260 clinicians, all volunteers with advanced degrees and clinical licenses, to provide therapy in Israel. (They also have a team of psychiatrists providing consultations and pharmacological treatments as needed.) According to Tadmor, not all of these therapists have formal psychedelic-assisted training. The majority of the therapists mobilized by SafeHeart and other activities were familiar with psychedelic and rave culture—which includes organized harm reduction—because of its long-standing ubiquity in Israel since the 1990s.

The initiative has, as of May 6, 2024, provided 5,200 hours of psychotherapy and psychiatric consultation for more than 2,500 survivors (SafeHeart newsletter, May 6, 2024). They've placed 750 survivors in long-term psychotherapy, coordinated seven group therapy retreats for more than 250 survivors, and recruited 820 survivors to join their in-depth research project with the University of Haifa, under the supervision of Professor Roy Salomon, head of the Lab of Consciousness and Self in the Department of Cognitive Sciences, and Professor Roee Admon of the Stress & Psychopathology Research Laboratory. In collaboration with SafeHeart, Saloman and Admon began a large-scale study examining the impact of acute trauma under the influence of psychedelics in the peritraumatic and long-term periods. The project used behavioral, cognitive, physiological, and neural (fMRI) measurements of the participants—all of whom are Nova survivors—to better understand clinical trajectories and mechanisms of trauma experienced while under psychedelics (Elliman, 2024).

On its website, SafeHeart (n.d.) defines itself as an "emergency mental health project that is operated by a network of psychologists, psychiatrists, clinical social workers, psychotherapists and licensed clinical supervisors, who all have experience working with severe trauma and the field of psychedelic harm reduction." While SafeHeart offers its services to all survivors of the Nova Festival massacre, one of its strengths is supporting rave attendees who were under the influence of psychedelics and therefore had intensified experiences. Their protocol is to match each survivor with a therapist who provides at least 24 individual therapy sessions. The treatments are provided by licensed and vetted clinicians who specialize in treating trauma and reducing risks related to consumption of psychedelics. It has also created a community that offers the opportunity for mutual support, alongside dedicated group therapy for the family members of survivors.[7]

Safe Spaces

Immediately after October 7, physical spaces were created and specifically designed to give Nova survivors a place to come together to grieve, connect, and receive support in a trauma-informed setting. These "safe spaces," such as Adama Tova and Kfar Izun, served as centers for survivors to meet, connect, integrate their personal stories, and receive various treatments such as psychotherapy, massage, breathwork, and music therapy.[8] Many musicians, artists, members of the Nova Festival production crew, and therapists volunteered at these initiatives, which remained available for survivors for months after the attacks.

Merhav Marpeh is an emergency mental health complex established in Rishpon by Dr. Lia Naor to provide immediate care for the thousands traumatized by the attacks at the Nova Festival. The initiative mobilized dozens of therapists—psychologists, psychiatrists, clinical social workers, psychotherapists and certified clinical instructors—to create a "healing space" within days of the attack. Dr. Naor stressed that the efforts were not meant as a full course of treatment, but rather to offer an "immediate and integrative response to trauma" (Koplewitz, 2023). Merhav Marpe provides a holistic, integrative, community approach to trauma treatment that ranges from psychotherapy to yoga.

IsraAID's Secret Forest Retreat

IsraAID is an international non-governmental humanitarian aid organization based in Israel, founded in 2001, that traditionally works in emergency and long-term development settings in more than 60 countries around the world (IsraAID, n.d.). However, after the October 7 attacks it applied its expertise to Israel's needs (Y. Polizer, CEO, personal communication, February 19, 2024). One of its activities became the training of local mental health specialists on emergency-specific psychosocial support, so they can best meet the urgent needs of affected people from Israel's south. IsraAID also funded and ran retreats at Secret Forest near Paphos in Cyprus for survivors of the Nova attack (Secret Forest, n.d.). Secret Forrest, a kosher farm-to-table retreat facility at the site of an old village owned by Israeli Yoni Kahana, offered IsraAID the location for free to help survivors heal (S. May, press officer, personal communication, July 30, 2024). Two thousand individuals signed up to attend the retreats and 1,090 eventually participated, end-

---

7 SafeHeart partnered with Brothers in Yoga (BY) and Maccabiah World Union (MWU) on retreats hosted in glamping tents set up at Kfar Maccabiah within weeks of the October 7th attacks. MWU is the world's largest Jewish sports and education organization, reaching 450,000 people in over 70 countries across six continents. BY is an organization launched in 2022 to help Israeli veterans in search of healing for war trauma. BY began operating at Maccabi alongside SafeHeart to help rave victims, then shifted their work to focus on soldiers with PTSD. BY's work focuses on a critical point (pre-PTSD) to reduce the risk of survivors and veterans suffering lingering PTSD. The campus mobilized quickly to provide retreat facilities to organizations working with victims from the attack on music festivals, displaced Israelis, and later soldiers cycling out of the reserves. MWU CEO Amir Gissin and BY founder Netta Margalith discussed how this war is perhaps the first to see mental health as a concern since day one (personal communication, interview February 21, 2024).

8 Adama Tova English page [website]: https://www.adamatova.org/englishpageadamatovaen
Izun English [website]: https://www.izun.org.il/izun-english/

ing each day with a party in which they were the DJs. IsraAID staffed the retreats with therapists that had experience with trauma (experts in different modalities) and emphasized the creation of a support network for the survivors given that the rave and Tribe of Nova communities are diffuse and the community could aid in the healing process.

II. Community & Artistic Activations

Israel's creative community members, ranging from artists, gallerists, musicians, and DJs, acted swiftly to create or adapt activations to honor the events of October 7 and support survivors. A few examples include the following:

Neve Schechter Gallery

Established in 2015, the Schechter Gallery in Tel Aviv serves as a vital bridge between the profound realm of Judaism's knowledge and the transformative power of artistic expression (Neve Schechter, n.d.). The exhibit *Mycelium* by Sharon Glazberg opened coincidentally the same week of the attacks and explored the relationship between art and its audience by using mycelia, the network of fungal hyphae usually found underground (Glazberg, 2024). This installation bridged the concepts of art and medicine, fostering relationships between humans and fungi that are akin to the patient-therapist or provider-nourishment connection. *Mycelium* transformed the gallery into a nurturing environment, with edible and medicinal mushrooms growing from wooden structures designed to resemble treatment beds (Dayan, 2023). Glazberg conducted sessions focused on therapy, healing, art, and ritual in the gallery alongside professionals spanning various fields such as psychotherapy, creativity, mind-body-spirit connections, philosophy, art, and music. During the first weeks of the war, the gallery provided the public free access to a team of therapists ready to treat primary and secondary trauma (Bar Yerushalmi, director & curator, personal communications, October 2023-February 2024).

Nova 6.29

The Nova Festival founders—Omri Sassi, Yoni Feingold, Ofir Amir, and Yagil Rimoni—organized a memorial exhibit curated by Reut Feingold that premiered in Tel Aviv and has since begun to tour internationally. *Nova 6.29* opened to the public at the Expo Tel Aviv International Convention Center on December 7, 2023, and was named for the exact hour on October 7 that Hamas' attacks began (Kershner, 2023). Its goal was to memorialize the nearly 364 people who lost their lives during the attack by showcasing items salvaged from the festival. The display includes video footage of people dancing in their last moments, WhatsApp exchanges capturing the fear and terror of the attendees, portraits of those who never made it home, and many items such as shoes and burnt-out cars. Israeli President Isaac Herzog attended the opening and described it as "a hallowed space" (Kershner, 2023). All proceeds from the exhibit go towards assistance for Nova Festival survivors coordinated by the Tribe of Nova Foundation. The Nova Festival founders, together with U.S. partners then brought this large-scale installation to New York and Los Angeles "with the objective to create a powerful, educational, and emotional exhibit that allows others to bear witness to the horrors of what occurred on that day at The Nova Music Festival" (Nova Exhibition, n.d.).

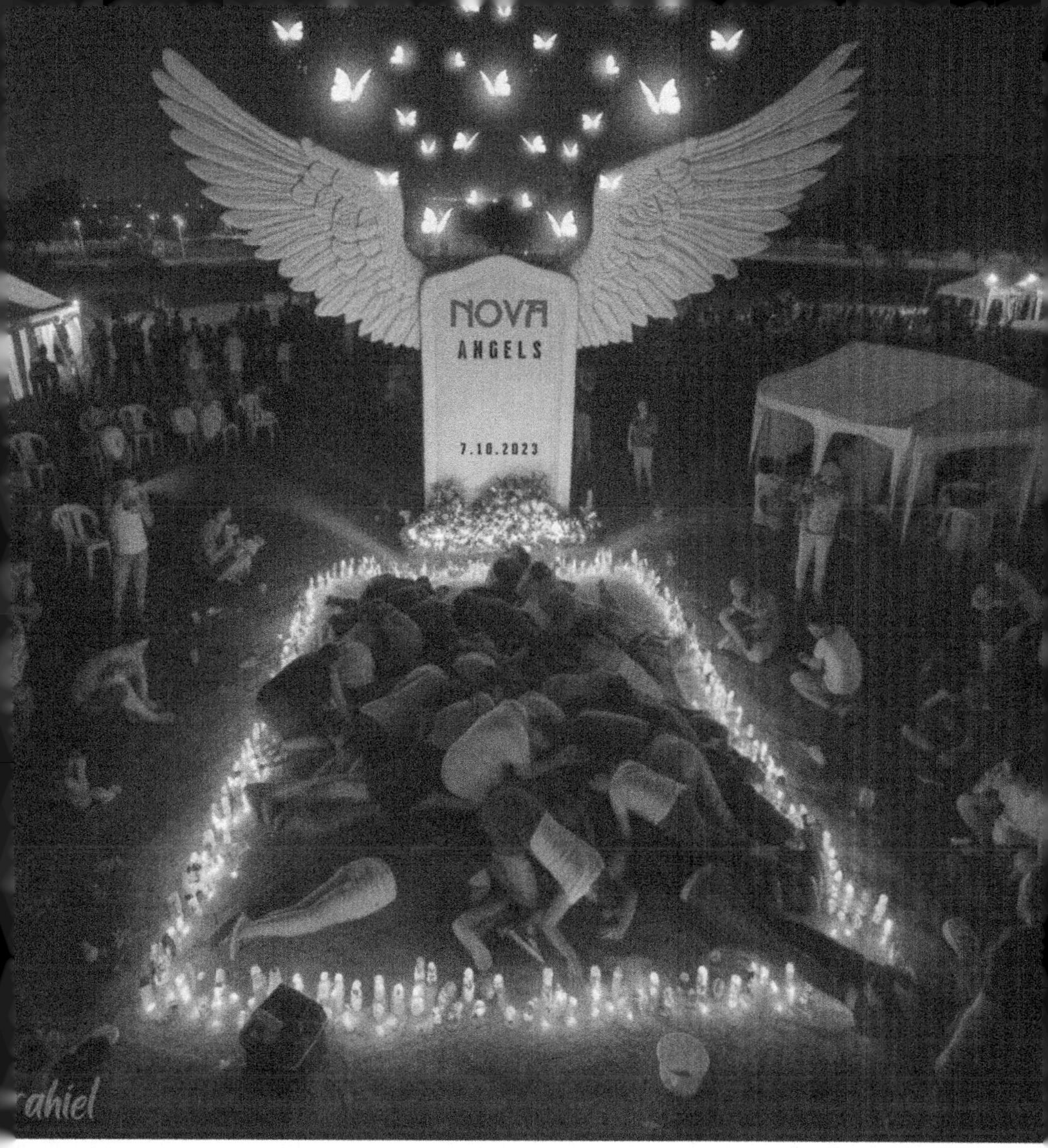

Nir Ahiel, *Untitled*, AI-generated art, Nov 6, 2023

Music-Related Activations

In addition to healing spaces and emergency mental health activations, a number of DJs, community leaders, and musicians have also taken it upon themselves to host events in honor of the Nova Festival survivors, helping to cultivate healing environments and raise money for support. For example, during an evening in Jerusalem, DJ Yaakov Babani (founder of Tribal Events) played ambient electronic music while musician Yosef Wildes led meditation and breathwork. The artist Merchav Mugen (Hebrew for "safe space") has created a YouTube series featuring multidisciplinary artists and creators who gathered for recordings at Kitsch Studios in Tel Aviv. "Out of the terrible pain," wrote Mugen in the text related to the first video in the series, "we searched for a way to express what cannot be expressed in words, and to offer comfort and hope through what connects us all: Israeli culture" (Mugen, n.d.). Ecstatic Dance Israel hosted a fundraising campaign and has adjusted the programming of the organization's nine centers to accommodate survivors and their sensitivities. The Tribe of Nova has been holding commemorative performances and fundraisers for victims of the attack who were injured (rehabilitation services, psychological treatments, and professional aid) and for the families of those killed, kidnapped, or deemed missing. The funds raised by the Tribe of Nova are also used to provide emotional and financial support for the individuals working at the Nova Festival who have been financially, physically, or emotionally impacted. Other popular musicians including DJ Freedom Fighters and DJ Inor Roni Kogno have been involved in commemorative events to honor and raise money for the survivors of October 7. Even the Israeli jazz community, distinct from the DJ scene, has stepped up to organize an online jazz festival to create unity and support PTSD prevention and treatment among survivors.

Various music and psychedelic arts parties have been happening all over Israel with the goal of bringing together survivors of the Nova Festival, building solidarity and uplifting the community. As described by one such party goer via WhatsApp to an acquaintance:

> We went to a wedding hall that has been transformed into a place of gathering and healing for survivors of the Nova party, from which 364 beautiful souls were murdered by Hamas terrorists, so many people were injured and dozens kidnapped and taken into captivity. Last night there were hundreds of young Israelis there. There was food, music, stations for different kinds of healing treatments and a stage on which musicians performed and spoke. On the far wall of the hall it said in English in blue lights, "We will dance again." (personal communication)

III. Psychedelic-Assisted Therapy Activations

In addition to initial harm reduction and expressions of artistic solidarity, more formal psychedelic-assisted therapeutic activations have been implemented in response to the trauma of October 7th.

MAPS Israel

MAPS Israel is an affiliate of the Multidisciplinary Association of Psychedelic Studies (MAPS) drug development company now known as Lykos Therapeutics. MAPS Israel operated clinical trials of MDMA for PTSD and is now fundraising for a new initiative named Healing October 7 that would treat or prevent post-traumatic stress disorder (PTSD) in survivors of the October 7 attacks (MAPS Israel, 2023). Healing October 7 would consist of two components: therapeutic programs aiming to prevent PTSD, as well as MDMA group therapy for survivors and soldiers with PTSD.[9] The initiative would be a breakthrough, multi-site group MDMA-assisted psychotherapy

9 The PTSD prevention initiative includes three non-psychedelic components: psychotherapy for residents of Kibbutzim Sufa, Ein Hashlosha, Re'im, and the city of Sderot (including Kitot Konenut); psychotherapy program for 40 Eilat residents who survived the Nova Festival; and programs for young residents (ages 20 to 35) of "otef aza" (the area enveloping Gaza) out of the Marpe Yami farm in Eilat. These programs are working independently now, and MAPS Israel supports some with consultation (K. Tzarfaty, CEO & Co-Founder of MAPS Israel, personal communication, July 31, 2024 and August 13, 2024).

study that would include various patient groups.[10] The goal of this study is to provide 15 weeks of group and individual therapy for the survivors inside five major hospitals in Israel. Group therapy was chosen for its ability to foster collective healing (leveraging shared experiences from a collective trauma) and for being cost-efficient. MAPS Israel's research aims to pioneer effective large-scale trauma treatment in group settings (K. Tzarfaty, CEO & Co-Founder of MAPS Israel, personal communication, April 18, 2024, and August 13, 2024).

Access Center for Psychedelic Therapy

Access Center for Psychedelic Therapy (ACPT) is an Israeli nonprofit organization founded by Pinchas Baumol[11] and Shaun Lacob in 2022 dedicated to increasing access to safe and legal psychedelic therapy options (ACPT, 2023). Immediately after the attack, ACPT reached out to trauma and ketamine experts around the world, as ketamine is the only legal psychedelic currently available for use in Israel (other substances are only available within the context of clinical trials or are illegal). ACPT created a protocol for treating acute stress disorder (ASD) within days of the attack. The protocol has been disseminated amongst Israeli mental health professionals who are using it to treat ASD among survivors and first responders who were on site at Nova Festival and other initial attacks.

Clinic in Lev Hasharon Hospital

Lev Hasharon Mental Health Center (LHMHC) started a public integrative-psychedelic clinic in response to the immediate need for psychiatric and psychological treatment that recognizes the special needs of those who were traumatized during their escape from the October 7 terror attack while under the influence of psychedelic substances. This clinic drew on information and volunteer support from harm reductionists and psychedelic therapists. LHMHC mobilized quickly and started treating survivors within days of the attack, recruiting them from support networks and initiatives dedicated to victims of the attack to the Nova Festival. This was done in tandem with the work LHMHC has done to offer psychological and psychiatric aid to refugees from settlements surrounding the Gaza Strip.

Conclusion

The Israeli psytrance scene, marked by its dynamic evolution, has faced a defining moment in the wake of the October 7th massacre. The tragedy prompted a profound shift in the discourse around harm reduction, emphasizing the need for community-driven initiatives grounded in the community's own values of peace, love, unity, and respect. The different responses showcase the transformative potential of harm reduction beyond substance use, serving as a vital instrument of communal healing and resilience.

---

10 The various patient groups would include 400 survivors suffering from moderate to severe PTSD as a result of the October 7th attack in Israel (in partnership with Sheba Medical Center and Lev Hasharon Mental Health Center), survivors of the southern Israel massacre (in partnership with Be'er Sheva Hospital), and soldiers who have developed PTSD (in partnership with Sheba and HaEmek Medical Center) (Tzarfaty, personal communication, July 31, 2024 and August 13, 2024).

11 Pinchas Baumol is one of the authors of this article.

As the Israeli rave scene navigates the complexities of recovery, the synthesis of cultural values, harm reduction principles, and community solidarity emerges as a beacon of hope amidst the shadows of tragedy.

The October 7th massacre at the Nova Festival serves as a poignant backdrop to the ongoing discourse on harm reduction within the Israeli psytrance community. The challenges faced by harm reduction teams during this tragedy are intrinsically linked to the broader patterns of substance use and attitudes identified in recent studies. In navigating the complexities of harm reduction within the Israeli psytrance subculture, it is imperative to weave together insights from recent studies. The substance use patterns, harm reduction attitudes, and law enforcement dynamics elucidated in these studies provide a comprehensive framework for understanding the challenges and opportunities in harm reduction efforts.

By and large, the Jewish psychedelic community has been supportive of the global efforts to address the trauma of October 7, while the greater mainstream psychedelic community has been largely quiet. The trauma of October 7 has had a ripple effect around the world, affecting not only Israelis but also the global Jewish community, now facing the surge in anti-Semitism that began with celebrations of the October 7 massacre. Many Jews are feeling insecure, unsafe, or activated, and to address this, communities across America and elsewhere are holding healing psychedelic ceremonies, song and prayer circles, vigils, and community discussions.

The global Jewish psychedelic community is diverse in levels of observance, Jewish practice, politics, and demographics. The community ranges from those who are holding space in ceremony, over Shabbat or other holidays, to those who are less involved in practicing Judaism but relate to psychedelics through secular culture and nonetheless bring their Jewish identities with them to their entheogenic work. A large portion of the Jewish psychedelic community relates to this topic via prayer and song circles (sometimes absent substances), integration gatherings, online courses and workshops, WhatsApp chat groups, and in person community.[12] There are also companies that sponsor events and projects focused on Jewish psychedelia.[13] Indeed, the conversation in the larger psychedelic Jewish community has been shifting toward a heavily trauma-informed focus—even before October 7—and now that lens has come into even greater relevance and need. Questions of inherited trauma, especially regarding the Holocaust, as well as the somatic expressions of trauma in the body, and the way in which global narratives affect the collective Jewish body and soul, are now begging for answers and resolution as Jews around the world grapple with the aftermath of the deadliest day in

12 Leading organizations include the nonprofit Shefa: Jewish Psychedelic Support (Bay Area, www.sheflow.org/); the Jewish Psychedelic Summit (virtual, www.jewishpsychedelicsummit.org), an online conference that brought together various speakers on May 2-3, 2021 and had an in-person gathering during the Psychedelic Science conference convened by MAPS in Denver in June 2024; Darkhei Rephua (New York, https://rephua.wordpress.com), a nonprofit that hosts events and Shabbatons; Casa Somati (upstate New York, https://www.instagram.com/casasomati), a private home that hosts Jewish prayer circles and other events; and JewWhoTokes, an Instagram account founded in 2016 that profiles Jewish individuals who partake and/or work in the psychedelic and cannabis industries, which since the October 7 attacks has been hosting weekly pre-Shabbat calls and in-person events. Co-author Madison Margolin is one of the founders of the Jewish Psychedelic Summit, and Adriana Kertzer is the founder of JewWhoTokes.

13 For-profit entities that have supported the Jewish psychedelic ecosystem include Plant Medicine Law Group, Nushama, DoubleBlind, and Ayin Press. Adriana Kertzer is the founder of Plant Medicine Law Group, and Madison Margolin was a co-founder of DoubleBlind and a contributor to Ayin Press.

Jewish history since the Holocaust.

The attacks on people attending a psychedelic music festival brought out a range of responses from international psychedelic and harm reduction organizations. Some were explicit in their condemnation of the attacks and organized fundraisers. For example, the Colorado-based Center for Medicinal Mindfulness founded by Daniel McQueen and Psychedelic Sitters School started a GoFundMe page to help fund support for survivors of the Supernova Sukkot Gathering attack. A volunteer with the German harm reduction team Eclipse donated funds to Anashim Tovim.[14] The psytrance festivals Apsara (Hungary) and Universo Paralello (the Brazilian festival entity that co-organized the festival) condemned the attacks through posts on Instagram and Facebook. MAPS did not specifically acknowledge the Nova Festival massacre, nor its psychedelic relevance, but it did issue a statement highlighting the organization's work in Israel and the need for continued healing for Israelis and Palestinians. However, large international psytrance festivals popular among Israeli ravers (e.g., Boom and Ozora), as well as major American harm reduction organizations (e.g., Zendo and Fireside) have not issued public statements as of this writing, potentially contributing to the sense of isolation and vulnerability experienced by the victims and the volunteers who have helped them.

The speed with which Israeli society mobilized to address the needs presented by the October 7 attacks is astonishing.[15] Treating the people who were on psychedelics at the Nova Festival with appropriate care meant that individuals from the Israeli harm reduction community and rave scene had to teach mental health professionals and the government how to deal with persons in altered states—and the potential exacerbated harm the attacks had on these individuals.

The history of psychedelic use among Jews in Israel and the diaspora is a rich one, as is a culture of early adoption, cultural exploration, and affinity with mental health education, presumably facilitating the swift, innovative, and multifaceted response. It is our hope that the mobilization described here will influence the larger conversation unfolding around the world about humans' desire to alter consciousness through psychedelics, the wisdom cultivated in the psychedelic underground, and the particular forms of trauma that can be experienced by individuals when they are on substances that are consumed in order to facilitate wonder, human connection, exploration, and delight.

14 This individual reached out to Pinni Baumol through mutual contacts inquiring how he could provide support after the attacks.

15 The fact that civil society came together after months of intense political protests related to the judicial reform measures led by Prime Minister Netanyahu, and mobilized largely without government support, merits credit.

Disclaimer

The views and opinions expressed in this article are those of the authors and do not necessarily reflect the views or positions of any organizations with which they are associated.

Acknowledgment

A version of this material was published by *Tablet Magazine* on August 6, 2024 under the title "The Worst Trip Ever" (https://www.tabletmag.com/feature/psychedelic-mental-health-nova-october-7-terrorist-attacks-israel).

References

ACPT. (2023). *ACPT's Forum: Shaping the Future of Psychedelic Therapy in Israel.* The Access Center for Psychedelic Therapy & Treatment. [Website]. https://acptisrael.com/en/therapist-forum/

Bonny-Noach, H. (2019). Harm reduction drug policy in Israel: What has been accomplished and what still needs to be done? *Israel Journal of Health Policy Research, (8)*75. https://doi.org/10.1186/s13584-019-0343-3

Bonny-Noach, H., Shapira, B., Baumol, P., Tadmor, N., Rosca, P., Shoshan, S., Harel-Fisch, H., & Caduri, A. (2023, August 9). Substance use, harm reduction attitudes and behaviors among attendees of nature rave parties in Israel. *Harm Reduction Journal, 20*(108). https://doi.org/10.1186/s12954-023-00845-3

Dayan, L. (2023, October 25). *We all need therapy now: The Tel Aviv gallery offering breathing space from the war.* Haaretz.com. https://www.haaretz.com/israel-news/2023-10-25/ty-article-magazine/.premium/we-all-need-therapy-now-the-tel-aviv-gallery-offering-breathing-space-from-the-war/0000018b-6722-d979-a3bb-ef77d3650000

ELEM. (2024). ELEM website. https://elem.org/who-we-are/about-us/

Elliman, W. (2024, April 18). *Trauma under the influence.* Haaretz.com. https://www.haaretz.com/haaretz-labels/power/2024-04-18/ty-article-labels/.premium/trauma-under-the-influence/0000018e-edaa-d240-a19f-fdab2c7c0000

Gavrielov, N. (2023, December 27). Hamas and other militant groups are firing rockets into Israel every day. *The New York Times.* https://www.nytimes.com/2023/12/27/world/middleeast/israel-hamas-gaza-rockets.html

Gettleman, J., Schwartz, A., Sella, A., & Shaar-Yashuv, A. (2023, December 28). Screams without words: How Hamas weaponized sexual violence on Oct. 7. *The New York Times.* https://www.nytimes.com/2023/12/28/world/middleeast/oct-7-attacks-hamas-israel-sexual-violence.html

Ghermezian, S. (2024). *Nova music festival massacre 'being forgotten and ignored,' says Jewish music executive after NY exhibit opens.* The Algemeiner. https://www.algemeiner.com/2024/05/06/nova-music-festival-massacre-being-forgotten-ignored-says-jewish-music-executive-ny-exhibit-opens/

Gifford, M.E. (2023, October 30). *After 260 killed at psychedelic-trance festival in Israel, trauma healing for survivors underway.* Lucid News. https://www.lucid.news/after-260-killed-at-psychedelic-trance-festival-in-israel-trauma-healing-for-survivors-underway

Gillet, F., & Cuddy, A. (2023, October 9). *Israeli music festival: 260 bodies recovered from site where people fled in hail of bullets.* BBC News. https://www.bbc.com/news/world-middle-east-67047034

Glazberg, S. (2024, January 3). *Mycelium* [Video]. YouTube. https://www.youtube.com/watch?v=JzxM6k82Bkg

IsraAID. (n.d.). [Website]. https://www.israaid.org

Kershner, I. (2023, December 15). As Israel weighs how to honor Oct. 7 victims, festival exhibit serves as 'hallowed space.' *The New York Times.* https://www.nytimes.com/2023/12/15/world/middleeast/israel-hamas-nova-festival-exhibition.html

Koplewitz, G. (2023, November 18). They survived Hamas's attack on a trance party. An ad hoc center with art and music is helping them heal. *The New York Times*. https://www.nytimes.com/2023/11/18/world/middleeast/hamas-attack-survivors-healing.html

MAPS Israel. (2023). *Healing October 7*. MAPS Israel [Website]. http://www.maps-israel.org

Morris, L., Piper, I., Sohyun Lee, J., and George, S. (2023, October 8). How a night of dancing and revelry in Israel turned into a massacre. *The Washington Post*. https://www.washingtonpost.com/world/2023/10/08/israel-festival-attack-gaza-militants/

Mugen, M. (n.d.). Safe Space Sessions: שלומי שבן - מודה אני (מאיר אריאל). https://www.youtube.com/watch?v=yZCewacTQ5w.

Neve Schechter. (n.d.). Contemporary Jewish Culture and Arts Center. Neve Schechter [Website]. https://neve-schechter.org.il/en/homepage/

Nova Exhibition. (n.d.) [Website]. https://www.novaexhibition.com/about-the-exhibit

Reuters. (2024, January 12). *Israeli hostage families shout their love to the captives across Gaza fence*. Reuters. https://www.reuters.com/world/middle-east/israeli-hostage-families-shout-their-love-captives-across-gaza-fence-2024-01-11/.

Rubin, S. (2023, November 25). Israel investigates an elusive, horrific enemy: Rape as a weapon of war. *The Washington Post*. https://www.washingtonpost.com/world/2023/11/25/israel-hamas-rape-sexual-violence

SafeHeart. (n.d.). [Website]. https://www.safeheartil.com/en

Secret Forest. (n.d.). [Website]. https://secretfo.rest/en

Shapira, B., Caduri, A., Baumol, P., Tadmor, N., Rosca, P., Shoshan, S., Harel-Fisch, Y., & Bonny-Noach, H. (2023). Attitudes and views regarding law enforcement activity at large outdoor raves in Israel: A cross-sectional survey. *Policing and Society, 33*(7), 784–801. https://doi.org/10.1080/10439463.2023.2200250

Supernova. (2023). *The Tribe of Nova Presents SUPERNOVA*. Ticketing website for the Nova Festival. https://www.eventer.co.il/novaparalellotranslate

Tabachnick, C. (2023, October 8). *Israelis search for loved ones with posts and pleas on social media*. CBS News. https://www.cbsnews.com/news/israelis-search-loved-ones-posts-pleas-social-media-hamas-attack/

Tadmor, N. (2024, June 7). *Providing psychedelic-informed therapy for the survivors of October 7th* [Conference Presentation]. Interdisciplinary Conference on Psychedelic Research, June 6-7, 2024, Haarlem, The Netherlands.

The Times of Israel. (2023, November 17). Death count from Re'im music festival massacre reportedly updated to 364—a third of Oct 7 fatalities. *The Times of Israel*. https://www.timesofisrael.com/liveblog_entry/death-count-from-massacre-at-reim-music-festival-reportedly-updated-to-364-a-third-of-oct-7-deaths/

Stephanie Ezust, PhD

Decatur, Georgia
drezust@comcast.net

Book Review

A Really Good Day: How Microdosing Made a Mega Difference in My Mood, My Marriage, and My Life
By Ayelet Waldman
Alfred A. Knopf,
New York, 2017, 229 pages

If the words, "life, liberty, and the pursuit of happiness" don't include the right to experiment with your own consciousness, then the Declaration of Independence isn't worth the hemp it was written on.
—Terence McKenna (Epigraph to Waldman's book)

This book came out in 2017, so a lot of the information Waldman provides has been updated since then, but it is still a fascinating read, which I highly recommend (let's start with my conclusion!).

Ayelet Waldman is a novelist and essayist, as well as a former federal public defender. She taught at Loyola Law School and the UC Berkeley School of Law, where she developed and taught courses on the legal implications of the war on drugs. This was particularly important as she contemplated and undertook 30 days of microdosing with LSD.

She is married to one of my favorite novelists, Michael Chabon. Chabon and Waldman (2017) edited a book that I also highly recommend: *Kingdom of Olives and Ash: Writers Confront the Occupation*, a collection of 26 essays by different writers. They collaborated with the Israeli NGO Breaking the Silence and present a picture of what it means to be a Palestinian in Israel and the occupied territories. This book predates the current tragedy and offers compelling context.

Waldman has a history of mental challenges and had gone through years of therapy and medication, yielding a number of different diagnoses, including bipolar disorder II and premenstrual dysphoric disorder (PMDD). As she describes it, she has been on a shitload of medications over the years. Her mood swings made her relationships with her husband and four children difficult and challenging. Her decision to try microdosing did not come easily. She did a great deal of research and soul searching, which she delineates, before taking the plunge. She was painfully aware that what she was doing was illegal, and this was the biggest challenge for her. In addition to the threat of being caught, there was no way for her to compare her experiences with trustworthy professionals or other users.

Waldman acquired a cobalt blue bottle containing 30 days' dosage from an anonymous person called "Lewis Carroll," whom she found through discretely inquiring among her acquaintances. Along with the bottle there was a note explaining how to take the drug over the course of the experiment. The following poem was included:

> Our lives may be no more
> Than dewdrops on a summer morning,
> But surely,
> It is better that we sparkle
> While we are here. (p. 14)

The book is organized as a journal around her 30-day doses. The microdoses are taken every third day. She begins each day with brief descriptions of the following categories: physical sensations, mood, conflict, sleep, work, and pain. The first of each 3-day cycle is "microdose day," the second "transition," and the third "normal day." Each day, she provides stories about her experience and information about the history of drug usage, both recreational and clinical, the history of the war on drugs, and current usage of different psychedelics.

A good part of what makes this book an entertaining read, in addition to its educational value, is her trenchant sense of humor. Here's an example:

> I've done mindfulness-based therapy, which required me to spend tortuous minutes meditating, and many more torturous hours discussing with my therapist why I hate meditating so much. I responded to a crisis in a friend's marriage by forcing my long-suffering husband into an infuriating kind of couples therapy that involved repeating back each other's words, theoretically in a tone not dripping with passive-aggressive fury. ("I hear that it upsets you when I criticize how you load the dish washer, but I feel sad when you insist on putting the glasses on the bottom rack, and I feel rage because, despite your vaunted intelligence, you can't seem to learn that that's how they get broken." Oops.). We might still be frantically using "I" language with one another had my husband not pointed out that it was the therapy that was the most serious threat to our marriage. "I" had to agree. (p. xii)

Her entry for Day 15 includes a blow-by-blow description of a couple's session that made me laugh out loud and then cry—you might consider reading this book just for this entry!

Waldman tells us that psychedelic microdosing was popularized by psychologist and psychedelic researcher James Fadiman (2011), quoting from his book:

> A microdose of a psychedelic drug is a subtherapeutic dose of a drug administered at a quantity low enough to elicit no adverse side effects yet high enough for a measurable cellular response. A microdose of a psychedelic drug is approximately one-tenth of a typical dose. (p. ix)

Throughout her journal, Waldman provides a history of the prohibition of drugs, going back to 1914 with the Harrison Narcotics Act. She talks about what made her decide to try the experiment, as well as the many reasons she was frightened by her decision. She describes how LSD works on the brain, comparing it with how antidepressants work, including the many side effects that antidepressants manifest. She also notes that, despite the bad press and distortions, there has never been a death reported as a result of taking LSD. She tells us that Fadiman (2011) cited the overwhelmingly positive reports he received from people microdosing, which he separated into four categories: emotion (such as reduction in anxiety, mood elevation, increased happiness), intellect (improved focus, increased creativity, more effective problem solving), relationships (general improvement, reduced conflicts), and physical (menstrual cycles became more regular and less painful; some people found themselves exercising more regularly and eating more healthy diets).

Waldman concludes the book saying that if microdosing were legal, she would continue doing it indefinitely, but her fears of the consequences of using the illegal drug outweighed the benefits she experienced.

The book includes an extensive bibliography.

I should mention in closing her reason for talking about "a really good day." Prior to this experiment, her really good days were few and far between. She reports that she has experienced more good days since, and that's a really good reason to applaud her experiment!

References

Chabon, M. & Waldman, A. (Eds.). (2017). *Kingdom of olives and ash: Writers confront the occupation.* New York: Harper Collins.

Fadiman, J. (2011). *The psychedelic explorer's guide: Safe, therapeutic, and sacred journeys.* Rochester, VT: Park Street Press.

McKenna, T. (1992). *Food of the gods: The search for the original tree of knowledge: A radical history of plants drugs and human evolution.* New York: Bantam Books.

Just say know.

—Timothy Leary

Mary Gresham, PhD

Atlanta, Georgia
docgresh1@gmail.com

Book Review

Psychedelic Integration: Psychotherapy for Non-Ordinary States of Consciousness.
By Marc Aixalà
Synergetic Press,
2022, 410 pages.

I HAVE JUST FINISHED MY SECOND READING of what seems to me to be the best book written on the topic of psychedelic integration. Marc Aixalà is well qualified to write this book, having been the primary therapist working in integration and support services for the International Center for Ethnobotanical Education, Research, and Service (ICEERS), a well-respected non-profit group in Spain. He has overseen the services there for more than 10 years and has worked on many hundreds of cases. He is also a facilitator for Holotropic Breathwork and has a deep understanding of the processes involved in non-ordinary states. His clarity of thinking is particularly useful in that in psychedelic integration we need to clarify from the outset whether we are working to maximize the benefit of the person's experience or to reduce the adverse effects of a psychedelic experience.

The section of the book that seems most valuable to me is the material on intervention to reduce the harm of an adverse reaction. Here Aixalà follows some of the principles of Grof, Watts, and the Palo Alto school. The case material is rich and specific in the use of interventions and also the clinical course followed. He delineates the difference between integration and psychotherapy. Integration is a short-term process—up to 10 sessions—that will maximize the client's sense of being resourced, autonomous, and in control. Descriptions of the most common adverse events are as follows: lack of preparation; unresolved difficult experiences; emergence of new traumatic memories; trauma with dissociative symptoms including derealization, depersonalization, flashbacks, numbing, or hyperarousal; facilitator abuse; repetitive use without integration; and prior mental disorders.

This is a treasure trove of clinical wisdom and thought-provoking theory from a wise and experienced practitioner. ▼

Call for Papers

Links in the Chain: Tradition and Innovation in Psychotherapy

Voices, 2025

Deadline for submission: April 15, 2025

Direct questions and submissions to the editors:

Molly Donovan
drmollyd@aol.com
Jonathan Farber
Jonathan.farber@gmail.com
Hallie Lovett
hallielovett@gmail.com
Penelope Norton
penelope.norton@gmail.com
and Barry Wepman
bjwep@aol.com

See Submission Guidelines on the AAP website: **www.aapweb.com** or in any issue of *Voices*

WE LIVE IN A TIME OF RAPID CHANGE: that would be trite, were it not so piercingly true. As practicing psychotherapists "of a certain age," we five have been reading, writing for, or editing Voices for over five decades. Today, we find ourselves, our readers, and our contributors facing a new challenge: obsolescence or evolution. Where might we go next as spokespersons and storytellers for the art and science of psychotherapy?

In considering *Voices'* evolution, our thoughts turned to our Academy and its origin story: How a group of traditionally trained therapists, frustrated by the segmentation and rigidity of psychoanalytic practice, conceived an organization grounded in the centrality of the person of the therapist. When we think of the chain of therapists, beginning with our founders, some of whom we knew personally, and continuing in our mentees and trainees, we celebrate that blend of tradition and innovation embodied in the generations of the Academy. Help us add links to this chain! Ultimately, Voices' (and the Academy's) evolution can be traced through its stories. We have five experienced editors for this issue, and we welcome contributions from new or struggling writers. Tell us your story; we will gladly help you write it. Tell us about how you copied and how you differed from your teachers. Tell us about the ways newer therapists learn from and differ from you. Tell us how you evolved as a therapist and a person. Tell us about your link in the chain.

Our field has taken many turns in the past several years, as theory and practice have expanded and even been turned on their heads. The Relational turn in psychoanalysis, for example, has reconceptualized the implications of therapist and patient being fully in the room, with conscious and unconscious elements at play. Strides in understanding the brain have led to techniques, such as EMDR which stimulates memory, and the recognition that trauma is physiological has challenged us to integrate specific attention to the body with our verbal psychodynamic approaches – the body as an avenue to the unconscious. We have become more aware of cultural, gender, and racial factors in development and in the treatment room. What stories from your life and work reflect foundation or innovation in psychotherapy?

Special section: Mentoring Moments

In addition to our regular articles (up to 4,000 words) we are looking for brief (one or two paragraphs) first person accounts of adding links to the chain. Tell us about a memorable encounter when you learned something from a mentor, or taught something about psychotherapy to a mentor or colleague? Don't think too hard about this, just write it and send it along to us. ▼

Voices welcomes submissions in the form of personal essay, research- and case-based inquiry, poetry, art, cartoons and photography.

The American Academy of Psychotherapists invites you to be a part of an enlightening journey into...

VOICES

Voices is a uniquely rewarding publication providing a meeting ground with other experienced psychotherapists. A theme-oriented journal, *Voices* presents personal and experiential essays by therapists from a wide range of orientations. Each issue takes you on an intimate journey through the reflections of therapists as they share their day-to-day experiences in the process of therapy. *Voices'* contributors reveal insights inherent in our lives, our culture and our society.

As a subscriber, you'll have the opportunity to experience contributions from noted luminaries in psychotherapy. Using various styles from articles to poems, *Voices* is interdisciplinary in its focus, reflecting the aims and mission of its publisher, the American Academy of Psychotherapists.

VOICES SUBSCRIPTION

Please start my one-year subscription to AAP's journal *Voices* at $65 for individuals PDF only; $85 for individuals PDF & print copy. Institutional subscriptions may be reserved directly through the AAP office or through the traditional subscription agencies at $249 per year. *Voices* is published electronically three times per year and is delivered to your email address as an ePublication.

Name ....
Address ....
City .... State .... ZIP ....
Telephone .... Fax ....
Email ....

☐ My check made payable to AAP *Voices* is enclosed.
☐ Please charge to my credit card, using the information I have supplied below:
Form of payment: ☐ Master Card ☐ Visa
Account # .... Expiration: ....
Signature ....

Address all orders by mail to:
Voices
230 Washington Ave Ext, Suite 101
Albany, NY 12203
You may also fax your order to (518) 240-1178.
For further information, please call (518) 694-5360

Voices: The Art and Science of Psychotherapy, is the journal of the American Academy of Psychotherapists. Written by and for psychotherapists and healing professionals, it focuses on therapists' personal struggles and growth and on the promotion of excellence in the practice of psychotherapy. The articles are written in a personalized voice rather than an academic tone, and they are of an experiential and theoretical nature that reflects on the human condition.

Each issue has a central theme as described in the call for papers. Manuscripts that fit this theme are given priority. Final decision about acceptance must wait until all articles for a particular issue have been reviewed. Articles that do not fit into any particular theme are reviewed and held for inclusion in future issues on a space available basis.

Articles. See a recent issue of *Voices* for general style. Manuscripts should be double-spaced in 12 point type and no longer than 4,000 words (about 16 to 18 pages). Do not include the author's name in the manuscript, as all submissions receive masked review by two or more members of the Editorial Review Board. Keep references to a minimum and follow the style of the *Publication Manual of the American Psychological Association, 5th ed.*

Submit via email, attaching the manuscript as a Word document file. Send it to the editor indicated on the call for papers. Put "Voices" in the email's subject line, and in the message include the author's name, title and degree, postal address, daytime phone number, manuscript title, and word count. Please indicate for which issue of *Voices* the manuscript is intended.

If a manuscript is accepted, the author will be asked to provide a short autobiographical sketch (75 words or less) and a photograph that complies with technical quality standards outlined in a PDF which will be sent to you.

Neither the editorial staff nor the American Academy of Psychotherapists accepts responsibility for statements made in its publication by contributors. We expect authors to make certain there is no breach of confidentiality in their submissions. Authors are responsible for checking the accuracy of their quotes, citations, and references.

Poetry. We welcome poetry of high quality relevant to the theme of a particular issue or the general field of psychotherapy. Short poems are published most often.

Book and Film Reviews. Reviews should be about 500 to 750 words, twice that if you wish to expand the material into a mini-article.

Visual Arts. We welcome submissions of photographs or art related to the central theme for consideration. Electronic submissions in JPEG or TIFF format are required. Photographs should be in high resolution format, preferably original size. Images are non-returnable and the copyright MUST belong to the submitting artist.

Copyright. By submitting materials to *Voices* (articles, poems, photos or artwork), the author transfers and consents that copyright for that article will be owned by the American Academy of Psychotherapists, Inc.

Vision Statement

Our vision is to be the premier professional organization where therapeutic excellence and the use of self in psychotherapy flourish.

Mission Statement

The mission of the American Academy of Psychotherapists is to invigorate the psychotherapist's quest for growth and excellence through authentic interpersonal engagement.

Core Values

- Courage to risk and willingness to change
- Balancing confrontation and compassion
- Commitment to authenticity with responsibility
- Honoring the individual and the community

Full Membership

Full Membership in the Academy requires a doctoral or professional degree in one of the following mental health fields: psychiatry, clinical or counseling psychology, social work, pastoral counseling, marriage and family therapy, counseling, or nursing, and licensure which allows for the independent practice of psychotherapy.

- Specific training in psychotherapy with a minimum of 100 hours of supervision.
- At least one year of full-time post graduate clinical experience (or the equivalent in part-time experience) for doctoral level applicants, at least two years for others.
- A minimum of 100 hours of personal psychotherapy.

A person who does not fulfill the above requirements but who is able to document a reasonable claim for eligibility, such as a distinguished contributor to the field of psychotherapy, may also be considered for full membership.

Other Categories of Membership

In the interest of promoting the development of experienced psychotherapists, one category of associate membership is offered for those with the intent of becoming full members. These members will be working with a mentor as they progress to Full Membership.

Associate Membership

- has completed a relevant professional degree
- is currently practicing psychotherapy under supervision appropriate to the licensure
- has recommendations from at least three faculty, supervisors, and/or Academy members
- has completed or is actively engaged in obtaining 100 hours of personal psychotherapy
- agrees to work with an Academy member mentor
- may be an associate for no more than five years

Student Affiliate

For students currently enrolled in a graduate degree program. Application includes acceptable recommendations from two faculty, supervisors or Academy members.

For information regarding membership requirements or to request an application, contact the Central Office. Membership information and a printable application form are also available on the Academy's Web site, www.aapweb.com.

Executive Offices

aap@caphill.com
230 Washington Ave Ext, Suite 101
Albany, NY 12203
Phone (518) 240-1178
Fax (518) 463-8656

Made in the USA
Monee, IL
05 November 2026

67812845R00164

Founded in 1964 by John Warkentin, PhD, MD and Thomas Leland, MD

Voices: *Journal of the American Academy of Psychotherapists*

VOICES: THE ART AND SCIENCE OF PSYCHOTHERAPY (ISSN 0042-8272) is published by the American Academy of Psychotherapists, 230 Washington Ave Ext , Suite 101 / Albany, NY 12203.

Subscription prices for one year (three issues): $65 for individuals PDF only; $85 for individuals PDF & print copy; $249 for institutions. Orders by mail payable by check: 230 Washington Ave Ext, Suite 101 / Albany, NY 12203. Orders by MasterCard or Visa: call (518) 240-1178 or fax (518) 463-8656. Payments must be made in U.S. dollars through a U.S. bank made payable to *AAP Voices.* Some back volumes may be available from the *Voices* Business Office.

Change of Address: Please inform publisher as soon as a change to your email address is made. Send change of email address to aap@caphill.com.